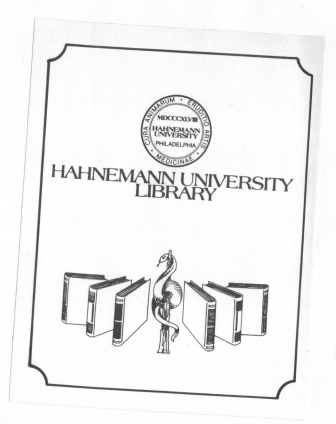

Renal Disease in Children

Amin Y. Barakat
Editor

Renal Disease in Children

Clinical Evaluation and Diagnosis

With a Foreword by Roscoe R. Robinson

With 70 Figures in 108 Parts and 95 Tables

Springer-Verlag
New York Berlin Heidelberg
London Paris Tokyo Hong Kong

Amin Y. Barakat
Clinical Professor of Pediatrics
Division of Pediatric Nephrology
Georgetown University School of Medicine
Washington, DC 20007, USA

(formerly Associate Professor of Pediatrics, Division of Pediatric Nephrology, and Director, Child Kidney Disease Prevention Program, Vanderbilt University School of Medicine, Nashville, Tennessee 37232, USA)

Cover: The color of the kidneys in the cover drawing resembles that of the precious stone jade, and a form of it, called *nephrite,* is said to have been worn as amulets by American Indians to protect themselves against kidney disease and calculi.

Library of Congress Cataloging-in-Publication Data
Renal disease in children: clinical evaluation and diagnosis/Amin
   Y. Barakat, editor; with a foreword by Roscoe R. Robinson.
      p.   cm.
   Includes index.
   ISBN 0-387-97036-3
   1. Pediatric nephrology.   I. Barakat, Amin Y.
   [DNLM: 1. Kidney Diseases—in infancy & childhood. WS 320 R392]
RJ476.K5R437 1989
618.92'61—dc20
DNLM/DLC   89-19664

Media conversion by Impressions, Inc., Madison, Wisconsin.
Printed and bound by Arcata Graphics/Halliday, West Hanover, Massachusetts.
Printed in the United States of America.

9 8 7 6 5 4 3 2 1

ISBN 0-387-97036-3 Springer-Verlag New York Berlin Heidelberg
ISBN 3-540-97036-3 Springer Verlag Berlin Heidelberg New York

To my wife, Amal,
and children, Rana, Nadim, and Zena

Foreword

The clinical specialty of adult nephrology has enjoyed spectacular growth during the past three decades. Such a statement is no less true for pediatric nephrology. This book stands in quiet testimony to that fact. Practitioners of pediatric nephrology are now concerned with the diagnosis and treatment of young patients with a widened spectrum of primary and secondary diseases of the kidneys and urinary tract, hypertension and disorders of water, electrolyte and acid-base metabolism. Their science, deriving from an exciting blend of physiology, morphology, pathology, immunology, biochemistry, microbiology, genetics and pharmacology, must also include an understanding of human developmental biology—an insight that colleagues who practice adult nephrology require to a somewhat lesser extent.

Dramatic, continuing advances in our understanding of the pathogenesis, pathophysiology, diagnosis and treatment of kidney diseases has led to a cascade of books and monographs on various aspects of the subject. Nevertheless, in view of the clear emergence of pediatric nephrology as a distinct medical specialty, it is most appropriate that a practical book, which focuses almost exclusively on approaches to the evaluation and diagnosis of young patients with kidney disease and related disorders, should appear. In that sense this book is unique. It provides an easily accessible, practical compendium or guide to the clinical investigation of all facets of kidney disease in children. Its special and unique emphasis is directed toward various approaches to the evaluation of such patients and the interpretation of associated laboratory or radiographical data. It avoids extensive discussion of disease mechanisms, pathophysiology or therapy. As an aid to diagnosis, the book will be particularly useful to those who participate in the daily care of children with disturbances of renal structure or function, whether the readers be students, house officers, family physicians, general pediatricians or pediatric nephrologists.

The editor and the authors have brought forth a volume that is easily read. It reflects a timely, highly useful and wonderfully concise, yet comprehensive view of an integrated and practical approach to the nephrological evaluation of children and adolescents. The book can serve as an introduction to diagnostic pediatric nephrology for students or as a ready bedside reference for the more experienced practitioner. The authors are noted and experienced clinicians whose individual contributions have been blended together by the editor in such a manner as to minimize unnecessary overlap and duplication among the various chapters. A clear and refreshing approach of practical utility without sacrifice of scholarship is a major hallmark of the text. The narrative progresses logically and sequentially from introductory chapters dealing with relevant diagnostic methods through later sections that offer descriptive approaches to the study of specific disorders. Timely and special reminders are conveyed in the three concluding chapters: 1) prenatal evaluation is useful and important to the diagnosis of certain types of kidney or urinary tract abnormalities; 2) early diagnosis and treatment are essential determinants of successful outcome in many circumstances and 3) clinical practice will be influenced increasingly by the use of sophisticated information systems and their clinical databases as we approach and enter the twenty-first century.

This writer takes great pride in the fact that both pediatric and adult nephrology are alive and well at Vanderbilt University Medical Center. The appearance of this book offers one more bit of evidence that this is so. The twelve Vanderbilt contributors and their valued colleagues from other institutions can be congratulated on the quality of their effort.

Nashville, Tennessee   ROSCOE R. ROBINSON

Preface

Our fundamental knowledge in nephrology has advanced significantly in the past three decades. Thanks to basic research, we are now closer to understanding the pathophysiology and molecular basis of many renal diseases as well as the transport, metabolic and endocrine functions of the kidney. DNA linkage has made possible the identification of autosomal dominant polycystic kidney disease, Lowe's oculocerebrorenal syndrome and Wilms' tumor-aniredia complex. Identification of the gene in polycystic disease and possibly in other genetic diseases of the kidney is imminent.

The clinical workup and diagnosis of patients with renal disease, however, continue to be the main concern of physicians and practicing nephrologists. Physicians caring for children should be familiar with the clinical aspects of acid-base and electrolyte disturbances, proteinuria, hematuria, urinary tract infection, glomerular and tubular diseases, acute and chronic renal failure, hypertension and renal involvement in systemic disease. They should be able to initiate the workup on a child with renal disease, interpret urinalysis and other laboratory findings and know when to refer a patient to a pediatric nephrologist.

The purpose of this book is to provide pediatricians, family physicians, nephrologists, urologists, residents, clinical fellows and medical students with a complete compendium on the clinical evaluation of renal disease in children. The book is meant to be a desk reference and a bedside manual for all those managing children with kidney problems, to help them in the diagnosis of disease and the interpretation of relevant clinical laboratory data. It is not designed to be a textbook. The depth and detail of the different chapters vary according to the complexity of the subject discussed. The versatility of the material presented makes this book equally useful to the specialist consultant, the generalist and the house officer.

The book covers pediatric nephrology problems classified by mode of investigation (urinalysis, imaging, kidney biopsy, etc.) or presentation (hematuria, proteinuria, urinary tract infection, renal failure, etc.). Detailed discussions of pathophysiology and management of different renal conditions have been omitted to save space, and to concentrate on workup and diagnosis. Pathophysiology and therapy are sometimes briefly presented to the extent that they have an impact on the workup. Other disciplines that contribute to the diagnosis of renal disease, such as pathology and urology, are also presented. Prenatal diagnosis, prevention and use of the computer in renal disease are briefly discussed. Many tables, algorithms and formulas are included to assist the reader in the differential diagnosis and workup.

Because of space limitations, an exhaustive list of references is not provided; rather, a limited number of specific references and a few general key ones are included to allow the interested reader to pursue certain problems in depth. Formulas and reference intervals are also referenced. Extensive cross-referencing avoids repetition and redundancy. A detailed appendix includes 1) reference intervals, 2) formulas used in the diagnosis and treatment of various renal conditions, 3) nomograms and 4) a table of over 400 conditions and syndromes associated with renal involvement, which presents main clinical features, renal abnormalities and inheritance. This table will help the practicing physician and consultant to identify the nature of renal involvement for different conditions.

The editor would like to thank Doctors Iekuni Ichikawa, Robert C. MacDonnell, Jr., Valentina Kon and Aida Yared of the Division of Pediatric Nephrology, Vanderbilt University Medical Center for reviewing parts of the manuscript, and Doctor Marshall Summar for his help with the art work. Special thanks also go to the staff of Springer-Verlag for their help and support.

I owe a great debt to the contributing authors who spent much time and effort in this endeavor to help physicians provide better care to children with kidney disease.

AMIN Y. BARAKAT

Contents

Contributors

BILLY S. ARANT, JR., M.D.
Professor and Director, Division of Pediatric Nephrology, University of Texas Southwestern Medical Center at Dallas, Dallas, TX 75235-9063, USA

AMIN Y. BARAKAT, M.D., F.A.A.P.
Clinical Professor of Pediatrics, Division of Pediatric Nephrology, Georgetown University School of Medicine, Washington, DC 20007, USA

JEAN-PIERRE DE CHADARÉVIAN, M.D.
Professor of Pediatrics (Pediatric Pathology), Temple University School of Medicine and Director, Department of Anatomical Pathology, St. Christopher's Hospital for Children, Philadelphia, PA 19133, USA

JAMES C.M. CHAN, M.D.
Professor and Vice-Chairman, Department of Pediatrics and Director, Division of Pediatric Nephrology, Children's Medical Center, Medical College of Virginia, Richmond, VA 23298-0498, USA

RUSSELL W. CHESNEY, M.D.
Le Bonheur Professor and Chairman, Department of Pediatrics, The University of Tennessee Memphis College of Medicine, Le Bonheur Children's Medical Center, Memphis, TN 38103, USA

ROBERT B. ETTENGER, M.D.
Professor of Pediatrics and Director, Pediatric Renal Transplantation Program and Transplantation Immunology Laboratory, UCLA School of Medicine, Los Angeles, CA 90024, USA

LEONARD G. FELD, M.D., PH.D.
Associate Professor of Pediatrics, SUNY at Buffalo School of Medicine and Chief, Division of Pediatric Nephrology and Director, Children's Kidney Center, Children's Hospital of Buffalo, Buffalo, NY 14222, USA

ROBIN A. FELDER, PH.D.
Assistant Professor of Pathology and Associate Director, Clinical
Chemistry and Toxicology, University of Virginia Health Sciences
Center, Charlottesville, VA 22908, USA

ROBERT D. FILDES, M.D.
Assistant Professor of Pediatrics, Division of Pediatric Nephrology and
Director, Pediatric End-Stage Renal Disease Program, Georgetown
University School of Medicine, Washington, DC 20007, USA

AGNES FOGO, M.D.
Assistant Professor of Pathology and Pediatrics, Vanderbilt University
School of Medicine, Nashville, TN 37232, USA

JOHN W. FOREMAN, M.D.
Associate Professor of Pediatrics, Medical College of Virginia,
Richmond, VA 23298, USA

RAYMOND M. HAKIM, M.D., PH.D.
Associate Professor of Internal Medicine and Director of Clinical
Services, Division of Nephrology, Vanderbilt University School of
Medicine, Nashville, TN 37232, USA

MANFRED HANSMANN, M.D.
Professor of Obstetrics and Gynecology, University of Bonn,
University Women's Hospital, 5300 Bonn, FRG

RICHARD M. HELLER, M.D.
Professor of Radiology and Radiological Sciences and Pediatrics,
Vanderbilt University School of Medicine, Nashville, TN 37232, USA

IEKUNI ICHIKAWA, M.D.
Professor of Pediatrics and Director, Division of Pediatric Nephrology,
Vanderbilt University School of Medicine, Nashville, TN 37232, USA

PHILIPPE JEANTY, PH.D., M.D.
Assistant Professor of Radiology and Radiological Sciences, Vanderbilt
University School of Medicine, Nashville, TN 37232, USA

ROBERT D. JEFFS, M.D., F.R.C.S.(C)
Professor and Director, Division of Pediatric Urology, The James
Buchanan Brady Urological Institute, The Johns Hopkins Hospital,
Baltimore, MD 21205, USA

PEDRO A. JOSE, M.D., PH.D.
Professor of Pediatrics, Physiology and Biophysics and Director,
Division of Pediatric Nephrology, Vice-Chairman, Department of
Pediatrics, Georgetown University School of Medicine, Georgetown
Children's Medical Center, Washington, DC 20007, USA

GAD KAINER, M.B., B.S., F.R.A.C.P.
Visiting Scholar, Department of Pediatrics, Medical College of
Virginia, Richmond, VA 23298, USA

BERNARD S. KAPLAN, M.D.
Professor of Pediatrics, University of Pennsylvania and Director of
Pediatric Nephrology, Children's Hospital of Philadelphia,
Philadelphia, PA 19104, USA

SANDRA G. KIRCHNER, M.D.
Professor of Radiology and Radiological Sciences, Vanderbilt
University School of Medicine, Nashville, TN 37232-2675, USA

VALENTINA KON, M.D.
Assistant Professor of Pediatrics, Division of Pediatric Nephrology,
Vanderbilt University School of Medicine, Nashville, TN 37232, USA

ROBERT L. LYNCH, M.D., PH.D.
Associate Professor, Division of Pediatric Nephrology, St. Louis
University School of Medicine, St. Louis, MO 63104, USA

ROBERT C. MACDONELL, JR., M.D.
Associate Professor of Pediatrics and Medicine, Assistant Professor of
Surgery, Vanderbilt University School of Medicine, Nashville, TN
37232, USA

MITSURO NAKANO, M.D., PH.D.
Visiting Scholar, Department of Pediatrics, Medical College of
Virginia, Richmond, VA 23298, USA

ZOE L. PAPADOPOULOU, M.D.
Professor of Pediatric Nephrology, University of Ioannina, Greece, and
Director, Division of Pediatric Nephrology, Saint Sophia Hospital,
Thessaloniki, Greece

ROSCOE R. ROBINSON, M.D.
Professor of Medicine and Vice-Chancellor for Health Affairs,
Vanderbilt University Medical Center, Nashville, TN 37232, USA

ROBERT C. ROCK, M.D.
Associate Professor and Director, Department of Laboratory Medicine,
The Johns Hopkins Hospital, Baltimore, MD 21205, USA

JUAN RODRIGUEZ-SORIANO, M.D.
Chairman, Department of Pediatrics, Hospital Infantil de Cruces,
Cruces, Bilbao, Spain

MOUIN G. SEIKALY, M.D.
Assistant Professor of Pediatrics, Division of Pediatric Nephrology,
University of Texas Southwestern Medical Center at Dallas, Dallas,
TX 75235-9063, USA

ZIAD M. SHEHAB, M.D.
Clinical Associate Professor of Pediatrics, Section of Infectious
Disease, Arizona Health Sciences Center, Tucson, AZ 85724, USA

JAMES E. SPRINGATE, M.D.
Assistant Professor of Pediatrics, Division of Pediatric Nephrology,
Children's Hospital of Buffalo, Buffalo, NY 14222, USA

SHARON M. STEIN, M.D.
Fellow, Department of Radiology and Radiological Sciences,
Vanderbilt University School of Medicine, Nashville, TN 37232, USA

MARSHALL SUMMAR, M.D.
Fellow, Division of Genetics, Department of Pediatrics, Vanderbilt
University School of Medicine, Nashville, TN 37232, USA

LETICIA U. TINA, M.D.
Associate Professor of Pediatrics, Division of Pediatric Nephrology,
Georgetown University School of Medicine, Washington, DC 20007,
USA

BRENT F. TREIGER, M.D.
Resident, The James Buchanan Brady Urological Institute, The Johns
Hopkins Hospital, Baltimore, MD 21205, USA

ELLEN G. WOOD, M.D.
Assistant Professor and Director, Division of Pediatric Nephrology, St.
Louis University School of Medicine, St. Louis, MO 63104, USA

AIDA YARED, M.D.
Assistant Professor of Pediatrics, Division of Pediatric Nephrology,
Vanderbilt University School of Medicine, Nashville, TN 37232, USA

1
Introduction to the Diagnosis of Renal Disease and Guidelines for Patient Referral

Amin Y. Barakat

I. Introduction

Renal disease is a major cause of morbidity and mortality. The primary physician should be familiar with the modes of presentation of different renal conditions and should have a high index of suspicion for patients with asymptomatic disease. Early diagnosis of these conditions in children is important in the prevention of renal failure and end-stage renal disease.

II. Presentation of Patients with Renal Disease

Patients with renal disease may present with 1) signs and symptoms of renal disease, 2) abnormal urinalysis, 3) urinary tract infection (UTI), 4) glomerular disease, 5) tubular disease, 6) electrolyte and acid-base disturbances, 7) decreased renal function, 8) hypertension, 9) congenital abnormalities of the kidney or urinary tract or 10) renal involvement in systemic disease. These complaints or findings should prompt a thorough history and physical examination including blood pressure determination (Chapter 2). A few simple laboratory and radiological studies may suggest the diagnosis or lead to a prompt referral. Often, renal diseases may be asymptomatic; therefore, a yearly urinalysis and blood pressure determination should be an integral part of routine medical care of children.

III. Signs and Symptoms of Renal Disease

Urinary symptoms such as frequency, urgency, dysuria, hesitancy and urinary retention may suggest UTI, obstructive uropathy or urinary calculi. Abdominal, loin or suprapubic pain may be present also.

Physicians should be familiar with the normal voiding pattern of children at various ages. The normal frequency and amount of urine at different ages are presented in Chapter 2 and Appendix I. Nocturnal *enuresis*, particularly the primary form, is associated with a positive family history, is usually idiopathic and initially requires no other investigation than a urinalysis and urine culture. Secondary and diurnal forms of enuresis, as well as enuresis beyond the age of 10 years, may require a renal sonogram (ultrasound) and voiding cystourethrogram. The physician should differentiate between *frequency* (usually suggesting UTI) and *polyuria,* which is the passage of larger amounts of urine than normal. Polyuria indicates a decrease in urine concentrating ability and may be seen in diabetes mellitus, diabetes insipidus and chronic renal failure. A random urine specific gravity (sp gr) of >1.020 rules out a urine concentration defect. A child with polyuria and decreased random urine sp gr should have a fasting sp gr or a water deprivation test (Chapter 12). Decreased concentrating ability with evidence of other renal disease may be due to chronic pyelonephritis, hydronephrosis, renal cystic disease or renal dysplasia, nephronophthisis-medullary cystic disease or sickle cell nephropathy. Referral to a pediatric nephrologist is necessary if these conditions are suspected.

It is important to keep in mind that renal disease in children may present in a subtle manner, and physicians should have a high index of suspicion of a renal cause for any child who fails to thrive or who has unexplained fevers, vague pains, gastrointestinal symptoms, anemia, acidosis, an abdominal mass, edema or hypertension. Physicians should be generous in performing urinalyses and urine cultures on children, particularly those below the age of five years, since UTI at this age often presents with signs and symptoms not related to the urinary tract. Younger children with a UTI may have a normal urinalysis and a urine culture is necessary to make the diagnosis. Children with a documented

UTI should be worked up radiologically to rule out structural abnormalities of the kidney and urinary tract (Chapter 9).

In general, most renal diseases are painless. Flank pain may be due to infection or inflammation of the renal parenchyma or stretching of the renal capsule. When associated with nausea, vomiting and fever, acute pyelonephritis should be suspected. Renal calculi may present with colicky abdominal or flank pain of rapid onset (Chapter 18). Passed stones are very valuable in diagnosis and should be analyzed.

Renal and bladder injury following trauma may also present with pain. *Dysuria*, or pain on urination, is a symptom of UTI or urethritis. The pain of cystitis or prostatitis is usually suprapubic and gradual in onset.

Abdominal masses of renal origin may be due to a multicystic dysplastic kidney, polycystic kidney disease, hydronephrosis, renal vein thrombosis, Wilms' tumor or neuroblastoma (Chapter 6). A pediatric nephrologist and urologist may be consulted, preferably in that order, when further workup is indicated.

IV. Abnormal Urinalysis

Patients may also present with abnormal urinary findings. A urinalysis performed in the physician's office on a freshly voided specimen is considered an integral part of the physical examination of every child with suspected renal disease (Chapter 3), and a yearly urinalysis should be performed on every child. The commonest urinary abnormalities are hematuria and proteinuria (Chapter 8). *Hematuria* may be gross, or microscopic, which is discovered on routine urinalysis. Persistent hematuria should be investigated. Some of the workup for a child with suspected renal disease is easily done by the primary physician. This includes history and physical examination including blood pressure determination, urinalysis with red blood cell morphology, urine culture, blood studies, quantitative urine protein determination, creatinine clearance, audiogram, renal sonogram and voiding cystogram (Chapter 8). Urinalysis and, when indicated, an audiogram on the immediate family members should be performed. Recurrent benign hematuria is probably the most common cause of familial hematuria; however, Alport's syndrome, IgA nephropathy and other forms of glomerular disease may be familial also. In general, the presence of persistent and recurrent gross hematuria should be taken seriously and the nephrologist should decide the sequence of further investigations. IgA nephropathy, membranoproliferative glomerulonephritis, Alport's syndrome, recurrent benign hematuria and various renal and urinary tract abnormalities may present with gross hematuria.

Persistent *proteinuria* should also be investigated. The primary physician may quantitate the proteinuria and exclude the orthostatic type (Chapter 8). Significant proteinuria (>1 g/1.73 m^2), or proteinuria associated with glomerular hematuria, decreased renal function, hypertension, decreased serum complement level or manifestations of systemic disease, is suggestive of glomerular involvement, and is an indication for renal biopsy (Chapters 7, 10 and 19).

Pyuria usually indicates UTI, although it may be seen with any inflammatory process of the kidney and urinary tract, renal calculi and abnormalities of the urinary tract. When pyuria is present, a urine culture should be performed. The persistence of pyuria after adequate treatment of the UTI should raise the possibility of infection with unusual organisms such as tuberculosis or anaerobic bacteria or viruses, as well as renal calculi and congenital abnormalities of the kidney or urinary tract with or without obstructive uropathy. Abnormal urine color and smell, crystalluria and the significance of casts are discussed in Chapter 3.

V. Urinary Tract Infection

Refer to sections III and IV (this chapter) and Chapter 9.

VI. Glomerular Disease

The majority of children with glomerulonephritis present with proteinuria and hematuria on routine urinalysis, hypertension or edema. Children with systemic diseases associated with glomerular abnormalities may present with arthritis, rash, hypertension, hematuria or proteinuria (Chapter 19). The most commonly encountered glomerular disease in practice is poststreptococcal acute glomerulonephritis. This disease may be treated on an ambulatory basis; however, the presence of hypertension, oliguria, hyperkalemia, other electrolyte abnormalities and cardiac overload are usual indications for admission to the hospital. A kidney biopsy may be indicated in patients who have an atypical course of the disease, prolonged oliguria or anuria or gross hematuria, a persistently low complement or associated nephrotic syndrome. Obviously, a nephrology consultation should be obtained on patients who have atypical signs and symptoms and those who require hospitalization and/or kidney biopsy. Other glomerular diseases are discussed in Chapters 10 and 19.

Nephrotic syndrome is characterized by proteinuria ≥ 40 mg/m^2 for a one hour collection and serum albumin <2.5 g/dL. By far, the most common type of nephrotic syndrome in children is minimal change nephrotic syndrome which is characterized by a response to corticosteroids and a good prognosis, although most patients have one or more relapses. Patients with this type of nephrosis may be treated by the primary physician. Those who are steroid resistent or dependent and those in whom a structural glomerular abnormality is suspected should be referred to the nephrologist, since they require a complex differential diagnosis, knowledge of current therapeutic regimens and a close follow-up (Chapters 7, 8 and 10).

VII. Tubular Disease

Renal tubular diseases include renal glucosuria, Fanconi syndrome with or without cystinosis, cystinuria and other aminoacidurias, renal tubular acidosis, nephrogenic diabetes insipidus, Bartter's syndrome and other conditions. The patient presents with failure to thrive, acidosis, urinary findings of glucosuria, aminoaciduria and phosphaturia, rickets and inability to concentrate the urine. Patients with metabolic acidosis and a persistently alkaline urine should be investigated for renal tubular acidosis (Chapter 13). Patients with glucosuria should have a serum glucose determination to rule out diabetes mellitus. The primary physician should be familiar with these rare hereditary disorders and should consider such a diagnosis when confronted with a patient who fails to thrive and who has other suggestive findings and a positive family history. Because renal tubular diseases are rare and complex, the help of a pediatric nephrologist is usually needed. Evaluation of children with renal tubular disorders is discussed in detail in Chapter 11.

VIII. Electrolyte and Acid-Base Disturbances

Vomiting, diarrhea, decreased intake of fluids, irritability, lethargy, acute weight loss, dry skin and mucous membranes, elevated pulse, seizures and coma may be accompanied by an electrolyte or acid-base disturbance. Severely affected patients should be referred immediately to a hospital where expert care can be delivered (Chapters 12 and 13). Physicians who handle such conditions should be familiar with the intricacies of their diagnosis and management.

IX. Decreased Renal Function

A distinction should be made between *azotemia* (elevated serum urea nitrogen), *renal failure* (reduction in renal function) and *uremia,* which refers to the syndrome that encompasses the overt consequences of chronic renal failure such as anemia, osteodystrophy, central nervous system (CNS), and gastrointestinal disorders and other manifestations.

Acute renal failure is an abrupt severe reduction in glomerular filtration and is characterized by oliguria (urine <0.5 ml/kg in a one-hour collection) and azotemia (Chapter 14). A patient presenting with the above findings and with hypertension, gross hematuria, electrolyte disturbances (particularly hyperkalemia and acidosis) and volume overload should be referred to a nephrologist immediately. The etiology of acute renal failure should be identified promptly, since workup, management and prognosis of this condition vary with the specific etiology. Additionally, some causes of acute renal failure are reversible. Acute renal failure may be prerenal (renal ischemia resulting from intravascular volume depletion due to gastroenteritis, hemorrhage, and heart failure), renal (chemical injury, glomerular/vascular disease, interstitial nephritis) or postrenal (urinary tract obstruction). Common renal causes include the hemolytic uremic syndrome, acute tubular necrosis, acute postinfectious glomerulonephritis and interstitial nephritis. Retardation of growth, anemia, a history of an underlying renal disease, renal osteodystrophy or small contracted kidneys suggest the presence of *chronic renal failure*, which is defined as the stage at which the kidneys are irreversibly damaged and unable to maintain homeostasis (Chapter 15). Once the diagnosis of chronic renal failure is suspected or documented, the patient should be referred to the nephrologist, since these patients invariably progress to *end-stage renal disease* requiring chronic dialysis and ultimately transplantation. Chapter 20 deals with the workup of the doner and recipient of a kidney transplant. Since many conditions leading to end-stage renal disease in children are potentially preventable (hereditary and congenital abnormalities of the kidney and UTI), early diagnosis and treatment of these conditions is of utmost importance (Chapter 22). The dose of various drugs that are excreted by the kidney including some antibiotics, analgesics, diuretics and others must be adjusted in renal failure.

X. Hypertension

Blood pressure should be measured routinely in every child over the age of three years, and when indicated. Hypertension in children is usually secondary to renal or vascular causes, but it often may be essential. Severe persistent hypertension should be investigated promptly and thoroughly in children, since treatable secondary causes are common in the pediatric age group (Chapter 16). The primary physician may initiate the workup on children with persistent mild to moderate hypertension. Children presenting with severe or malignant hypertension requiring a comprehensive workup and initiation of antihypertensive therapy should be referred to a nephrologist. Every patient with documented and persistent hypertension should be seen by a nephrologist at some stage.

TABLE 1-1. Role of the Primary Physician in the Workup of the Child with Renal Disease

1. Take history and perform physical examination including blood pressure determination
2. Take family history
3. Do urinalysis on patient and, when indicated, on family members
4. Culture urine
5. Direct laboratory testing including BUN, creatinine, electrolytes, quantitation of proteinuria and creatinine clearance
6. Order imaging studies including renal sonogram and voiding cystourethrogram on patients with UTI, suspected congenital abnormalities and renal calculi
7. Evaluate the general state of health and exclude other systemic diseases
8. Screen for orthostatic proteinuria, tubular disorders and other conditions
9. Treat UTI, uncomplicated acute glomerulonephritis, conditions not associated with acute or progressive deterioration of renal function such as minimal change nephrotic syndrome, mild abnormalities and others that the physician is comfortable with

TABLE 1-2. Role of the Pediatric Nephrologist in the Workup of the Child with Renal Disease

1. Repeat the steps listed in Table 1.1
2. Perform fine renal function studies—glomerular, tubular, concentration
3. Evaluate renin-angiotensin-aldosterone system
4. Request and interpret secondary imaging studies—renal scan, CT, MRI, arteriogram
5. Perform and interpret specialized studies such as renal biopsy
6. Consult urologist when needed
7. Treat and follow patients with renal failure, severe hypertension, renal transplantation, complicated urogenital abnormalities and those conditions the primary physician does not feel comfortable with
8. Treat and follow patients with complicated genetic renal disorders and rare tubular diseases such as Fanconi syndrome and cystinosis
9. Coordinate efforts between primary physician, urologist, geneticist, social worker, dietician and all others concerned with the care of the patient

XI. Congenital Abnormalities of the Kidney and Urinary Tract

Congenital abnormalities of the kidney and urinary tract occur in 5 to 10% of the general population. Some of these abnormalities are minor and are discovered incidentally; others are major, leading to obstruction, renal scarring, pyelonephritis and renal failure. These abnormalities should be suspected in any child with UTI, congenital anomalies of other organ systems (cardiovascular, gastrointestinal, CNS and others), chromosomal aberrations, various malformation syndromes and in children with a single umbilical artery or supernumerary nipples (Chapter 2). The prenatal diagnosis of renal and urinary tract abnormalities is the subject of Chapter 21.

TABLE 1-3. Some Guidelines for Patient Referral to the Pediatric Nephrologist

 1. Persistent unexplained hematuria
 2. Persistent, nonorthostatic proteinuria
 3. Persistent hypertension
 4. Decreased renal function
 5. End-stage renal disease
 6. Renal tubular disease
 7. Nephrotic syndrome, particularly steroid dependent or resistant
 8. Atypical or persistent glomerulonephritis
 9. Unexplained acid-base and electrolyte abnormalities
10. Systemic diseases associated with progressive renal involvement such as systemic lupus erythematosus (SLE) and diabetes mellitus
11. Genetic and congenital abnormalities likely to cause progressive renal damage
12. When invasive studies, e.g. kidney biopsy, are indicated
13. When prenatal diagnosis is indicated
14. Renal disease that is likely to progress, e.g. focal glomerulosclerosis, IgA nephropathy, diabetes mellitus, cystinosis and conditions associated with acute complications, e.g. hypertension, caculi, hemolytic uremic syndrome
15. When team work is required (urologist, dietician, social worker, geneticist)

XII. Renal Involvement in Systemic Diseases

Physicians should be aware of renal involvement in systemic diseases and various conditions and syndromes (Chapters 19 and 22, Appendix IV). In general, renal involvement should be ruled out in any individual with such multisystem diseases as collagen disease, diabetes mellitus and storage diseases. Findings suggesting renal involvement in systemic disease include hematuria, proteinuria, hypertension, decreased serum complement levels, decreased renal function, large kidneys (leukemia, lymphoma, amyloidosis) and other conditions. Often, a renal biopsy contributes significantly to the diagnosis of certain systemic diseases.

XIII. The Role of the Primary Physician and Guidelines for Patient Referral

It is difficult to delineate the responsibilities of the primary physician and to list indications for referral to the specialist. In general, the primary physician may initiate workup to the extent he/she feels comfortable with. An attempt to separate the role of the primary physician, outlined in Table 1-1, from that of the pediatric nephrologist, outlined in Table 1-2 has been made. An outline to screen children with suspected renal disease is presented in Chapter 22. Some guidelines for patient referral to the pediatric nephrologist are presented in Table 1-3.

2
History and Physical Examination of the Child with Renal Disease

AIDA YARED and AMIN Y. BARAKAT

I. Introduction

In the pediatric patient, especially the younger child, serious renal disease may present with findings that are nonspecific or unrelated to the urinary tract such as irritability, diarrhea and failure to thrive. Thus, the clinician should always have a high index of suspicion for occult renal dysfunction whenever a child with symptoms or signs of unclear etiology is assessed. History and physical examination are the most important clues to the presence of renal disease. A simple urinalysis, performed by the examiner on a freshly voided urine specimen, is considered an integral part of a complete physical examination, and will be the subject of Chapter 3.

II. Clinical Presentation

The patient with renal disease usually presents with or is referred for evaluation of 1) abnormal voiding pattern, 2) abnormal urinalysis, 3) pain or 4) systemic signs and symptoms.

A. Abnormal Voiding Pattern

About 90% of newborn infants pass urine in the first 24 hours of life, and 98% do so within 48 hours. In the first year of life, when fluid intake is high, and the infant's urine concentrating ability is limited as compared to the older child and adult, voiding is frequent, and is both diurnal and nocturnal. Beyond school age, after sphincter control is mastered, voiding is usually diurnal, occurs four to six times a day and is voluntary. At all ages, voiding is effortless and painless, involves passage of an adequate volume of urine and leads to complete emptying of the bladder.

1. Timing

Nocturia is, in the older child, the awakening at night to pass urine. Occasional nocturia can be a normal occurrence, especially following copious intake of water around bedtime; this can be easily inferred if withholding of fluids at bedtime dramatically improves the condition. Otherwise, nocturia can indicate loss of urinary concentrating ability.

2. Volume

The volume of urine normally passed during a single void (bladder capacity) in ounces is equal to age (years) + 2, and plateaus by 9 years of age (1). Urine volume in full term babies varies between 15 and 60 mL/day in the first two days of life, rising to about 200 mL by the 10th day. Beyond the neonatal period, the total volume of urine voided in 24 hours roughly represents half of the daily fluid intake. In the infant, whose daily intake averages 100 mL/kg, the hourly urine output averages 2 mL/kg body weight. Age-related daily urine output values are presented in Appendix I.

The newborn can come to medical attention because of a *delay in the passage of urine.* If the physical examination demonstrates the presence of two kidneys of normal size, and the bladder contains urine by percussion, delay in the passage of urine is likely to be normal. However, renal agenesis and obstructive uropathy should be considered.

Oliguria is defined, in the newborn, as the passage of <0.5 mL/kg of urine hourly. In the sick neonate, it is most frequently prerenal in origin, and would respond to appropriate fluid administration. However, acute tubular necrosis, congenital renal anomalies, a renal vascular accident (renal vein thrombosis) or a drug-related toxicity should be kept in mind. A urinalysis and blood chemistry values should be obtained. In the older child, oliguria is defined as a 24-hour urine output <300 mL/m², and anuria <50 mL/m². This decrease in urinary flow rate can occur by two mechanisms: 1) elaboration of a more concentrated urine while the glomerular filtration rate (GFR) remains normal, and 2) a decrease in the renal clearance ability, which is classically divided into prerenal, renal and postrenal (obstructive).

Polyuria is the passage of a larger than normal urine volume. It should not be confused with *frequency* of urination, when the patient often feels the need to void, but passes only a small amount of urine. If it is unclear whether the child has polyuria or frequency of urination, a 24-hour urine collection is indicated.

Polyuria is often accompanied by *polydypsia,* i.e. an increased intake of water. Acute onset of polyuria/polydypsia suggests two conditions in which urine concentrating ability is lost: diabetes mellitus, and diabetes insipidus (DI). DI may be central (inadequate production or release of antidiuretic hormone, ADH), or nephrogenic (inability to concentrate the urine in the presence of ADH). Nephrogenic DI can be due to congenital or aquired unresponsiveness of the distal nephron to ADH; it can also be an early sign of chronic renal failure due to a variety of causes (chronic pyelonephritis, hydronephrosis, renal cystic disease or dysplasia). Rarely, polydypsia and polyuria have a psychogenic origin in children, as part of a pattern of attention-seeking behavior.

3. The Act of Voiding

The infant who exhibits symptoms of urinary retention, or who has difficulty initiating voiding may be suffering from a serious underlying disease. Retention, in the child with neurological deficits, suggests a neurogenic bladder. In the otherwise normal male child, the physician should always be alert to the possibility of bladder outlet obstruction (bladder neck obstruction, posterior urethral valves, urethral stricture or severe meatal stenosis). Acute difficulty in voiding can also occur with urethritis or cystitis; here, other signs and symptoms of inflammation are usually present. The urinary stream can also be abnormal. A weak urinary stream, or dribbling of urine, can be the presenting sign of an obstructive uropathy.

Dysuria, or pain on urination, is highly suggestive of urinary tract infection (UTI); it is often accompanied by *frequency* of urination (the child feels the need to pass urine, but only passes small amounts) as well as *urgency*, i.e. the inability to hold urine voluntarily for a reasonable amount of time. In the younger infant, the parents might report that the child invariably screams when passing urine.

4. Voluntary Control

Enuresis is absence of voluntary control of urination. It can be primary (the child has never been toilet trained) or secondary (the child had bladder sphincter control for a period of time, then started wetting again). Enuresis is very common in pediatrics. About 19% of children between 4 and 5 years of age, 8% at 8 years, and 5% at 10 years have enuresis. Nocturnal enuresis is most commonly benign. Diurnal enuresis, especially if secondary, is more likely to indicate underlying pathology, whether infectious, anatomical or emotional. Enuresis is a frequent accompaniment of UTI in the toddler age group, and can be its only manifestation in about 10% of boys (2). Urgency incontinence may be secondary to acute or chronic cystitis or uninhibited bladder contraction. Overflow incontinence is most often seen with neurological problems, such as myelodysplasia. Diurnal enuresis or incontinence is an indication for a thorough urological, neurological and psychosocial investigation. Persistent dampness of the underwear in a child who is toilet trained and continent suggests ureteral ectopia.

B. Abnormal Urinalysis

Frequently, children are referred for investigation of an asymptomatic abnormal finding on urinalysis, discovered upon pre-school screening or a general checkup. Newborns and infants can also come to medical attention because of an unusual urine color or odor. A detailed review of urinalysis is presented in Chapter 3.

1. Abnormal Urine Color

Hematuria is rare in the newborn. A pink color to the urine due to the presence of large amounts of uric acid crystals is a benign and transient finding in the newborn. Physiological vaginal bleeding, which can occur in female newborns due to withdrawal of high levels of maternal hormones, can be confused with hematuria. Substances that change the color of urine are presented in Table 3.1.

2. Abnormal Urine Odor

An unusual odor is often the sign of an underlying metabolic disorder involving organic or amino acids. Such finding warrants immediate investigation (see Chapter 3).

3. Hematuria and Proteinuria

Most commonly, children are referred for investigation of asymptomatic hematuria and/or proteinuria. These findings are discussed in detail in Chapter 8.

4. Crystalluria

Uric acid crystals are common and normal in the urine of the newborn. The evaluation and treatment of urolithiasis in children is the subject of Chapter 18. Although stones and renal calculi are unusual in the pediatric age group, recent attention has been drawn to their increased occurrence in premature infants due to prolonged furosemide administration; they are more likely to form if the infant is on a calcium supplement, either orally or intravenously (see Chapter 18).

C. Pain

Most diseases of the urinary tract are painless. Pain most often relates to an acute process, usually inflammation or distension of a hollow viscus. It is noteworthy that hydronephrosis is not accompanied by pain. When pain is present, the examiner should inquire about its location (flank, suprapubic), possible radiation, nature (dull or colicky) and severity.

Flank pain of renal origin most commonly results from infection, or inflammation, of the renal parenchyma, which leads to stretching of the renal capsule. When accompanied by fever, nausea and vomiting, flank pain strongly suggests acute pyelonephritis, even in the absence of other symptoms of UTI. It can also be a prominent feature of IgA nephropathy (Berger's disease), in which 35 to 50% of the episodes of gross hematuria are accompanied by flank pain that resembles that of acute pyelonephritis. Flank pain can also occur in 5% of patients with acute poststreptococcal glomerulonephritis. In both pyelonephritis and glomerulonephritis, the pain is described as persistent and dull, with little or no radiation, and is often accompanied by tenderness to percussion. Colicky pain is usually due to the presence of a stone. Although renal stones are relatively rare in children, they should be kept in mind, especially in a child with a positive family history for stones. The pain, in this condition, is typically described as colicky and excruciatingly severe, radiating to the groin or migrating along the course of the ureter. Such a classic picture, however, is rare in children with urolithiasis, who are much more likely to present with nonspecific symptoms such as anorexia, nausea or vomiting and, in about 16%, generalized abdominal pain (3).

Abdominal, flank or back pain is the most frequent presenting symptom of autosomal dominant (adult) polycystic kidney disease (APKD), occurring in about 60% of cases. The pain is described as dull, nagging or aching and occasionally colicky. Radiation to the epigastric or suprapubic area is common.

Suprapubic pain, associated with suprapubic tenderness, is highly suggestive of acute cystitis, a common condition in childhood. Typically, it is accompanied by urinary frequency and urgency. Cystitis can be of bacterial or viral etiology and is often associated with hematuria.

In the child with abdominal pain, inquiry should be made for a history of recent trauma, and the child examined for the presence of skin bruises. Renal or bladder injury (hematoma or rupture) have been reported to occur in children who have been severely abused; however, it would be unusual to have injury to the urinary tract in the absence of other findings.

D. Systemic Signs and Symptoms

The systemic signs and symptoms of renal disease may be unrelated to the urinary tract. Thus, nausea, vomiting and failure to thrive occur with uremia, acidosis, or UTI. Metabolic acidosis is often associated with weakness and growth retardation. The three most commonly encountered physical signs that strongly suggest renal pathology are edema, hypertension and abdominal mass.

1. Edema

Edema can occur by three possible mechanisms, two of which directly relate to renal pathology: 1) Decreased oncotic pressure of plasma, due to decreased plasma protein concentration. In children, most edema/

hypoproteinemia is due to renal protein loss, which occurs in the nephrotic syndrome. Nephrotic edema tends to be most prominent in the periorbital area due to the low tissue turgor; anasarca, or generalized edema, is more frequent in the younger infant. 2) Increased venous pressure. Volume overload can occur when GFR is decreased while intake of fluids is not curtailed. Typically, edema is present in 75% of children with acute postinfectious glomerulonephritis. 3) Increased vascular permeability, such as that due to prematurity or allergic reaction. Although this mechanism of edema formation does not involve the kidney, it is noteworthy that many cases of nephrotic syndrome in children are initially misdiagnosed as allergies.

The parents might report that the child has a spontaneous tendency to remove his or her shoes or that socks leave their imprint when taken off. Edema typically changes position, being more prominent in the periorbital area in the morning, and in the dependent areas such as lower extremities after prolonged standing.

2. Hypertension

The belief that almost all cases of hypertension in children are secondary is probably erroneous. With better definition of what normal, age-related blood pressure values are, and more widespread screening for hypertension, "essential" hypertension is increasingly recognized, especially in the second decade of life. Most hypertension in infants under one year of age is of vascular etiology. A history of placement of umbilical lines in the neonatal period should be sought, since the incidence of thrombosis in such a line is extremely high, especially if it is left in place for a long time. Such thrombosis is the most common cause of hypertension in the sick newborn. Coarctation of the aorta is the other common cause; thus, special attention should be paid to perfusion of the extremities, including temperature, pulses and blood pressure. Simultaneous assessment of capillary filling time in an upper and a lower extremity is also helpful.

Beyond the first year of life, most cases of severe hypertension in children are due to renovascular or renal parenchymal disease. Renovascular hypertension involves reduction in blood flow to the whole kidney or a portion of it, which activates the renin-angiotensin system. Common causes are stenosis of the renal artery or a branch or extrinsic compression by a tumor, lymph node, cyst, etc. Renal parenchymal causes of hypertension can be congenital (polycystic kidney disease), acute (acute glomerulonephritis) or chronic (chronic renal failure). Thus, the finding of hypertension in a child always should prompt investigation of the kidney. The extent and invasiveness of the diagnostic procedures largely depends on the age of the child and the severity of hypertension, and will be the subject of Chapter 16.

3. Abdominal Mass

A large proportion (55%) of abdominal masses in newborns are of renal origin. Most of these masses are benign; the majority represent a non-functioning multicystic dysplastic kidney, polycystic kidney disease, or hydronephrosis. Beyond the neonatal period, over 50% of all children presenting with an abdominal mass have a nonsurgical condition. The majority of the remaining masses are retroperitoneal and renal in origin. An abdominal flank mass may represent a wide variety of conditions, including enlarged kidneys (polycystic kidney disease, multicystic dysplasia, hydronephrosis), a tumor (Wilms' tumor or neuroblastoma) or a renal vascular accident (renal venous thrombosis). A suprapubic mass can be a distended bladder. The incidence of malignant conditions, namely Wilms' tumor and neuroblastoma, increases with age to peak at two to three years of age, when they become the leading cause of abdominal masses in a child.

III. History

A. Family History

A history of consanguinity should be obtained if an autosomal recessive disorder is suspected, such as the infantile form of polycystic kidney disease or the Finnish type of congenital nephrotic syndrome. Family history of death in infancy due to renal problems can suggest the infantile form of polycystic kidney disease.

In the child with isolated hematuria, a similar finding in other family members can help suggest the diagnosis of benign familial hematuria, and thus avoid the expense of a more thorough investigation. However, various causes of hematuria, including polycystic kidney disease, Alport's syndrome and sickle cell disease or trait, are genetically transmitted. Family history of hearing loss, with or without renal impairment, should alert the physician to the possibility of Alport's syndrome, an inherited condition (autosomal dominant or X-linked) characterized by high frequency sensorineural hearing loss and chronic renal failure. It is more likely to be clinically manifest in males. A family history of chronic renal failure, dialysis or kidney transplantation raises the possibility of a genetic form of nephropathy.

A family history of renal calculi points out the possiblity of a metabolic disorder underlying stone formation. Children with idiopathic nocturnal enuresis commonly have a positive family history. The family history is also important in various forms of renal tubule dysfunction. Cystinosis, an autosomal recessive disease with excessive intracellular accumulation of cystine, is a disease characterized by Fanconi syndrome (multiple proximal tubule transport defects, including bicarbonaturia, glucosuria, phosphaturia and aminoaciduria), and gradual loss of renal function. A family history of hypertension should be sought in the child with a mild elevation in blood pressure, since essential hypertension is often familial. Ureter-ovesical reflux occurs in more than one third of asymptomatic siblings of affected children (4). Family history is important in various genetic renal disorders (see Table 2.1 and Appendix IV).

B. Perinatal History

In taking the history of a newborn with renal disease, attention should be paid to pre- and postnatal events. Obviously, the history of drug intake in the mother could predispose the newborn to a variety of congenital anomalies. Maternal diabetes can predispose the newborn to renal vein thrombosis, which can present in the neonatal period with hematuria, abdominal mass and renal insufficiency. During delivery, the placenta and abdominal cord should be carefully examined. The presence of am-nion nodosum should alert the examiner to the possible occurrence of renal agenesis or severe obstructive uropathy. A single umbilical artery is associated with genitourinary anomalies (27%). Oligohydramnios is suggestive of bilateral renal agenesis, or severe bilateral renal obstruction, since urine contributes to the formation of amniotic fluid. Because the presence of a normal volume of amniotic fluid is essential for adequate pulmonary development, these conditions are often associated with pul-

TABLE 2-1. Most Common Genetic Renal Disorders

Autosomal dominant
  Polycystic kidney disease—adult type[a]
  Benign familial hematuria
  Distal renal tubular acidosis
  Alport's syndrome
  Uric acid urolithiasis
Autosomal recessive
  Polycystic kidney disease—infantile type[a]
  Cystinosis[a]
  Finnish type nephrotic syndrome[a]
  Cystinuria[a]
  Hereditary xanthinuria
X-linked
  Alport's syndrome
  Proximal renal tubular acidosis
  Nephrogenic diabetes insipidus
Unknown
  Aniridia/Wilms' tumor
  Vesicoureteral reflux[a]
  IgA nephropathy
  Focal segmental glomerulosclerosis

[a] Prenatal diagnosis possible

monary hypoplasia. Polyhydramnios may suggest gastrointestinal tract atresia, which is commonly associated with renal and urinary tract abnormalities. A history of infusion of oxytocin to the mother during the course of labor, usually with the administration of a large amount of hypotonic fluids, places the newborn baby at risk for significant hyponatremia and fluid overload. Obviously, a history of hypotension, neonatal depression, hemorrhage or shock can predispose the newborn baby to acute tubular necrosis.

C. Patient's History

In addition to the signs and symptoms detailed earlier in this chapter, several points should be stressed in the child's history and system review.

1. Growth

Growth retardation is a common finding in children with chronic renal failure, and growth arrest is often the first clue to the condition. Failure to thrive in a younger child can also be the manifestation of recurrent or chronic UTI, especially if accompanied by poor feeding or chronic diarrhea. Growth failure is a frequent finding of diabetes insipidus (DI) in the infant; developmental delay is often seen as well, due to recurrent bouts of dehydration and hypernatremia. Failure to thrive can also be the sole manifestation of renal tubular acidosis.

2. Congenital Anomalies

Various surface anomalies suggest the presence of concomitant congenital renal anomalies. Of infants with a single umbilical artery, 20 to 30% have associated urinary tract abnormalities (5). Malformations of the external ears, the presence of preauricular pits (usually with proteinuria) (6) or the presence of supernumerary nipples (7) should alert the clinician to the possibility of renal malformations. The absence or severe laxity of the abdominal musculature, especially in the presence of undescended testes, suggests the "prune-belly" syndrome. In its complete form, this syndrome consists of the triad of bilateral cryptorchidism, absent abdominal muscles, and complex malformations of the upper urinary tract; partial forms of the syndrome are also known to occur (8).

Major internal anomalies are associated with renal abnormalities (9), and will be considered below under each system. Several genetic syndromes (Appendix IV) are associated with an extremely high incidence of urological anomalies, and imaging studies of the urinary tract should be performed as part of their initial investigation. Various congenital anomalies, including aniridia, hemihypertrophy and ambiguous genitalia, are associated with Wilms' tumor.

a. Cardiovascular

Congenital heart disease, particularly ventricular septal defect, is associated with a high incidence of renal anomalies (10). The incidence of urological anomalies in patients with cardiac defects is sufficiently high to warrant investigation; this is most easily done by visualizing the kidneys in the course of cardiac catheterization, at the time the contrast is concentrated and excreted by the kidneys.

Along with the eyes and kidneys, the heart is primarily targeted by hypertension; cardiomegaly suggests long-standing hypertension. Congestive heart failure or arrythmias can accompany acute severe hypertension.

Obviously, any cardiac problem leading to a reduction in cardiac output can reduce the GFR. In addition, congestive heart failure presenting in the child with no previous cardiac problems should prompt a good look at the urine sediment in search of red blood cell casts, since fluid overload is a common presentation of acute poststreptococcal glomerulonephritis.

b. Respiratory

The respiratory tract is rarely involved in childhood renal disease. It should be noted, however, that tachypnea or dyspnea can be signs of congestive heart failure. In addition, pulmonary pathology, such as pneumonia or assisted ventilation, can predispose to the syndrome of inappropriate ADH secretion (SIADH).

c. Gastrointestinal

The incidence of genitourinary anomalies is higher in children with gastrointestinal anomalies, such as imperforate anus, and esophageal or rectal atresia. The incidence is also increased in children with tracheoesophageal fistulae.

Anorexia, nausea and vomiting can be nonspecific symptoms of renal disease, such as uremia, urolithiasis or renal tubular acidosis. Diarrhea is a prominent symptom of urinary tract infection in the younger infant. Conversely, severe fluid deficits due to increased fluid losses or poor fluid intake can predispose to prerenal impairment in glomerular filtration.

d. Genital

Hypospadias, hydrocoele, undescended testes and other genital abnormalities are common, easily detected conditions. Since they are not associated with underlying upper urinary tract abnormalities, there is some controversy over whether these findings should prompt imaging of the upper urinary tract (11,12). It is generally agreed that children with coronal hypospadias do not need imaging, whereas children with perineal hypospadias do. Severe epispadias can be accompanied by exstrophy of the bladder, and occurs more commonly in girls. Ambiguous genitalia are one of the components of abnormal gonadal differentiation, nephropathy and Wilms' tumor (Denys-Drash) syndrome. Patients with ambiguous genitalia and nephropathy should be followed up closely for the possible development of Wilms' tumor.

e. Skeletal

Patients with kyphosis or scoliosis have been reported to have a higher incidence of genitourinary anomalies than the general population. Skeletal malformations, such as bowing of the legs, can be consequent to renal tubular acidosis accompanied by renal phosphate loss, or to the renal osteodystrophy of chronic renal failure. Orthopedic manipulation or traction has been reported to trigger hypertension.

f. Neurological

Meningomyelocele with agenesis of the sacral segments predisposes the patient to a neurogenic bladder, with consequent urinary retention and infection. The patient with a shunt for the treatment of hydrocephalus is at risk for shunt nephritis, usually concomitant with an active shunt infection. Frontal headache can be a sign of hypertension. Bell's palsy or extraocular palsies may also accompany hypertension. Any CNS pathology, including meningitis or intracranial tumor, can produce SIADH.

3. Infection

Parents should be questioned for a history of recurrent UTI or unexplained fevers. Such a history is of extreme importance for the child with decreased renal function, since the majority of pyelonephritic scars occur at an early age and can lead to loss of functional renal mass. In addition, a child with recurrent UTI should be investigated for a predisposing anomaly, such as obstruction, ureterovesical reflux, urinary stasis or a renal stone.

A history of a recent or an ongoing infection outside the urinary tract is also a clue, since at least three forms of renal pathology are associated with acute infection: postinfectious glomerulonephritis (which most commonly follows streptococcal pharyngitis or impetigo), shunt nephritis (which accompanies infection of a ventriculoatrial shunt) and the glomerulonephritis of subacute bacterial endocarditis.

4. Psychosocial History

Evaluation of family dynamics is of primary importance in enuresis and suspected psychogenic DI.

5. Dietary History

Dietary intake is important in the evaluation of the child with polyuria/polydypsia. Excessive intake of foods that generate a large osmolar load (such as milk or peanut butter) can lead per se to these symptoms in small infants, since their urinary concentrating ability is limited; in such children, these signs will abate with dietary readjustment. The child with genuine DI, however, will often spontaneously curtail his or her intake of protein and favor carbohydrates. A history of anorexia and decreased intake, also associated with spontaneous avoidance of protein foods, characterizes the child with chronic renal failure. A dietary review to determine approximately daily sodium intake is important in the child with hypertension.

6. Drug History

Various drugs are nephrotoxic, producing a decrease in GFR. The most commonly used drugs are furosemide and the aminoglycoside antibiotics. In the patient suspected of having aminoglycoside nephrotoxicity, a review of drug levels reached during the course of therapy is essential, since nephrotoxicity is often related to elevated trough levels. On the other hand, semisynthetic penicillins, such as methicillin, are notorious for causing interstitial nephritis, which is manifested primarily as hematuria and decreased GFR. Such patient often have other findings suggesting a drug reaction, such as fever, skin rash or eosinophilia (see Chapter 10).

It is important to keep in mind that, although renal prostaglandins play a minor role in determining renal function in the normal patient, they are of major importance in preserving renal function in conditions associated with renal hypoperfusion. Thus, prostaglandin inhibitors, such as aspirin or nonsteroidal antiinflammatory drugs, can lead to an acute decrease in GFR in the patient with preexisting renal dysfunction.

Drugs that lead to renal dysfunction should be kept in mind in the evaluation of the child undergoing treatment for a malignancy. Chemotherapy given to a child with a large tumor mass can lead to hyperuricemia and a consequent acute obstructive uric acid nephropathy with renal failure. Vincristine is known to cause SIADH. Amphotericin B, used to treat various systemic fungal infections, often leads to hypokalemia and a dose-dependent decrease in GFR.

IV. Physical Examination

A. General Appearance

The name *Potter syndrome* was initially used to describe bilateral renal agenesis. The facies typically consist of a flattened mid-portion of the face, with wide-set eyes, a beaked nose, low-set ears and a prominent fold originating at the inner canthus of the eye (Figure 2-1). It may be more appropriately renamed renal nonfunction syndrome, as suggested by Potter herself.

Height and weight should be measured, and plotted on appropriate growth charts (Appendix III). Assessment of hydration is obviously of

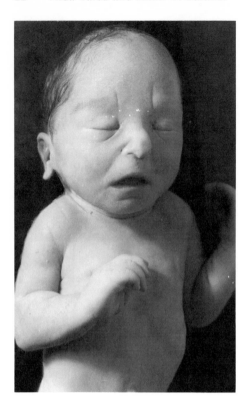

FIGURE 2-1. A newborn with "Potter" facies and bilateral renal agenesis. Courtesy of E.L. Potter, M.D. Reproduced with permission from Barakat AY, et al (1986) The Kidney in Genetic Disease. Churchill Livingstone, Edinburgh, p 24.

importance; dehydration in a child with azotemia would suggest a prerenal etiology. Edema should be noted, since it may indicate hypoproteinemia or fluid overload. Congenital anomalies, such as hemihypertrophy and ambiguous genitalia, should be noted.

B. Vital Signs

Fever in the younger child may be the only sign of UTI, and when unaccompanied by localizing findings of infection, should prompt the search for UTI by urinalysis and urine culture. About 7% of female infants with unexplained fever may have a UTI (13).

Blood pressure (BP) measurement is often neglected in the pediatric age group. However, it should be an integral part of a complete physical examination, even in younger infants (Chapter 16). The readings should be interpreted in relation to age, on a nomogram. Hypertension is defined as a reading above the 95th percentile for age. It is important to use the appropriate cuff in measuring BP. A very small cuff will give a high BP reading, whereas too large a cuff will give a low reading. The wrong size cuff is a very common cause of alarming BP readings in pediatrics. Numerous studies have shown the Doppler technique to be reliable in children.

Recently, the use of the Dinamap monitor, an oscillometric device, is gaining popularity in hospitals because of its ease of use, especially with a small uncooperative child (14). Although this method is fairly reliable for general screening and monitoring, values outside the normal range should be confirmed by the auscultatory method. If an elevated reading is obtained, BP should be measured in all four extremities, because aortic coarctation is a very common cause of hypertension in younger children.

Tachycardia, as a sign of congestive heart failure, should be noted in evaluating an azotemic child, since prerenal failure can occur because of low cardiac output. An increased respiratory rate suggests metabolic acidosis with respiratory compensation through hyperventilation. Deep rapid breathing, although typically present in diabetic ketoacidosis, can also be observed with other causes of metabolic acidosis, such as chronic renal failure.

C. Skin

Patients with chronic renal failure may have pallor due to anemia or a yellowish skin. Various other skin changes or rashes can accompany renal disease. Alopecia, lanugo hair or a malar rash in the child being investigated for hematuria of proteinuria suggest SLE. A purpuric elevated rash localized over the buttocks or lower extremities is typical of Henoch-Schönlein (anaphylactoid) purpura, as is localized edema over the scalp, face, scrotum or extremities. Impetigo (a vesiculopustular lesion containing a yellowish serous fluid that dries to a thick, honey-colored crust) is, together with pharyngitis, a common infecting site of nephritogenic streptococci.

Adenoma sebaceum in a butterfly distribution around the nose is a common finding in tuberous sclerosis, a condition often accompanied by renal tumors. Neurofibromas or *café-au-lait* spots (Von Recklinghausen's disease) in a hypertensive child raise the suspicion of vascular hypertension as well as pheochromocytoma, this latter condition being otherwise very rare in the pediatric age group.

D. Eyes and Throat

Aniridia, or absence of the iris, has been associated (in conjunction with mental retardation and ambiguous genitalia) with the occurrence of Wilms' tumor. Eye abnormalities primarily involving the lens, such as cataracts, can be observed in the older patient with Alport's syndrome, as well as in the patient with Lowe's oculocerebrorenal syndrome (Fanconi syndrome with mental retardation and ocular anomalies). Slit-lamp examination of the eye is mandatory in the child with Fanconi syndrome:

here corneal or retinal deposition of cystine crystals is diagnostic of cystinosis. Fundoscopic examination helps to differentiate acute from chronic hypertension and to assess its significance in terms of end-organ damage. Hypertensive changes are classified into four grades: Grade I, increased arteriolar light reflex; Grade II, arteriovenous nicking; Grade III, cotton wool exudates and flame-shaped hemorrhages; Grade IV, papilledema. Grades I and II suggest a chronic hypertension, whereas Grades III and IV usually accompany acute increases in arterial pressure; papilledema occurs in malignant hypertension.

The tonsils should be examined in the child with suspected poststreptococcal glomerulonephritis, although pharyngitis would often have subsided by the time renal manifestations occur.

E. Heart

Congenital heart disease, particularly ventricular septal defect, is associated with a high incidence of renal anomalies. The presence of a hemic murmur can suggest anemia, a frequent finding in chronic renal failure. Careful cardiac examination should be performed especially in the child with hypertension: a murmur best heard at the second or third intercostal space along the sternal edge and radiating to the back, or a soft systolic murmur of collateral flow heard around the left scapular area, suggest aortic coarctation, a common cause of hypertension in the younger child. The femoral pulses should be palpated. In the child with hypertension, cardiomegaly, signs of congestive heart failure due to increased afterload, or cardiac arrythmias should be sought. A sudden "heart failure" in a previously healthy child should suggest the possibility of acute glomerulonephritis.

A decreased cardiac output can be the cause of prerenal failure. In the child with azotemia, signs of congestive heart failure should be noted, including accessory heart sounds, a gallop rhythm or venous congestion (prominent neck veins, hepatomegaly or peripheral edema).

F. Lungs

The lungs should be examined for the presence of rales, which suggest congestive heart failure due either to a primary cardiac problem or to fluid overload. Signs of pleural effusion (decrease in breath sounds and dullness to percussion around the base of the lung) can often be detected in the edematous patient with nephrotic syndrome.

G. Abdomen

In the newborn, a patent urachus can be suspected from passage of urine from the umbilicus; it is easily ligated surgically. The abdomen should be examined for absence or laxity of the abdominal muscles. Absence of such muscles ("prune-belly") is usually obvious; their laxity can be revealed by watching the newborn crying, and by asking the older child, while recumbent, to lift the head against pressure (the examiner's hand applied over the forehead). Such maneuvers will increase the intraabdominal pressure and cause the abdomen to bulge and the umbilicus to become prominent.

Abdominal masses, while manifesting as abdominal enlargement if very large in size, should be sought by palpation. In the newborn, the unimanual technique is preferred (Figure 2-2) (15), and will permit the examiner to ascertain, in addition to the presence of masses, the presence of kidneys and their size. It is most reliably performed in the first three days of life, when the abdominal muscles are still hypotonic and the abdominal cavity is easily palpated. The abdomen is relaxed by flexing the legs of the prone infant while lifting the buttocks off the bed. The fingers of the opposite hand support the matching loin posteriorly while the thumb searches that side of the abdomen systematically, first superficially and then deeply. Deep palpation is performed by applying a gentle, steadily increasing presssure subcostally in a superior and cephalad direction. The thumb is then slid downward without reducing the posteriorly applied pressure. Usually, the upper pole of the kidney is felt between the descending thumb and the posteriorly placed fingers. While mild traction is exerted on the kidney, it slips cephalad under the thumb,

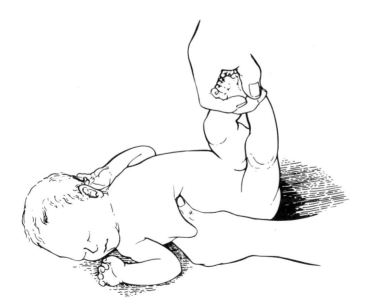

FIGURE 2-2. Unimanual technique of abdominal palpation in the newborn. The legs of the prone infant are flexed while the buttocks are lifted off the bed to relax the abdomen.

and during this passage, its shape and size can be ascertained. The opposite side of the abdomen is examined by changing hands and repeating the above maneuver. Using this technique, about 0.5% of newborn infants are found to have a renal anomaly, which can be confirmed by ultrasonography. Obviously, early detection of asymptomatic anomalies allows early treatment in patients with congenital renal anomalies, which would otherwise remain asymptomatic until later in life. The presence of meningomyelocoele or anal atresia should be noted. In the older child, abdominal palpation is best carried out by using light pressure and a bimanual technique.

The location of an abdominal mass, as well as its surface characteristics, can help determine its etiology. Upper abdominal masses most likely arise from the kidneys, adrenals, liver or spleen. In the older child, polycystic kidneys can sometimes be palpated as bilateral flank masses. It is often mentioned that the mass of hydronephrosis is smooth and cystic, while that of Wilms' tumor is smooth and firm and that of neuroblastoma is nodular. In the younger child, transillumination of the abdomen can be invaluable in differentiating a cystic mass (such as hydronephrosis) from a solid mass. A pelvic mass in a boy suggests an enlarged bladder with outlet obstruction; in a girl, it is more likely to be a hydrocolpos.

The abdomen should be examined for ascites. Its presence is suggested by bulging flanks, with dullness to percussion, while the periumbilical area remains tympanic. A fluid wave is obtained with difficulty in children; it is elicited by tapping a flank sharply with one hand, while the other hand receives the impulse against the opposite flank. Shifting dullness is easily demonstrated by percussing and delineating the area of dullness in the flank when the child is supine, then following a one-minute change to a decubitus position. These maneuvers detect the presence of a large amount of free fluid. A small amount of fluid is difficult to detect by physical examination, and ultrasonography of the abdomen may be necessary. In the child with nephrotic ascites, the abdominal girth should be measured; this is best done with the child standing, and always at a fixed distance from a landmark such as the umbilicus. Flank tenderness should be elicited, on both sides, by gently tapping the costovertebral angle with a closed fist.

Auscultation of the abdomen is likely to be unrevealing in the child with renal disease. However, in the presence of hypertension, a flank bruit should be sought by listening over the flank with the bell of the stethoscope in a quiet room. Its presence suggests a renovascular etiology of the hypertension. A bruit heard over the kidney area following a needle biopsy suggests the presence of an iatrogenic arteriovenous fistula or aneurysm.

The suprapubic area should be examined. Exstrophy of the bladder is obvious. The bladder is normally unpalpable in the normal child. A palpable bladder with a thickened wall suggests hypertrophy due to an anatomical obstruction such as posterior urethral valves or severe reflux. Suprapubic tenderness is often present in the child with cystitis of bacterial or viral etiology. Bladder fullness can be assessed by percussion. Urinary retention in the child with a neurological problem (meningomyelocoele) can predispose to a UTI. In the infant, a suprapubic bladder tap for diagnostic purposes should be performed only if the bladder is full.

H. Extremities

The extremities should be examined for pitting edema. When pressure is exerted by a finger, the edematous area leaves a characteristic pit. This is most easily apparent over a bony area, such as the tibial surface or just above the medial malleolus. In the bedridden patient, edema is more easily observed in the presacral area. The finding is elicited by applying pressure over the sacrum, and looking for pitting. Arthritis suggests a connective tissue disease such as SLE, and is a component of Henoch-Schönlein purpura, the most common vasculitis of childhood. Skeletal abnormalities, such as bowing of the legs, can be a sign of renal osteodystrophy in the child with chronic renal failure or renal tubular disease.

I. Genitalia

Wet underwear in the toilet-trained child can be a sign of urinary urgency due to a UTI. Examination of the external genitalia is of importance in the evaluation of the child with abnormal urinary findings, such as hematuria or pyuria. The urethral meatus should be examined for ulcerations, erosions or prolapse that would explain the presence of red blood cells in the urine. Poor hygiene, especially in the uncircumcised boy, or vulvovaginitis in the girl, can lead to the presence of white blood cells or squamous cells in the urine. Signs of sexual abuse should also be sought. Cryptorchidism, hypospadias and the presence of ambiguous genitalia should be noted.

J. Voiding

The physical examination of the infant or child with a reported voiding abnormality is incomplete if the child is not actually observed voiding. This is particularly important in boys, because of a higher incidence of bladder outlet obstructive lesions. Children with posterior urethral valves will strain to urinate, and exibit a weak stream or dribbling. A child with meatal stenosis, however, will have a strong but very thin stream. Retention should be suspected in the child who is able to void a sizable amount of urine soon after emptying the bladder.

K. Rectal Examination

Rectal examination can be useful in evaluating an abdominal mass. It is also important to assess the rectal sphincter in a child with new onset incontinence. Eliciting the bulbocavernosus reflex (squeezing the glans and observing rectal sphincter contraction) is indicated when a neurological deficit is suspected.

L. Neurological Examination

Hearing assessment by audiometry should be performed in the child with unexplained hematuria or decreased renal fuction suspected of having Alport's syndrome. High frequency sensorineural loss is the typical finding in this condition; hearing impairment is often not noted clinically, since it does not involve the speech range. Sensorineural hearing loss can also result from the use of two common otonephrotoxic drugs, namely furosemide and aminoglycosides. Various cranial nerve palsies, including facial (VII) and ocular (III) nerve palsies can result from severe hypertension.

References

1. Berger RM, Maizels M, Moran GC, et al (1983) Bladder capacity (ounces) equals age (years) plus 2 predicts normal bladder capacity and aids in diagnosis of abnormal voiding patterns. J Urol 129:347–349
2. Burbige KA, Retik AB, Colodny AH, et al (1984) Urinary tract infection in boys. J Urol 132:541–542
3. Walther PC, Lamm D, Kaplan GW (1980) Pediatric urolithiases: a ten-year review. Pediatrics 65:1068–1072
4. Van den Abbeele AD, Treves ST, Lebowitz RL, et al (1987) Vesicoureteral reflux in asymptomatic siblings of patients with known reflux: Radionuclide cystography. Pediatrics 79:147–153
5. Leung AKC, Robson WLM (1989) Single umbilical artery. A report of 159 cases. Am J Dis Child 143:108–111
6. Lachiewicz AM, Sibley R, Michael AF (1985) Hereditary renal disease and preauricular pits: Report of a kindred. J Pediatr 106:948–950
7. Varsano IB, Jaber L, Garty B-Z, et al (1984) Urinary tract abnormalities in children with supernumerary nipples. Pediatrics 73:103–105
8. Woodhouse CRJ, Ransley PG, Innes-Williams D (1982) Prune-belly syndrome—report of 47 cases. Arch Dis Child 57:856–859
9. Barakat AY, Seikaly MG, Der Kaloustian VM (1986) Urological abnormalities in genetic disease. J Urol 136:778–785
10. Barakat AY, Dakessian B (1986) The kidney in heart disease. Int J Pediatr Nephrol 7:153–160
11. Noble MJ, Wacksman J (1980) Screening excretory urography in patients with cryptorchidism or hypospadias: A survey and review of the literature. J Urol 124:98–100

12. Noe HN, Patterson TH (1978) Screening urography in asymptomatic cryptorchid patients. J Urol 119:669–670
13. Roberts KB, Charney E, Sweren RJ, et al (1983) Urinary tract infection in infants with unexplained fever: A collaborative study. J Pediatr 103:864–867
14. Park MK, Menard SM (1987) Accuracy of blood pressure measurement by the Dinamap monitor in infants and children. Pediatrics 79:907–914
15. Perlman M, Williams J (1976) Detection of renal anomalies by abdominal palpation in newborn infants. Br Med J 2:347–349

Additional Reading

Barakat AY, Der Kaloustian VM, Mufarrij AA, et al (1986) The Kidney in Genetic Disease. Churchill Livingstone, Edinburgh
Barness LA (1981) Manual of Pediatric Physical Diagnosis (5th edition). Yearbook Medical Publishers, Chicago
Kelalis PP, King LR (1985) Clinical Pediatric Urology (2nd edition). Saunders, Philadelphia

3
The Urine and Urinary Sediment

Agnes Fogo and Amin Y. Barakat

I. Introduction

It has been known for centuries that abnormalities in urine may indicate disease. The science of urinalysis has progressed greatly since the days of the medieval "Pisse Prophets" who, by visual examination of the urine, claimed to diagnose disease and see into the future. A carefully performed urinalysis using physical, chemical and microscopic examination offers very important information regarding the kidney. The results of any urinalysis depend on proper collection, preservation and careful examination. Numerous specific tests are also available for specific diagnoses when indicated by the initial routine screening tests (1-6).

II. Specimen Collection and Preservation

Proper specimen collection is the first, and perhaps most important step for accurate urine examination. The urine should be collected in a clean, dry container. Preservation methods are necessary if the urine is not tested within one hour of collection. Continued bacterial growth will otherwise lower the glucose and pH, and the cellular elements and casts may decompose or lyse. Adequate preservation for 24 hours without interference with routine dipstick tests may be achieved by refrigeration or the use of chemicals. There is no adequate method for prolonged preservation of red blood cells, bilirubin or urobilinogen. Preservatives increase the specific gravity (sp gr) when added to a small volume of urine. One formaldehyde-releasing tablet per 30 mL of urine results in a 0.005 increase in sp gr. Stabilur tablets decrease pH and urobilinogen slightly due to direct interference.

Thymol crystals do not inhibit bacterial growth sufficiently, and a urine thus preserved may give a false positive nitrite test. Furthermore, the proper amount of crystals must be added to the specimen (100 mg/50 mL urine); a large amount may give a false positive test for protein. Sodium fluoride thymol tablets (SFT, 1 tablet/50 mL urine) are easy to use and they inhibit bacterial growth. These tablets, however, inhibit the reagent strip glucose test, but the glucose hexokinase and copper reduction tests are not affected. Formalin prevents bacterial growth and allows better preservation of formed elements in the urine compared to other methods of preservation. Formaldehyde (40%) (1 drop/10 mL urine) directly interferes with dipstick tests for ketones, blood and urobilinogen. Too much formalin may precipitate protein. Other preservatives may also interfere with tests as follows: toluene elevates Diastix strip glucose levels; merthiolate may cause false negative glucose results with both Diastix and Clinistix strips (Ames Division, Miles Laboratories, Inc., Elkhart, IN 46515); chlorhexidine gluconate, which preserves glucose in 24-hour collections, may give a false positive protein test by reagent strip.

Culture of urine requires a "clean-catch" specimen collected into a sterile, covered container. The area around the urethral meatus should be cleaned with an antiseptic solution in a front-to-back fashion in females and with the foreskin retracted in noncircumcised males. The first few milliliters of the voided specimen are voided outside before the clean-catch sample is collected. For infants and small children, special plastic bags with adhesive may be used. The entire perineal area covered by the bag is cleaned to avoid fecal contamination. The bag should be checked every 15 minutes to ensure a clean urine collection. One-third of infants will produce a urine specimen within the first hour. An alternative method, especially in infants and young children, is suprapubic needle aspiration, which, in experienced hands, can be done safely and without complications. The procedure should be performed on a full bladder, and it should not be attempted if it is less than one hour since the last voiding. The success rate of suprapubic tap under these conditions is as high as 90%. Transient gross hematuria is seen in less than 1% of patients when the aspiration is properly performed. Bladder catheterization, which may be indicated with a history of urinary retention and suspected pelvic or vaginal infection, carries a risk of iatrogenic infection of approximately 2 to 4%.

The timing of the urine specimen collection is an important consideration. First morning voided specimens yield the most concentrated urine and are more likely to show formed elements and to allow detection of bacteria because of the overnight incubation in the bladder. Postprandial specimens are more likely to show elevated glucose.

For routine urinalysis, 10 mL of urine are needed, although a much smaller sample (2.5 mL) is sufficient to perform multiple reagent strip, copper reducing, bilirubin and sp gr tests. A timed, usually 24-hour urine collection is necessary for quantitation of many substances. To start the collection, the bladder is emptied and the inital urine voided is discarded. The time is noted and all urine for the next 24 hours is collected. For accurate results, the sample must be complete and the container should be refrigerated during the collection. Special precautions are necessary for some collections. The most commonly used procedures are outlined below, but should be verified with the reference laboratory utilized, since methods may vary.

Urine for vanillylmandelic acid (VMA) analysis requires a 24-hour specimen with 20 mL of 6 N HCl added to the container. Porphyrin requires a 40-mL aliquot of a 24-hour collection with 5 g Na_2CO_3 added as a preservative; the container should be opaque or stored away from bright light. Urine urea, nitrogen and uric acid may each be determined from separate 10-mL aliquots of a 24-hour urine collection, whereas calcium requires a 40-mL aliquot with 10 mL of concentrated HCl added to the container. Citrate requires a 100-mL aliquot with toluene as a preservative, steroids require 1 g of boric acid/100 mL urine and free cortisol requires 10 mL of 0.5% thymol in acetic acid as a preservative. Oxalate is preserved by acidifying the specimen to a pH <3.0 by adding 10 mL of 6 N HCl; the pH must be < 2 for heavy metal determinations.

The normal 24-hour volume increases from 15 to 60 mL in the term newborn to 250 to 450 mL at age two months, to an adult range of 700 to 1500 mL by age eight years. Adequacy of a 24-hour collection may be assessed by measuring the amount of creatinine excreted, and compared to expected ranges for age and body weight (usually 8 to 20 mg/kg/day).

III. Quality Control and Instrumentation

Quality control involves all aspects of specimen handling and ensures accurate results. Specimen identification is the most likely area for errors to occur. It is imperative that the container (not the lid) be properly labeled and that identification of the sample is maintained throughout transportation, specimen preparation and testing until the results are correctly recorded. Known positive and negative controls should be run routinely in the laboratory to ensure that test procedures and reagents give correct results. Corrective action should be taken if results do not fall within the known and expected range. Urine must be at room temperature during testing and the color change of reagent strips must be read at the right time interval. Any excess of urine must be properly drained off, since "run over" (reagent buffers from one area of the strip seeping over to another) may give false results.

Instruments in the clinical laboratory should be checked regularly to assure proper performance. Reagent strips must be stored in a cool, dry place, not refrigerated. A cap left loose on the container may result in deterioration of the reagents and cause false positive or negative results.

The TS (total solid) refractometer used to measure sp gr should be calibrated periodically against distilled H_2O (sp gr 1.000) and another solution of known higher sp gr, e.g. 71 mL xylene + 28 mL bromobenzene (sp gr 1.030). The urinometer must also be checked against such standards for accuracy. The TS meter is temperature compensated at normal working conditions. The urinometer requires a correction factor with the addition of 0.001 sp gr units for each 3°C increase in the working temperature above the calibration temperature.

IV. Physical Examination

Gross examination of the urine provides important information. The appearance may be altered by the presence of cellular or other material. Normal urine is clear, transparent and yellow due to the presence of the pigment urochrome and urobilin, a breakdown product of hemoglobin. Turbid, cloudy urine may be due to leukocytes, red blood cells, epithelial cells or bacteria. Large amounts of amorphous phosphates or carbonates in alkaline urine may also cause a turbid appearance that disappears if acetic acid is added to the specimen. A pink, turbid urine frequently occurs with excess urates. Milky urine may be due to chyle as a result of lymphatic obstruction or fat in patients with nephrosis. Spermatozoa may also cause cloudy urine.

Color is also affected by substrates in the urine. Dilute urine, which may be seen normally with increased fluid intake or pathologically with diabetes insipidus or diabetes mellitus, is pale or colorless. Concentrated urine, seen with decreased fluid intake, is dark yellow-orange. Substances changing the urine color and appearance are presented in Table 3-1.

The odor of urine reflects its components, although it is seldom diagnostic. Freshly voided normal urine has an aromatic odor due to volatile acids. On standing, a characteristic ammonia odor results from degradation of urea. In some diseases, the urine does have an unusual characteristic odor. The fruity odor due to acetonuria in the diabetic was noted by ancient Greek physicians. A foul or putrid odor is indicative of an infection. Maple syrup disease derives its name from the characteristic scent of the urine. Some other metabolic diseases may also cause an abnormal odor: phenylketonuria causes a musty odor, hypermethioninemia, a fishy odor; isovaleric acidemia or excess butyric or hexanoic acid, a "sweaty feet" odor. Any persistent unusual odor of urine in infants should alert the physician to the possibility of a metabolic disorder, and appropriate screening tests should be done (see below).

V. Specific Gravity

The sp gr of urine reflects the relative proportion of solutes in a given volume of urine; 70 to 90% of the sp gr is due to urea, creatinine, chlorides, sulfates, phosphates and bicarbonates, and the remainder reflects the presence of various organic compounds. Specific gravity may range from 1.003 to 1.030, but usually remains between 1.010 and 1.025. A sp gr of 1.023 or more in any random urine specimen indicates normal concentrating ability. Water diuresis can decrease the urine sp gr to 1.001. Ab-

TABLE 3-1. Urine Appearance

Appearance	Cause
Clear, colorless or pale yellow	Dilute—increased fluid intake, diabetes mellitus or diabetes insipidus
Turbid or cloudy	Amorphous phosphates or carbonates with alkaline pH, urates (pinkish), cells, bacteria, yeast, spermatozoa, mucin, X-ray media, fecal contamination
Milky	Fat (nephrosis), chyle (lymphatic obstruction), pus
Yellow-orange to yellow-brown	Concentrated, urobilin, bilirubin, pyridium, nitrofurantoin, dilantin, acriflavin (green fluorescence)
Red to red-brown	Hemoglobin, RBC, myoglobin, porphyrin, beet ingestion, aniline dyes (candy), rifampin, theophylline, iodine
Brown-black	Phenothiazines, methyldopa, metronidazole, phenols
Brown-black to brown-purple on standing	Porphyrins, melanins, homogentisic acid (alkaptonuria)
Red-pink	Phenolsulfonphthaleine, bromsulphalein, rhubarb
Blue-green	*Pseudomonas*, methylene blue, amitriptyline, methocarbomal, chlorophyll pigment (mouth wash), riboflavin
Yellow-green	Bilirubin, biliverdin

normally low values may be due to intrinsic renal loss of concentrating ability, central or nephrogenic diabetes insipidus or polydipsia. The most common causes of an increase in sp gr are dehydration and elevated urinary protein, glucose or contrast media. Specific gravity may also help in differentiating prerenal failure from acute tubular necrosis. In prerenal failure, the sp gr is elevated and urine sodium is low (<20 mEq/L); in acute tubular necrosis, the sp gr is low (<1.012), and urine sodium is elevated (up to 60 mEq/L). Preservatives increase the sp gr slightly (see above).

Three methods are commonly used to determine urine sp gr. The urinometer measures sp gr based on buoyancy. The bulb-shaped stemmed instrument floats at a level that depends on the density of the fluid, and sp gr can be read directly off the scale on the stem at the level of the fluid meniscus. This method requires a large enough volume of urine to allow the urinometer to float freely in the container without touching the sides or bottom. It is also important that the instrument be properly calibrated (see above).

The TS refractometer is a hand-held instrument that measures the refractive index of a solution; this value is directly proportional to the sp gr. The TS meter further has the advantage of requiring only one drop of urine and no temperature calibration between 60 to 100°F. The instrument must be washed and dried after each use. The sample is allowed to pass under the closed cover plate by capillary action. The TS meter is then held up to the light and the sp gr is read at the boundary of the light and dark shades. The meter should be calibrated daily with distilled water and adjusted if necessary to give a sp gr of 1.000. Both instruments will show an increased sp gr in the presence of increased glucose, protein or contrast media. The following should be added to the sg: 0.003 for each 1 g protein/100 mL, 0.004 for each 1 g glucose/100 mL; 0.001 for each 0.15 g NaCl/100 mL.

Recently, the Multistix 10 SG reagent strip (Miles Laboratories) has been used to measure urine sp gr. The pretreated polyelectrolytes of the reagent strip change pK_a in relation to the ion concentration in the specimen and therefore can change the color of an indicator. These changes are empirically correlated to sp gr levels and given as 0.005 increments between 1.000 and 1.030. Elevated glucose, urea or non-ionic contrast dyes will not influence the result, whereas increased protein (which may be ionic) may cause an elevated sp gr. Alkaline or highly buffered urine may give falsely low readings. Correction by adding 0.005 to the sp gr if the urine pH is >6.5 is therefore recommended.

The newest advance in sp gr measurement, the falling drop direct method, is available in some automated urinalysis instruments. Precisely measured drops of urine fall through a silicone-based oil column. The drop's fall time is measured by the breaking of two light beams at either end of the column, and this fall time is converted into sp gr units. The denser the drop, i.e. the higher the sp gr, the faster the drop falls.

Although both sp gr and osmolality reflect solute concentration, the latter is a measure only of the number of particles in a solution and is not affected by the weight of the solutes. Osmolality thus reflects the concentrating ability of the renal tubules. The normal range in a newborn is wide, 15 to 585 mOsm/kg, with a mean of 240 mOsm/kg. Regular diet and kidney maturation increase the normal range in children to 300 to 800 mOsm/kg. Neonates normally have some concentrating ability and are able to increase osmolality to a mean of 950 mOsm/kg after 12 to 14 hours of fluid deprivation. By age two years, the concentrating ability after dehydration approaches the adult range (1200 mOsm/kg). Osmolality of <800 mOsm/kg after water deprivation indicates a loss of concentrating ability. With advanced renal disease, urine osmolality approaches that of the plasma and the glomerular filtrate (285 mOsm/kg), indicating complete loss of diluting or concentrating ability of the renal tubule. In prerenal failure, urine osmolality remains higher than plasma osmolality, whereas in acute tubular necrosis they are similar. Osmolality is measured by freezing point depression or by vapor pressure depression; 1 osmole of any solute added to 1 kg of water lowers the freezing point of water by 1.86 °C.

VI. Chemical Examination

Routine chemical screening assays of urine are often done by reagent strip testing (4). These consist of a plastic strip with multiple pads, each impregnated with specific reagents, indicators and buffers. The reagent portion is immersed into the fresh, well-mixed urine specimen and immediately removed. The excess urine is removed by running the edge of the strip against the container rim and the strip is held vertically (Chemstrip, Boehringer Mannheim, Indianapolis, IN 46250) or horizontally (Multistix, Miles) and the color change compared, under adequate light at the appropriate reading time, with the color chart standards provided by the manufacturer. Proper storage and handling of reagent strips with appropriate quality control are imperative. Some substances (serenium, azo dye-containing drugs, pyridium, nitrofurantoin, riboflavin) that color the urine may interfere with or mask the reagent strip color reactions. Confirmatory or more specific tests are done by separate chemical assays. The characteristics of reagent strips used in urinalysis are presented in Table 3-2.

A. pH

Normal urine pH varies from 4.5 to 8.5; however, the urine is normally slightly acidic due to the acid produced by normal metabolism. The kidney normally excretes 50 to 100 mEq of hydrogen daily as titratable

TABLE 3-2. Characteristics of Reagent Strips Used in Urinalysis

Test	Chemostrip[a]	Multistix[b]	False positive results	False negative results
pH	5-9	5-8.5 visual 5-9 pH meter	None	None
Protein	6 mg/dL (albumin)	15-30 mg/dL (albumin)	Highly alkaline urine[b]; Phenazopyridine[a]; antiseptics and detergents[a,b]	Low levels of proteins other than albumin, very dilute urine, urine pH <4.5[a,b]
Glucose	40 mg/dL	75-125 mg/dL	Peroxide, oxidizing cleaning agents	Decreased sensitivity: high sp gr[a,b]; ketones > 40 mg/dL[b]
Ketones	9 mg/dL (acetoacetic acid) 70 mg/dL (acetone)	5-10 mg/dL (acetoacetic acid)	Phenylketones, phenolphthalein, (acetoacetic acid), levodopa metabolites (red reaction vs violet for ketones), highly pigmented urines, sulfhydryl-containing compounds[a,b]; high sp gr[b]	
Blood	0.03 mg/dL hemoglobin, 5 RBC/hpf	0.015-0.062 mg/dL hemoglobin, 5-20 RBC/hpf	Myoglobin, bacterial peroxidases, oxidizing cleaning agents, menstrual contamination[a,b]	Decreased sensitivity: high protein, ascorbic acid, high sp gr[b]
Bilirubin	0.5 mg/dL	0.4-0.8 mg/dL	Pyridium, Indican, other substances that color urine red, chlorpromazine?[a,b]	Ascorbic acid > 25 mg/dL, light exposure[a,b]; decreased sensitivity: high nitrite[a]
Urobilinogen	0.4 mg/dL	0.2 mg/dL	Phenazopyridine,[a] Ehrlich's reagent interfering substances (sulfonamides, p-aminobenzoic acid)	Decreased sensitivity: formalin > 200 mg/dL, light exposure[a,b]; nitrite > 5 mg/dL[a]
Nitrite	0.05 mg/dL	0.06-0.1 mg/dL	Substances coloring urine red[a,b]	Decreased sensitivity: high sp gr, short bladder incubation, ascorbic acid > 25 mg/dL[a,b]
Leukocytes	92.7% sensitivity correlates with > 10^5 bacteria/mL	5-15 WBC/hpf correlates with > 10^5 colonies/mL	Oxidizing cleaning agents, nitrofurantoin[b]	Cephalocin, gentamycin, albumin >500 mg/dL[a]; decreased sensitivity: glucose > 3g/dL, high sp gr, tetracycline, high concentration oxalic acid[b]; cephalexin[a,b]

acid and ammonium. Transient acidity may occur after eating cranberries or after a high protein meal. A persistent increase in urinary acidity may be present with respiratory or metabolic acidosis, fever, phenylketonuria, alkaptonuria, methanol intoxication, renal tuberculosis, severe diarrhea, starvation or uremia.

Alkaline urine is seen if the urine sample has been allowed to stand for a prolonged time interval due to the escape of CO_2 and the conversion of urea to ammonia. Postprandially, urine is normally alkaline. Diets high in citrate (citrus fruit) may also give an alkaline urine. Infection with urea-splitting organisms, respiratory or metabolic alkalosis, hyperaldosteronism, Cushing's syndrome and renal tubular acidosis also cause an alkaline urine.

Urine pH is usually determined by a reagent strip indicator sensitive to changes in pH. More precise measurements, when indicated, as in suspected cases of renal tubular acidosis, may be done on a freshly voided specimen using a pH meter with a glass electrode.

B. Protein

The urine contains small amounts of protein, normally ≤ 100 mg/m^2/ 24 hours. In children, two-thirds of the physiological urine protein consists of albumin and one-third represents a mixture of Tamm-Horsfall protein and globulin. This ratio is reversed in adults. Tamm-Horsfall protein, a large glycoprotein, is normally present at a concentration of 2 to 2.5 mg/dL.

Marked proteinuria (>4 g/1.73 m^2/day) may be seen in amyloidosis, severe glomerulonephritis, systemic lupus erythematosus (SLE), malignant nephrosclerosis or severe renal venous congestion such as renal vein thrombosis. Moderate proteinuria (0.5 to 4 g/1.73 m^2/day) may be seen in most renal diseases, including any of the ones listed above, diabetic nephropathy, preeclampsia, interstitial diseases or lower urinary tract disease. Mild proteinuria (<0.5 g/1.73 m^2/day) may be present in chronic glomerulonephritis, tubular diseases, polycystic kidney disease or nephrosclerosis without malignant hypertension. Proteinuria is nephrotic when it is ≥ 40 mg/m^2/hour.

Postural or orthostatic proteinuria is a benign form of proteinuria occurring only when the child is in the upright position. Nonrenal conditions, such as strenuous exercise, fever, emotional stress, cold or heat exposure or congestive heart failure, may all be associated with functional proteinuria.

Protein may be detected by reagent strips that use buffered tetrabromphenol blue (N-Multistix, Miles) or tetrachlorophenoltetrabromosulfophthalein (Chemstrip, Boehringer) indicators. At a constant pH, the binding of the protein to the reagent changes the color from yellow to green-blue with increasing protein concentrations (from 30 to >1000 mg/

dL). The reagent strips are much more sensitive to albumin than glob-ulins, hemoglobin or Bence-Jones protein (Table 3.2).

Qualitative protein testing may also be done by precipitation methods, by heating or by adding sulfosalicylic acid. The latter method is more sensitive, detecting as low as 5 to 10 mg/dL of all urine proteins including albumin, globulins, glycoproteins and Bence-Jones protein.

Quantitative protein determination on a timed, 24-hour collection is done by precipitation methods. The sample should be freed of debris by centrifuging at 1200 rpm for 10 minutes. Turbidity resulting from the precipitation reaction is measured by a photometer, nephelometer or by eye, and compared with known standards. Heat and acetic acid precip-itation are most sensitive, detecting protein levels as low as 2 to 3 mg/dL. Sulfosalicylic acid or concentrated nitric acid methods are less sen-sitive. False positive acid precipitation may occur with some radiographic contrast media. Tolbutamide metabolites, massive doses of penicillin, sulfonamides or other highly buffered alkaline urine may give false neg-ative results. A semiquantitative method is the urine protein/creatinine ratio (see Chapter 8).

C. Glucose and Reducing Substances

Reducing substances in the urine are normally very low in concentration (<100 mg/dL); most of this is contributed by glucose. The amount of glucosuria depends on the blood glucose level and the amount of tubular reabsorption. The normal renal threshold for glucose is 160 to 180 mg/dL. Some patients may have a benign, congenitally lowered renal glucose threshold. Significant glucosuria is usually an indication of diabetes mel-litus. Other possible causes of hyperglycemia and glucosuria, such as some endocrinopathies, glycogen storage diseases, thiazide diuretics or steroid drugs should be considered. Postprandially, glucose in blood and urine may be transiently elevated. Glucosuria without hyperglycemia is seen in some tubular defects, such as Fanconi syndrome, cystinosis and lead poisoning.

Spillover of carbohydrate in the urine occurs in disorders of carbo-hydrate metabolism (galactosuria, lactosuria, fructosuria, pentosuria), or may be physiological, due to increased ingestion of the sugar. The most significant in children is galactose, due to an inborn error of metabolism (galactose–1-phosphate uridyltransferase deficiency). Lactose may be seen in the urine of patients with lactase deficiency. Lactosuria is common in premature infants and newborns until three to four days of age, when the gastrointestinal flora is established. Pentosuria may rarely occur due to an inborn error of metabolism, but it is more commonly due to inges-tion of large amounts of cherries or plums.

Screening tests for sugars in the urine employ either glucose oxidase, which is specific for glucose, or copper reduction tests, which react with any reducing substance. The glucose oxidase test becomes less sensitive as the urine sp gr increases. High urine vitamin C levels may interfere with the oxidation of the chromagen because it is oxidized by the peroxide reagent, causing false negative results. When indicated, the specific non-glucose sugar in the urine may be identified by paper chromatography.

The commonly used multiple reagent strips N-Multistix and Chemstrip both utilize glucose oxidase and detect 75 to 100 mg/dL and 40 mg/dL, respectively. Moderately high ketones (40 mg/dL) may decrease sensitivity for trace glucose levels with the N-Multistix. Specific strips for monitoring urine glucose in diabetics that use the glucose oxidase technique include Diastix, Keto-diastix, Clinistix (Miles), Tes-Tape (Eli Lilly, Indianapolis, IN 46285) and Chemstrips. The Clinitest (Miles) tablets are based on the nonspecific copper reduction (Benedict's) test and give accurate quantitative results, as does the glucose-specific Diastix. The sensitivity of the Clinitest is 250 mg/dL. False positive Clinitest results may result from nalidixic acid, cephalosporins, probenicid, creatinine, uric acid and high levels of ascorbic acid or other reducing sugars. Large quantities of formaldehyde used as a preservative may also interfere with the test, since formaldehyde is a reducing substance. False negatives may result from high protein concentration. Some sulfa drug metabolites may interfere with detection of low ($<$500 mg/dL) glucose levels. The greater sensitivity of the Benedict's test (50 mg/dL) also results in a greater number of false positives. Other substances, such as salicylates, penicillin, streptomycin and oxytetracycline in high enough concentrations may also give false positive results.

D. Ketones

The ketone bodies acetoacetic acid, beta-hydroxybutyric acid and acetone are intermediates of fatty acid metabolism with normal proportions of 20%,78%, and 2%, respectively. Small amounts (2–4 mg/dL) are normally present in the blood, with increased amounts seen after the renal excretory capacity has been exceeded. Normal urine levels are up to 2 mg/dL of acetoacetic acid and 20 mg of total ketones. Ketosis may develop in any condition associated with abnormal or decreased carbohydrate metabolism, such as diabetes mellitus, low carbohydrate intake as in prolonged vomiting or starvation, low carbohydrate levels relative to increased metabolic demands seen in severe prolonged exercise or glycogen storage disease. Screening tests utilize the sodium nitroprusside or nitroferricyanide reaction to acetoacetic acid as an indicator of the presence of ketone bodies. Sensitivity is 5 to 10 mg/dL for Chemstrip (Boehringer) N-Multistix, Ketostix, Keto-diastix, and Acetest tablets (Miles). The latter two also detect acetone with a sensitivity of 40 to 70 mg/dL and 50 mg/dL, respectively.

E. Blood

Red blood cells (RBC) in the urine may originate from any site of the urinary tract, from glomerulus to urethra. Bleeding may be microscopic or gross. Hematuria may be seen in numerous diseases (see Chapter 8). When hematuria is renal in origin, proteinuria and casts are often seen also. The normal range of RBC excretion in the urine is wide. Quantitative studies indicate normal ranges of $\leq$ 240,000 RBC per 12 hours, with lower levels for females. In most laboratories, by standard methods, these values correspond to 1 RBC/2 to 3 high power fields (hpf) or approximately 500 RBC/mL; however, up to 3 RBC/hpf may be considered normal. Trace positive dipstick reagent test for blood should therefore be evaluated by microscopic examination. The detection of blood is based on the lysis of the RBC and the peroxide-like activity of the released hemoglobin. Intact RBCs produce a speckled pattern, in contrast to the smooth color change seen with hemoglobin (see below). When sp gr $\leq$ 1.004, RBCs will be almost completely lysed within two hours. In acid urine (pH <6), some lysis also occurs. Therefore, RBCs may not be detected on microscopic examination under these conditions, although the hemoglobin dipstick test will detect the hemoglobin released from lysis. None of the preservative reagents adequately preserve blood over a 24-hour period. Interference with the dipstick test is presented in Table 3-2 (2-6).

F. Hemoglobin and Myoglobin

Hemoglobinuria, like hematuria, produces a red discoloration of the urine, and gives a positive dipstick test for blood. A combination of chemical and microscopic examination on a freshly voided specimen is, therefore, necessary to differentiate the one from the other. Hemoglobinuria without hematuria is the result of excess free hemoglobin in the blood and is seen with hemolytic anemia, transfusion reactions, paroxysmal nocturnal hematuria, paroxysmal cold hemoglobinuria, severe infectious diseases and some prosthetic heart valves; it is also seen after severe burns, renal infarcts, poisoning with snake venom or mushrooms or strong acids and strenuous exercise. Myoglobin is derived from skeletal muscle and is a small, easily filtered molecule seen in the urine following muscular damage, such as trauma, convulsions, prolonged severe exercise, heat stroke, electric shock, myocardial infarction and other conditions. Acute renal failure may result from high levels due to renal tubular cell toxicity. Both hemoglobin and myoglobin are detected by their peroxidase-like activity. The Multistix and Chemstrip reagent pads cause lysis of intact RBC when they touch the reagent area. The result is that free hemoglobin or myoglobin gives a uniform green color, whereas the lysis of intact RBCs on the reagent pad causes a green spot or speckled reaction. The sensitivity ranges are 0.015 to 0.016 mg/dL of free hemoglobin or 5 to 20 RBC/hpf (Table 3-2). Myoglobin can be differentiated from hemoglobin, although both produce clear red urine, because the plasma remains colorless with increased myoglobin, in contrast to the red-pink plasma seen with hemoglobinemia. Additional tests, such as elevated serum creatine phosphokinase (CPK) levels to detect muscle injury, electrophoresis or ammonium sulfate tests (precipitates hemoglobin but not myoglobin) may also aid in the differentiation (see Chapter 8).

G. Bilirubin

Bilirubin is formed from hemoglobin breakdown, and becomes water soluble when conjugated in the liver to glucuronide. Most of the bilirubin is excreted in the bile and enters the enterohepatic circulation. Intestinal bacteria further break down bilirubin to urobilinogen, a portion of which is reabsorbed. Small amounts of bilirubin and urobilinogen are normally excreted in the urine (<0.02 mg/dL of bilirubin and <4 mg/day—0.1–1.0 Ehrlich units/dL of urobilinogen). Elevated urine bilirubin is seen with liver parenchymal disease. Detection of bilirubin is based on a diazo reaction. The Multistix reagent detects 0.2 to 0.4 mg/dL; Chemstrip 0.5 mg/dL; and Ictotest (Miles) reagent, 0.05 to 0.1 mg/dL.

Urobilinogen detection is based on the Ehrlich aldehyde reaction (Multistix) and detects 0.2 Ehrlich units/dL, whereas the Chemstrip reagent is based on an azo reaction and detects 1.0 Ehrlich units/dL. Normal random urines may therefore show trace positive reactions and clinical correlation is necessary to interpret these findings. Substances that interfere with these tests are presented in Table 3-2.

H. Bacteria

Chemical testing for microorganisms is based on the presence of nitrite formed by bacterial reduction of the nitrates normally present in urine. Neither bacteria nor nitrite is present in normal clean-catch urine samples. Testing should be done on a first-morning void, since the urine must be incubated with the bacteria for at least four hours to allow nitrite to form. The sensitivity of this chemical test in the culture-proven, early morning specimen is about 90%. A positive test indicates the presence of significant bacteria; a negative test does not rule out urinary tract infection. False negatives may be due to a short bladder incubation time, or because the bacteria lack the reductase enzyme to produce nitrite. False positive results may occur due to interference from agents that turn the urine red. Occasionally, further reduction of nitrite to nonreacting nitrogen may occur. Rarely, the diet, and thus the urine, may be devoid of nitrate. Due to these factors, the degree of positivity is not correlated with the number of bacteria in the urine. With either Chemstrip or Multistix reagent strips, high levels of ascorbic acid (>25 mg/dL) decrease the sensitivity or may cause false negative results with small amounts of nitrite.

A new dipstick test allows screening for leukocytes, using the presence of leukocyte esterase in these cells. Leukocytes in the urine are most commonly due to infection, although they may be seen with various other conditions presented later in this chapter. The test detects the leukocyte esterase from intact and lysed white blood cells (WBC). Sensitivity is 5 to 15 WBC/hpf for the Multistix, which correlates well with more than 10^5 bacteria/mL. The Chemstrip reagent has over 97% sensitivity for the detection of significant bacteria. Test sensitivity is decreased with high sp gr as well as elevated glucose, oxalic acid, albumin and certain antibiotics (Table 3-2).

I. Electrolytes

Electrolyte values in the urine normally vary widely in response to diet and fluid intake. Sodium (Na) excretion is useful for volume status assessment and evaluation of acute renal failure. Decreased urine Na (< 10 to 15 mEq/L) is most commonly seen with effective volume depletion. In acute renal failure due to acute tubular necrosis, Na is usually >20 meq/L, whereas in prerenal failure urine Na is usually <20 mEq/L. Urinary Na is also used to calculate the fractional excretion of Na, the most accurate renal failure index.

Chloride (Cl) excretion parallels that of Na and thus urine Cl usually adds little information to that given by urine Na. However, in cases of hypovolemia with metabolic alkalosis, since some excess HCO_3^- is excreted as $NaHCO_3$, the resulting elevated urinary Na concentration does not reflect the volume status. In this instance, urine Cl remains low and thus provides useful information.

Urine potassium (K) excretion reflects dietary intake. With K depletion due to extrarenal losses or to diuretic use, excretion may fall to very low levels. Higher levels associated with hypokalemia suggest the presence of renal K wasting. In renal failure, the ability to excrete K is impaired. Thus, urine K is inappropriately low and hyperkalemia is seen. Urine Na/K ratio may be of diagnostic value (Appendix I). Measurement of these electrolytes in the urine is performed by flame photometry without interference by other substances.

VII. Other Studies

A. Inborn Errors of Metabolism

When an inborn error of metabolism is suspected, specific diagnostic tests are performed. After routine urinalysis, a reducing substance test (e.g.

copper reduction test) or Clinitest (on fresh urine) will detect metabolic defects associated with increased carbohydrate excretion. If the glucose oxidase test is negative, the specific abnormal carbohydrates or reducing substances may be identified by specific enzymatic reactions, gas chromatography or thin-layer chromatography (TLC).

The mucopolysaccharidoses are a specific group of diseases of carbohydrate metabolism due to deficiency of one or more lysosomal enzymes. There is a resulting increase in urinary excretion of mucopolysaccharides and abnormalities due to accumulation within tissues. Screening on random or 24-hour urine samples is performed by precipitation, electrophoresis or TLC. The MPS strip test is based on the metachromatic reaction of a basic dye with the anionic mucopolysaccharides. The toluidine blue test is based on the same reaction. False positive results occur in the presence of heparin and numerous other substances.

The dinitrophenylhydrazine (DNP) test detects elevated ketoacids, which are seen in numerous conditions, among others, phenylketonuria, maple syrup urine disease and tyrosinosis. Comparison with routine urinalysis is necessary, since ketones also will give a positive result. Therefore a positive DNP test is common in the neonate who normally excretes increased ketones. The cyanide nitroprusside (CNP) test detects sulfhydryl-containing amino acids and thus is used to screen for cystinuria and homocystinuria. Dilute or highly acid urine may produce a false negative reaction. The nitrosonaphthol (NP) test detects tyrosine and its metabolites. False positive reactions may occur with gastrointestinal disease with bacterial overgrowth, resulting in increased amounts of p-hydroxyphenyl acetic acid.

Specific tests to identify the elevated amino acids or other compounds include enzymatic, spectrophotometric, thin-layer chromatography, gas liquid chromatography, ion exchange chromatography, and high pressure liquid chromatography, depending upon which substance is suspected on the initial screening. The ferric chloride reaction is not specific; it gives different color reactions with various metabolic diseases, medications and dyes.

Thin-layer chromatography with ninhydrin color development may also be used to screen for other amino acidurias (e.g. alkaptonuria, maple syrup urine disease, cystinosis). The normal range of total urinary amino acids in children from 2½ to 12 years of age is 3.3 to 6.2 mg/kg/hour, and in infants 3.8 to 6.5 mg/kg/hour. If increased levels are detected by TLC, individual amino acids can be identified by specific reaction or separation techniques. Several spot screening tests are also available. The DNP reagent strip will detect branched chain ketoacids in random urine samples if their blood level is >10 mg/dL and is therefore used also to screen for maple syrup disease.

Disorders of purine or pyrimidine metabolism (such as Lesch-Nyhan, xanthinuria, orotic aciduria and gout) are characterized by hyperuricemia and excess urates in the urine. The infant with these diseases may thus present with a red- or pinkish-tinged diaper due to excess urates. Examination of the urine identifies many of these abnormal crystals. Specific enzyme defects may be identified in some of these diseases.

Disorders of porphyrin metabolism may be detected by· screening for urinary porphobilinogen (Watson-Schwartz test). The urine may be deep red, which turns darker upon exposure to light. Other screening tests detect other urinary porphyrins (coproporphyrin, uroporphyrin, protoporphyrin) by their red flourescence under ultraviolet light after extraction. Specific quantification may then be done. Normal daily levels are 70 to 250 mg (coproporphyrins), 10 to 30 mg (uroporphyrin), 2 mg (porphobilinogen) and 1 to 7 mg (aminolevulinic acid).

B. Miscellaneous

Urine creatinine levels are used to assess renal clearance and adequacy of timed urine collections. The Jaffe reaction measures noncreatinine chromagens in the plasma which are not present in the urine. This offsets the overestimation of creatinine clearance caused by the low tubular secretion of creatinine. Thus the calculated creatitine clearance approximates the true glomerular filtration rate.

Urinary proteins may be specifically tested by radioimmunodiffusion, nephelometry, radioimmunoassay, or more commonly, electrophoresis and immunoelectrophoresis. Protein selectivity index and β-2 microglobulins are discussed in Chapter 8. Different drugs, such as opiates, amphetamines, acetaminophen and others may be detected in the urine by gas chromatography/mass spectrometry (7).

VIII. Microscopic Examination

The urinary sediment may normally contain some elements from the kidney and urinary tract such as crystals, low numbers of epithelial cells, RBC, white blood cells (WBC) and hyaline casts (Figure 3-1) (1-6). Although the methods in use lack standardization and automation and are difficult to quantitate, significant information can be obtained from careful preparation and examination of the urinary sediment. The fresh or properly preserved sample should be thoroughly mixed prior to centrifugation. Ten milliliters are centrifuged at 400 rpm for five minutes. The supernatant is decanted, leaving a standard, uniform urine volume of 0.5 or 1.0 mL. If a stain is used, it should be added before the specimen is gently resuspended. One drop of the resuspended sediment is placed on a clean labeled glass slide, covered with a 22 × 22 mm coverslip avoiding air bubbles and immediately examined. The entire slide must initially

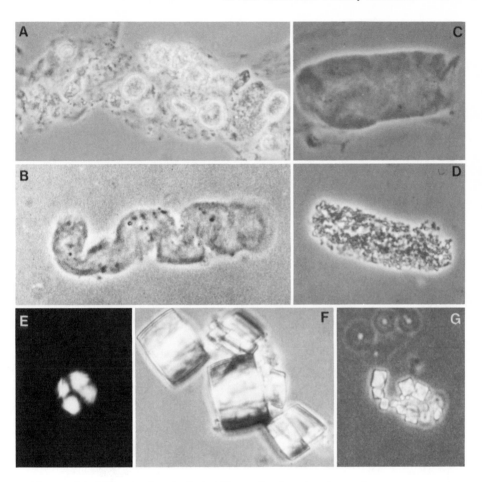

FIGURE 3-1. Microscopic urinalysis (all examinations by phase microscopy, except "E," which is polarized). (A) Cellular cast (× 200). (B) Waxy cast (× 200). (C) Hyaline cast (× 200). (D) Coarse granular cast (× 200). (E) Talc-"maltese cross" appearance (× 500). (F) Uric acid crystals (× 500). (G) Calcium oxalate crystals (× 500).

be examined at low power with special attention to the edges where formed elements tend to cluster. Findings are quantified over at least 10 low power fields. High power examination (40×) of 20 fields should be done and the urine elements counted. With conventional bright field microscopy, there is little contrast between urine and casts because of their similar refractive index. Optical contrast can be increased by a combination of shutting down the iris diaphragm, lowering the condenser and decreasing the light source brightness. Staining of the sediment may also help visualization and identification of formed elements. Phase-con-

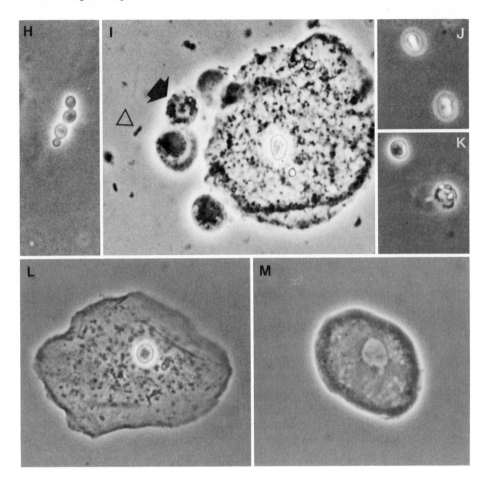

FIGURE 3-1. (H) Yeast (× 500). (I) Large squamous epithelial cell with adjacent, darkly granular polymorphonuclear leukocytes (arrow) and small, rod-shaped bacteria (triangle) (× 500). (J) Normal RBCs (× 500). (K) Dysmorphic RBCs (× 500). (L) Renal epithelial cell (× 500). (M) Renal tubular cell (× 500).

trast microscopy amplifies phase differences and translates these into intensity differences, which can be recognized by the human eye. Thus, excellent visualization of all elements of the sediment is possible without staining. With all techniques, continuous fine focusing is necessary to examine and detect the three-dimensional sediment elements. Polarized light allows easier identification of certain crystals and fat bodies. If a special polarizing microscope is unavailable, the use of two pieces of exposed X-ray film, one piece on top of the slide, the other over the light source and rotated until the field is polarized, may aid the examination.

This method does not, however, allow detailed examination under high power, since the film on the slide interferes with focusing.

The Sternheimer-Malbin stain is the most frequently used supravital stain and is commercially available as kova stain. White blood cells, epithelial cells and casts are stained. Sudan or oil red 0 staining methods make fat pink-red. Eosin is useful because it stains RBCs but not yeast. Hemosiderin is detected by the Prussian blue stain. The Papanicolaou stain, although it is more time consuming and requires the preparation of fixed permanent slides, is superior for the identification and study of nucleated cells.

A. Cells

Normal urine contains epithelial cells, WBCs and RBCs within a wide normal range. Based on laborious quantitative studies (Addis count) of urine collections from healthy patients, normal ranges for 24-hour excretion are up to 130,000 RBCs, 650,000 WBCs and epithelial cells and 2000 hyaline casts (1-6).

Red blood cells are biconcave, anucleate cells measuring 6 to 7 μ in diameter. Normally, the urine may show up to 3 RBC/hpf. The morphology of the RBC by phase microscopy or a simple Wright's stain may indicate the source of bleeding. Dysmorphic RBCs with irregular membranes, distortion and cell to cell variation indicate a glomerular origin whereas RBCs with normal morphology suggest a nonglomerular origin. Crenated RBCs seen in hypotonic urine are symmetrical and less variable than dysmorphic cells. A careful search for RBC casts is imperative, since their presence is diagnostic of glomerular hematuria.

The presence of increased WBCs in the urine is referred to as pyuria or leukocyturia. Polymorphonuclear leukocytes (pus cells) are larger than RBCs. They are round, have a characteristic multilobed nucleus and measure 12 to 15 μ in diameter. Large polymorphonuclear leukocytes with brownian movement of granules in their cytoplasm are called glitter cells; these are now considered not to be of special diagnostic significance. The upper limit of normal WBC excretion is 5/hpf, although most clean-catch specimens have <1 WBC/hpf. More than 10 WBC/mm^3 on a clean, midstream uncentrifuged urine using a counting chamber is also considered abnormal. Pyuria may originate from any part of the urinary tract. Although the commonest cause of pyuria is urinary tract infection (UTI), the absence of pyuria, particularly in preschool children, does not rule out UTI. Sterile pyuria may arise from various conditions including dehydration, fever, trauma from instrumentation, foreign body or calculus, chemical inflammation, gastrointestinal and respiratory infection, urogenital abnormalities, renal tubular acidosis and glomerulonephritis. Pyuria persisting after infection has cleared should suggest urinary tract obstruction due to a foreign body or congenital anomaly. Persistent pyuria requires adequate workup including cultures for anaerobic organisms and tuberculosis, renal sonogram, voiding cystourethrogram and cystoscopy.

Renal tubular cells are polyhedral cells, 15 to 24 μ in diameter, and frequently have eccentric nuclei. Increased numbers (>15 /hpf) are indicative of renal tubular damage, such as acute tubular necrosis, papillary tip necrosis or graft rejection. Slightly increased numbers are, however, normally seen in the newborn. Renal tubular cells that have degenerated or are filled with lipid show a maltese cross formation under polarized light. These cells, called oval fat bodies, are characteristically seen in patients with the nephrotic syndrome.

Bacteria, yeast, parasites and ova may be present in the urine. Bacteria are very small, rod shaped or round cocci. The presence of any number of bacteria on a nonspun clean-catch urine specimen correlates well with $>10^5$ colonies/mL and suggests a UTI. Culture defines the specific organism and its sensitivity to antibiotics. Yeast are 3 to 5 μ (smaller than RBC); they do not lyse with acetic acid and do not stain with eosin. Mycelial branching forms or budding yeast may be present, the most common of which are the *Candida sp.* Ova and parasites such as *Enterobius vermicularis* are due to fecal contamination.

B. Casts

Casts originate in the renal tubules and have a matrix composed of the Tamm-Horsfall mucoprotein. They are tubular in shape with rounded or blunted ends, depending on the site of formation. They may be curved, straight or convoluted. The absence of dark edges serves to differentiate them from fibers; artifacts that may appear cast-like. Cast formation is increased with acid urine and low urine flow. Casts are classified by their structure and components such as hyaline, cellular and mixed casts. Elements are added to the mucoprotein matrix before it is passed in the urine, thus the cast gives important information on processes occurring within the kidney at the site of formation (3-4).

The morphology of a cast is also dependent on how long it has been retained before passage, with a generally accepted progression from cellular to coarsely granular to finely granular to waxy. The cast diameter is dependent on the site and conditions of formation. Casts are usually uniform in diameter, being narrower in children than in adults. Narrow casts may indicate swollen tubular epithelium that has reduced the tubular lumen size. Broad casts, often measuring more than 150 μ in diameter, may be seen with any type of casts but are most commonly waxy. They are usually of greater prognostic importance, since they originate in collecting or abnormally dilated tubules and they are the result of urinary stasis in the lower portion of the duct. Broad casts are formed when entire groups of nephrons decrease in functional capacity, and they are often described as renal failure casts.

Hyaline casts are the most commonly found, and least diagnostic of the casts. Less than 1 cast/100 hpf, or 0 to 2/hpf, is considered within normal limits. They are formed by precipitation of protein in the tubular lumen and may have additional elements, cells and debris. They are found in increased number after physical exercise, diuretics, heat or de-hydration, and are also elevated in many types of renal disease. These casts are colorless, homogeneous and transparent. They have a refractile index similar to urine and therefore are more difficult to detect with bright-field microscopy. Phase microscopy greatly enhances the ease of identification. Hyaline casts dissolve in water and in an alkaline medium, and hence may not be seen in advanced renal failure in which the urine is dilute and alkaline.

Cellular casts may contain epithelial or blood cells. Epithelial casts are formed by conglutination of desquamated cells from the epithelial lining of the tubule. Red blood cell casts are always pathological and usually indicate glomerular bleeding. They may be present in any form of glo-merulonephritis, renal infarction, renal vein thrombosis or renal trauma. They appear as yellow to brown cylinders with variable numbers of RBC. Degeneration and cell lysis produce a more homogeneous yellow-brown cast. White blood cell casts indicate a renal origin of leukocytes and are indicative of pyelonephritis, interstitial nephritis, SLE or other inflam-matory diseases. They appear refractile and granular; the multilobed nu-cleus of the polymorphonuclear leukocyte is discernible unless the cast has degenerated; differentiation from epithelial cell casts may then be difficult. Occasional epithelial cells are expected within a cast, due to normal cell turnover. However, large numbers of these cells in a cast indicate tubular damage. Epithelial cell casts are often present with RBC and WBC casts in cases of glomerulonephritis or pyelonephritis. Staining, particularly with the Papanicolaou stain, facilitates differentiation be-tween WBC and epithelial casts, accentuating the epithelial cell's single, round central nucleus.

With time, cellular casts begin to disintegrate, forming coarsely gran-ular, finely granular and finally waxy casts. Waxy casts are yellow-tan, dense and homogeneous, and differ from hyaline casts by having a high refractive index. The progress of this cellular degeneration is slow and the presence of waxy casts is indicative of oliguria or anuria. Fatty de-generation of tubular epithelial cells produces fatty casts. These contain large amounts of fat globules and may be seen in the nephrotic syndrome. They appear transparent, with highly refractile fat droplets showing Maltese cross formation under polarized light.

Mixed casts may contain the above elements in combination. Their significance is determined by the dominant component, so that a hyaline granular RBC cast has the same significance as a RBC cast.

C. Crystals

Urine that has been allowed to stand for a while may show precipitation of many crystals, very few of which are of clinical significance. The type of crystals formed is dependent on the pH of the urine. Normal crystals seen in acid urine are uric acid, amorphous urates, calcium oxalate, or less commonly, calcium sulfate or hippuric acid.

Crystals that are always abnormal and appear in acid to neutral urine are cystine, leucine, tyrosine, cholesterol and those due to radiographic dye or antibiotics, such as sulfonamides. The appearance of the abnormal crystals is as follows: cystine is typically hexagonal and occurs with cystinosis or cystinuria. Leucine has regular concentric striations and is seen in maple syrup urine disease or severe liver disease. Tyrosine crystals look like sheaves of fine, highly refractile needles and are seen with inborn errors of tyrosine metabolism or severe liver disease. Cholesterol crystals consist of flat plates with notched corners and are indicative of nephritis, nephrotic syndrome or lymphatic obstruction. Crystals of sulfonamides produce brown or clear sheaves of needles, whereas radiographic dyes produce variable sized needles singly or in sheaves. The sp gr of the urine is usually very high with these dyes (>1.050).

In alkaline urine, one may normally see calcium phosphate, calcium carbonate or ammonium biurate. Uric acid characteristically forms a rhombic prism, which is diamond or rosette shaped and which shows many interference colors under polarized light. These crystals increase in number with increased cell turnover, especially during leukemia therapy, or in gout. Calcium oxalate is envelope or dumbbell shaped and shows a pathological increase in number with ethylene glycol intake, diabetes mellitus, liver disease, after small bowel resection or with Crohn's disease of the small bowel; these crystals also increase in number in the rare hereditary disease hyperoxaluria and in chronic renal disease or with ingestion of large amounts of vitamin C. Amorphous urates, calcium sulfate and hippuric acid have no diagnostic significance. Triple phosphate (ammonium magnesium phosphate) appears as prisms, often coffin-lid shaped, and may be implicated in urinary calculus formation. Other potentially stone-forming crystals include calcium phosphate. Amorphous phosphates and the thorn-applelike ammonium biurate crystals are of no diagnostic significance. Differentiation of specific crystals may thus be based on their presence in alkaline, neutral or acid urine, and specific solubility and heat precipitation tests (3-5). Most important, the presence of many of the commonly seen, nondiagnostic crystals should not obscure examination of the rest of the sediment for important diagnostic clues to renal disease. The characteristic appearance of the commonly seen crystals is illustrated in Figure 3-2.

Acknowledgment. The authors would like to acknowledge the expert technical assistance of Debra Ellis, M.T. (A.S.C.P.).

Acid Urine

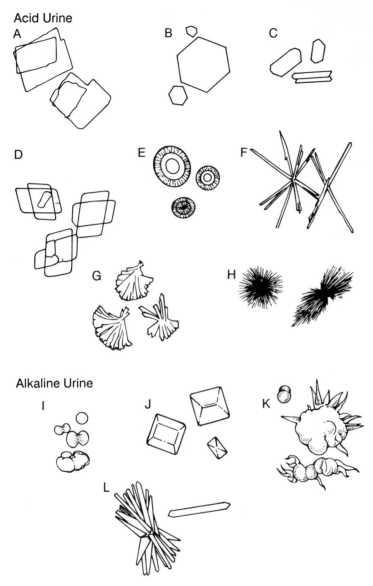

Alkaline Urine

FIGURE 3-2. Crystals seen in acid or alkaline urine (drawn at magnification 150–200). (A) Cholesterol. (B) Cystine. (C) Hippuric acid. (D) Hypaque. (E) Leucine. (F) Renograffin. (G) Sulfonamides. (H) Tyrosine. (I) Calcium carbonate. (J) Triple phosphate. (K) Ammonium biurate. (L) Calcium phosphate.

References

1. Addis T (1926) The number of formed elements in the urinary sediment of normal individuals. J Clin Invest 2:409–415
2. Sheets C, Lyman JL (1986) Urinalysis. Emerg Med Clin North Am 4:263–280
3. Graff L (1983) A Handbook of Routine Urinalysis. JB Lippincott, Philadelphia
4. Free HM (ed) (1987) Modern Urine Chemistry. Application of Urine Chemistry and Microscopic Examination in Health and Disease. Miles Laboratories, Elkhart, Indiana
5. Bradley M, Schumann GB (1984) Examination of the urine. In: Henry JB (ed) Todd, Sanford, Davidsohn Clinical Diagnosis and Management by Laboratory Methods, 17th edition. WB Saunders, Philadelphia, pp 380–458
6. Free AH, Free HM (1986) Urinalysis: its proper role in the physician's office. Clin Lab Med 6:253–266
7. Boeckx RL (1987) Urine drug screening by gas chromatography-mass spectrometry. Application to a pediatric environment. Clin Lab Med 7:401–414

4
The Role of the Chemistry Laboratory in the Clinical Study of Renal Disease

ROBERT C. ROCK

I. Introduction

A. Changes in Laboratory Technology

Chemical methods for pediatric specimens were originally developed as manual micromethods. Within the past 10 years, a number of automated instruments capable of handling microsamples in the range of 50 to 200 μL have become available, with individual analysis requiring as little as 5 to 10 μL.

Current automation thus allows any laboratory, whether in a children's hospital or in a facility serving both adult and pediatric patients, to perform rapid, precise microchemical determinations.

The accuracy of micromethods has also improved in the past 10 to 15 years. For example, the widespread use of enzymes as diagnostic reagents for more specific measurement of substrates such as glucose and uric acid has greatly reduced potential interferences from both drugs and endogenous metabolites.

B. Reference Intervals

Infant and child populations may have associated reference values for a number of constituents in serum and urine that differ appreciably from those found in adult populations (1–5). For example, healthy newborns may have glomerular filtration rates (GFR) that are only 20% to 30% of the values predicted by calculation and "correction" for surface area (6). A detailed table for pediatric reference intervals is presented in Appendix I.

C. Pediatric Specimens

1. Sample Collection and Handling

Skin puncture, rather than venipuncture, is preferred for newborns and small infants, to avoid iatrogenic anemia, to preserve venous access for treatment and to reduce the cumulative trauma of multiple sampling. In a typical U.S. children's hospital, approximately two-thirds of specimens were obtained from skin puncture and most of the remainder were drawn from in-dwelling catheters (7). Significant dilutional effects may be seen in plasma from specimens collected from long central lines, and clinical laboratories should work with the clinical staff to determine the actual void volume required to clear the line of parenteral fluid. For that reason, our laboratory prefers to receive samples collected by skin puncture, if possible.

A wide variety of containers are available for microsampling by skin puncture. Our laboratory uses glass microhematocrit tubes, polyethylene tubes, and a polypropylene collecting system (Microtainer, Becton-Dickinson and Co., Rutherford, NY). Heparin, either as the ammonium or lithium salt, is the preferred anticoagulant (2). Most studies have not shown any consistent major differences between serum and plasma for most common analytes.

Specimens from skin puncture should be mixed thoroughly with an anticoagulant immediately after collection. Small clots that form in both plastic and glass microsample containers may result not only in mechanical blockage of small-bore automated analyzers but also inaccurate results. Specimens for determination of pH, blood gases, ammonia, lactate and pyruvate should be transported to the laboratory in a container of ice, to prevent deterioration. Under optimum circumstances, these analytes should be measured within 20 to 30 minutes of collection.

Determination of urinary constituents in pediatric clinical chemistry is more often made on "spot" collections rather than on timed urine specimens, given the difficulties of patient compliance. For most analytes, no added preservative is necessary, provided that the specimen is stored at refrigerator temperature until transported to the laboratory.

2. Interferences with Methods

Some automated analyzers used in pediatric microchemistry appear to be affected by a variety of the substances in plasma. In addition to interference from hemoglobin, bilirubin and lipid in high concentrations, other unidentified substances (particularly in neonatal plasma) may cause inaccurate results in certain methods; these are discussed below.

3. Effects of Renal Disease

Both acute and chronic renal disease may produce substances that interfere with some chemical methods; presumably interference is due to retained metabolites, altered acid-based balance and abnormal shifts of fluid and electrolytes. The loss of metabolic homeostasis that accompanies chronic renal failure may result in increased intraindividual variation of a number of chemical analytes, including the majority of those described in this chapter (8).

II. Specific Individual Analytes

A. Electrolytes, Fluid and Acid-Base Balance

1. Sodium and Potassium

a. Serum, Plasma, and Whole Blood

Specimen: Although serum or plasma has been the traditional specimen for determination of sodium (Na) and potassium (K), some new microanalyzers are designed to accept whole blood. Heparin is the appropriate anticoagulant if plasma or whole blood is used.

Methods: Flame photometry, a traditional method, is gradually being replaced by nondestructive methods employing ion-selective electrodes (ISE). These systems are available in both manual and automated versions, and the new systems can accept whole blood. Analytical precision of measurement of Na and K with current techniques is approximately 1.5% for Na and 3.0% for K. The ISE instruments are of two types: "indirect," where the sample is diluted many-fold (typically 1:200), and "direct," without sample dilution. Indirect ISE methods (as well as flame photometry) are more susceptible than direct methods to what has been termed the "electrolyte exclusion effect," caused by electrolyte exclusion from the nonaqueous phase of plasma (4). This effect may produce falsely low results when a significant fraction of total plasma volume is replaced by nonaqueous components, such as lipids or proteins. The magnitude of this negative error is less than 5% until serum triglyceride concentrations are greater than 2500 mg/dL, and can be estimated using the following formula (9):

$$\% \text{ negative error} = (2.1 \times \text{triglycerides, g/dL}) - 0.6$$

Although massive increases in serum total proteins may also theoretically produce similar electrolyte exclusion effects, increases above 10 g/dL are rare in practice.

Interpretation: With few exceptions, measurement of Na in extracellular fluid provides a rapid and effective estimate of extracellular hypo- and hypertonicity, since Na accounts for no more than 90% of the osmotically active extracellular solute. Measurement of serum osmolality allows further categorization of hypo- and hypernatremias as hypertonic, isotonic and hypotonic (10). Concentration of K in plasma or serum does not consistently reflect total body stores of K. Interpretation of hyperkalemia is complicated by occasional spurious elevations, caused by release of K in leukocytosis (white blood cells $>100,000/mm^3$), thrombocytosis

($>750,000/mm^3$) and hemolysis during specimen collection and storage (10) (see Chapter 12).

b. Urine

Specimen: Random "spot" urine specimens are usually adequate for diagnostic purposes in infants and children, although accurate estimation of urinary losses of Na and K requires timed urine collections.

Methods: Both flame photometry and ISE are currently used to measure urinary Na and K. The newer automated ISE instruments have built-in calibration systems to allow rapid changeovers from plasma/serum to urine, thus improving turnaround time.

Interpretation (11): Urinary Na concentration is most useful in the differential diagnosis of volume depletion, acute oliguria or hyponatremia. When hypokalemia is present, urinary K concentration of greater than 10 mEq/L is evidence of excessive renal excretion. A more sensitive discriminator of prerenal azotemia may be the fractional excretion (FE) of Na (FE_{Na}) (see Chapter 12).

2. Chloride

Specimen: Quantitation of chloride (Cl) is most commonly performed on samples of plasma or serum, and less commonly on urine and sweat.

Methods: Pediatric samples are often analyzed by coulometricamperometric titration, and ISE are also available for Cl determination, and are increasingly used in automated instruments. All methods produce results with comparable reference intervals.

Interpretation: Hypochloremia may occur in a variety of chronic renal diseases and in association with loss of gastric secretion. Hyperchloremia may be present in renal tubular acidosis, as well as in acute renal failure.

3. Anion gaps

The most common equation for calculating the anion gap is

$$\text{Anion gap (mEq/L)} = [Na^+] - ([CO_2] + [Cl])$$

where the concentrations of Na, Cl and total CO_2 are expressed in milliequivalents per liter. Using this equation, the reference interval for ambulatory subjects is often stated to be 7 to 14 mEq/L (12). Metabolic acidosis may be due to an increased or a normal anion gap (see Chapter 13).

4. Osmolality

Specimen: Either serum or heparinized plasma is suitable; urine should be collected without preservatives and centrifuged promptly to remove particulate matter.

Methods: A variety of instruments have been developed to measure osmolality, and either of two principles are generally employed: 1) freezing point depression and 2) vapor pressure lowering. Vapor pressure osmometers have yielded less precise results than freezing point depression instruments in interlaboratory surveys, but they have the advantage of requiring smaller samples (7–10 μL) than freezing-point models (typically 50–100 μL). Osmolality is related to the number of solute particles per mass of solvent and, for serum and urine, is usually expressed as osmols per kilogram of water. Osmolality may also be calculated using the measured concentrations of Na, glucose and urea (13) (see Chapter 12 and Appendix II).

Interpretation: Serum osmolality is normally under tight homeostatic control, with a reference interval of 285 to 295 mOsm/kg. Urine osmolality, in contrast, has a wide dynamic range, varying from 50 mOsm/kg during the diuresis following water loading to 1200 mOsm/kg during severely reduced fluid intake. Normal individuals with their customary fluid intake have urinary osmolalities in the range of 300 to 1000 mOsm/kg.

Analogous to anion gaps, *osmolal gaps* can be estimated by subtracting the calculated osmolality (from the above formula) from the measured osmolality. The "normal" gap is less than 5 mOsm/kg.

Increased osmolal gaps may be associated with increased concentrations of endogenous osmotically active nonelectrolytes (e.g. in uremia and diabetic acidosis). Osmolal gaps of 10 mOsm/kg or greater may be found with ingestion of osmotically active solutes, such as ethanol, methanol and ethylene glycol.

Measurement of the osmolality of serum and urine can also be used to calculate *osmolal clearance*, the volume of plasma theoretically cleared of solute per unit time (mL/min) (see Chapter 5).

5. pH, pCO_2 and pO_2

Specimen: Arterial capillary blood collected anaerobically by skin puncture into heparinized microtubes is the most reliable specimen from neonates and infants; currently available blood-gas analyzers require 100 to 200 μL of whole blood for measurement of pH, pCO_2 and pO_2. The area of sampling is warmed for at least 10 minutes to achieve good perfusion before skin puncture. A common source of sampling error is the presence of air bubbles; pO_2 measurements in particular may be altered by equilibration with room air. For older children, arterial puncture with a gas-tight, all-glass syringe (1–3 mL, volume) containing 0.1 to 0.2 mg of liquid heparin anticoagulant is suitable. Specimens are unstable at room temperature; the pH of whole blood decreases by 0.03 pH units/hour, pO_2 decreases by 2 to 6 mm Hg/hour and pCO_2 increases by 2 to 4 mm Hg/hour (4). Specimens for blood gas analysis should be preserved on ice and analyzed within 30 minutes of collection. Inadequate mixing of specimens with anticoagulant is probably the most common cause of inaccurate results.

Methods (4,14): The majority of instruments used for in vitro analysis of blood gases and pH combine a sequence of individual electrodes for pH, pCO_2 and pO_2. Certain instruments also incorporate ISE for NA, K, Cl and calcium (Ca), thus allowing rapid determination of both blood gases and electrolytes on a microsample (75–150 μL) of whole blood. The current generation of blood gas instruments allows determinations to be made with a precision of 1 to 2%. For practical purposes, pH is usually reported to two decimal places; pCO_2 and pO_2 are reported to the nearest whole number (4).

In vivo transcutaneous monitoring can be carried out for pH, pCO_2 and pO_2 (15), utilizing electrode systems comparable to those used for in vivo analysis. Transcutaneous pCO_2 measurements with current devices are higher than in vitro pCO_2 (15). More experience is available with transcutaneous monitoring of pO_2; correlation between transcutaneous and arterial pO_2 values in one study was good except for infants under 24 hours old (16). Practical problems with the currently available transcutaneous systems are their high cost, the requirement to heat the skin to achieve hyperemia and the drift of electrode performance over time.

Carbon dioxide (CO_2) may also be measured in plasma or serum by a variety of methods. Total CO_2 content usually measures not only dissolved CO_2, but also CO_2 present as bicarbonate (HCO_3^-) or carbamino; released CO_2 may be quantitated by manometry. Most clinical laboratories measure total CO_2 by either colorimetric methods or by instrumentation that incorporates a pCO_2 electrode.

Plasma HCO_3^- may also be calculated from measured pCO_2, using the following equation (3):

$$[HCO_3^-] = 31.39 \times \frac{pCO_2}{pCO_2 + 12.95}$$

where pCO_2 = measured pCO_2 (mmHg). Because of the different principles of measurement, however, calculated HCO_3^- derived from pCO_2 measurements may not correlate well with measured total CO_2 content.

Interpretation: The metabolic acidosis that accompanies chronic renal failure is usually associated with retention of hydrogen and associated anions; pCO_2 is usually decreased in partial compensation for the decrease in HCO_3^- (reflected in the decrease in total CO_2 content as measured chemically) (see Chapter 13).

B. Other Inorganic Analytes

1. Calcium

Specimen: Either serum or plasma (with heparin or EDTA as anticoagulant) may be used for determination of total Ca. Prolonged venous stasis may produce spurious hypercalcemia. Urine specimens for quantitative studies of Ca excretion should be collected in containers with acid to prevent the precipitation of Ca salts (3).

Serum for the determination of ionized Ca requires collection and processing under anaerobic conditions, with preservation on ice during transportation. Heparinized plasma may also be used; newer instruments employing Ca-selective electrodes accept heparinized whole blood, which is the preferred specimen if skin puncture is to be used. The approximate volumes of specimen required are 50 to 100 μL for total Ca, and 100 to 500 μL for ionized Ca.

Methods: A variety of methods have been used for determination of total Ca (17). Atomic absorption spectrophotometry (AAS) is the generally accepted reference method for total Ca in both serum and urine. A number of colorimetric, spectrophotometric and fluorimetric methods have been used also. Many of these methods, however, are subject to interference from lipemia, hemolysis and hyperbilirubinemia.

Ionized Ca is measured using ISE with an ion exchanger membrane selective for Ca. Selectivity for Ca, however, is relative rather than absolute, and certain electrodes may also pick up high concentrations of magnesium (Mg) (which may appear in the course of chronic renal failure). Use of EDTA, oxalate, or citrate as anticoagulant interferes with the measurement of ionized Ca, due to the formation of nonionized complexes with Ca. Even heparin in excess may reduce the ionized Ca concentration by chelation.

Interpretation: Ionized Ca is the most important physiological fraction of total Ca in blood, and may correlate with neuromuscular function better than total Ca in the presence of hypoalbuminemia. Until recently, calcium-selective electrodes were difficult to maintain in a clinical laboratory setting. Newer instruments are more rugged, require smaller sample volumes and when combined with automated blood-gas analysis, may encourage the more widespread use of ionized Ca determinations.

2. Phosohorus

Specimen: Either serum or heparinized plasma should be used. Other anticoagulants may interfere with the phosphomolybdate reaction, which still serves as the basis for most methods (4). Phosphorus (P) in urine may be determined in the same acidified specimen used for Ca determination.

Methods: Almost all manual and automated methods for P involve some variant of the reaction of P with molybdate salts. Protein separation prior to the phosphomolybdate reaction minimizes interference from lipemia.

Interpretation: Hyperphosphatemia often develops in chronic renal failure when GFR decreases to less than 20 mL/1.73 m^2 a minute; under these conditions, serum P may increase to 5 to 10 mg/dL. In acute renal failure, hyperphosphatemia also may occur, especially in association with extensive muscle injury. Increased urinary excretion of phosphate may occur with certain inherited renal tubular defects, in vitamin D deficiency and in other types of renal tubular damage and may be associated with *hypophosphatemia.*

Estimation of the *tubular reabsorption of phosphate (TRP)* may allow assessment of damage to proximal tubular reabsorptive mechanisms. This calculation requires measurement of both P and creatinine in both serum and urine (see Chapter 11).

3. Magnesium

Sample: Either serum or heparinized plasma may be used. Methods in common use require 20 to 100 μL of sample. Hemolysis may result in spuriously increased Mg concentrations, due to contamination with high concentrations of Mg in red blood cells (RBC).

Methods: The generally accepted reference method is AAS. Fluorometric methods using fluorescent compounds are also used in both manual and automated instruments. Spectrophotometric and fluorimetric methods generally yield results that are comparable to those produced by AAS, although they may be more susceptible to interference from lipemia and hyperbilirubinemia.

Interpretation: Hypermagnesemia may occur when renal excretion is reduced to below 15% of normal (3). Excessive ingestion of Mg-containing compounds (e.g. laxatives and antacids) may also be a factor in patients with chronic renal failure, as may dialysis with "hard" water containing Mg salts (10).

C. Glucose and Metabolites

1. Glucose

Specimen: In terms of stability, the most appropriate specimen if there is any delay between collection and analysis is plasma obtained from blood collected with fluoride to inhibit glycolysis and oxalate to prevent coagulation. In whole blood, which is allowed to clot and stand at room temperature, glucose in serum decreases 5 to 10 mg/dL in an hour. Glucose values in whole blood are 10 mg/dL lower than values for plasma or serum. Current methods for glucose measurement require approximately 10 μL of the specimen.

Methods: The new enzymatic methods employ either hexokinase (the currently accepted reference method) or glucose oxidase. These methods are much less susceptible to interference from either exogenous compounds (such as drugs) or endogenous substances (such as retained metabolic products in uremia) than the older methods.

Interpretation: Repeated measurement of plasma glucose in appropriately collected specimens is the most appropriate initial strategy to establish the presence of hyperglycemia.

2. Pyruvate and Lactate

Specimen: Both pyruvate and lactate are very unstable in whole blood. Collection should be into evacuated tubes containing fluoride and oxalate; the sample is chilled immediately and the plasma is separated within 15 to 20 minutes of collection. Plasma is then deproteinized using phosphoric acid.

Methods: Pyruvate and lactate are measured spectrophotometrically. Although most procedures call for only 50 to 100 μL of deproteinized plasma supernatant, the extensive specimen processing usually requires that at least 500 to 750 μL of whole blood be collected.

Interpretation: Lactic acidosis may occur with a number of inherited inborn errors of metabolism such as glucose-6-phosphate dehydrogenase (G6PD) deficiency, carnitine deficiency and propionic acidemia. It is more common, however, as a consequence of severe circulatory and metabolic disturbances associated with tissue hypoxia. Under these conditions, lactate accumulates, and the lactate:pyruvate ratio is greater than 10:1.

D. Nitrogenous Compounds

1. Urea

Specimen: Serum is most commonly used for determination of urea. If plasma is to be used, heparin is the most suitable anticoagulant, since other anticoagulants may interfere with enzymatic urease methods.

Methods: Indirect methods involve initial hydrolysis of urea to release ammonia, followed by quantitation of ammonia by either a colorimetric or an enzymatic reaction.

Interpretation: Although urea measurements are determined with serum, references to BUN (blood urea nitrogen) persist. The original methods, now of historical interest only, measured the nitrogen in urea, although current methods quantitate urea itself. A number of nonrenal factors including dehydration and protein catabolism influence serum urea concentration, making it a less reliable indicator of renal function than serum creatinine.

2. Creatinine

a. Creatinine in Serum and Urine

Specimen: Serum is more commonly used than plasma for measurement of creatinine in the circulation. Hemolysis may produce spurious elevations of creatinine due to the release of noncreatinine chromogens from RBCs. Since creatinine in urine appears to be stable for two to three days at room temperature and for five days under refrigeration, no preservative is required for creatinine measurement itself (18,19). The reaction between creatinine and picrate ion formed in alkaline solution (the Jaffe reaction) serves as the basis for virtually all manual and automated methods. A large number of noncreatinine, Jaffe-reacting chromogens are found in serum, including protein, guanidine, ketoacids and drugs such as cephalosporins. Interference from these substances can be reduced by absorption onto aluminum silicate (Lloyd's reagent) and other methods. A potential reference method for determination of creatinine involves reverse-phase, high-performance liquid chromatography.

Interpretation: Although the clinical literature would suggest that pretreatment with Lloyd's reagent results in "true creatinine," in actual practice current automated methods produce results that are more precise and of the same order of accuracy as the older manual methods using Lloyd's reagent.

b. Creatinine Clearance

This correlates reasonably well with rates for glomerular filtration as estimated by the clearance of inulin, a carbohydrate that is neither secreted nor reabsorbed by the renal tubules. The continuously changing rate of creatinine excretion in children compared to the rate of excretion of other compounds makes normalization of their excretion relative to creatine less reliable than in adults (20). The clinical testing and evaluation of renal function is discussed in detail in Chapter 5.

c. Alternatives to Creatinine Clearance in Estimating Glomerular Filtration Rates

See Chapter 5 and Appendix II.

3. Uric Acid

Specimen: Serum, heparinized plasma, or urine may be used for determination of uric acid. Serum or plasma is stable for two to three days at room temperature, and three to seven days when refrigerated. Uric acid in urine is stable for several days when refrigerated.

Methods: Newer enzymatic methods that use uricase are much more specific than the older methods. Sample volumes required for these enzymatic methods are 10 to 50 μL.

Interpretation: Renal retention of uric acid during the course of chronic renal disease is one of the most common causes of secondary hyperuricemia; intrarenal deposition of urate under these conditions may exacerbate the underlying renal failure. Hypouricemia is rare; among the causes is decreased renal tubular reabsorption or uric acid associated with inherited or acquired tubular defects (e.g. generalized Fanconi syndrome).

4. Ammonia

Specimen: Plasma from specimens collected in EDTA or lithium heparin, chilled immediately with ice and rapidly separated from blood cells, is the only suitable sample. Ammonia is rapidly generated in vitro by deamination of amino acids, and prompt analysis is essential by more specific enzymatic techniques. The most commonly used enzymatic sequence involves the reaction of ammonium and oxoglutarate with glutamate dehydrogenase. Ammonia-selective electrodes have been developed, but their use is currently confined to research.

Interpretation: The increased serum urea concentration that may occur with chronic renal disease leads to increased excretion into the intestine, where microbial action converts urea to ammonia, which then may back-diffuse into the circulation.

E. Proteins

1. Total Proteins

a. Serum

Specimen: Serum rather than plasma, which contains fibrinogen, is the preferred specimen. Currently available automated instruments require approximately 10 to 50 μL of serum for this measurement. Hemolysis and lipemia may interfere with these methods.

Methods: The most common method is the reaction of protein peptide bonds with cupric ions in alkaline solution—the biuret reaction. Refractometry provides a quick semiquantitative estimate of serum total protein, but hyperglycemia and azotemia may significantly interfere. Other techniques such as precipitation with nephelometry or turbidimetry may work well with urine but are not accurate for use with serum.

Interpretation: Proteinuria in renal disease may lead to decreased concentration of total serum proteins, which is usually most marked in the albumin fraction.

b. Urine

Specimen: A 12- or 24-hour collection of urine, stored at 2 to 6°C during and after collection, is the preferred specimen for quantitative assessment of proteinuria. No preservatives should be used. Random samples may be used for qualitative screening purposes.

Methods: Application of the biuret technique to urine samples usually requires prior precipitation or concentration by other means and thus has not been used widely. The most common methods involve precipitation by acid (such as trichloroacetic acid) and quantitation by turbidimetry or nephelometry. Qualitative detection of proteinuria in a random "spot" urine sample involve the use of dipsticks (see Chapter 3).

Interpretation (see Chapter 8)

2. Albumin

Specimen: Serum is preferable to plasma. Lipemia interferes with most commonly used methods. Currently used manual and automated methods require 10 to 20 μL of sample.

Methods: Although specific antisera to albumin could be used as the basis for immunochemical assays for albumin, almost all currently used methods use one of a variety of dyes such as bromocresol green (BCG) or bromcresol purple (BCP). At the high concentrations (3–5 g/dL) of albumin normally present in serum, dye-binding methods are reasonably specific; however, binding to alpha and beta globulins produces a positive interference at serum albumin levels below 2.0 g/dL.

Interpretation: Hypoalbuminemia associated with albuminuria appears when hepatic synthesis of albumin can no longer compensate for renal loss.

3. Fractionation of Proteins by Electrophoresis

Specimen: Serum is preferable to plasma. Either random "spot" urine or timed quantitative urine samples may be used; at lower levels of proteinuria, concentration by techniques such as ultrafiltration is usually necessary.

Methods: A wide variety of media (cellulose acetate and agarose gel) are used for electrophoretic separation of proteins in serum, urine and other body fluids. The newest method, immunofixation (IFE), which combines electrophoresis in agarose gel with immunoprecipitation in the gel using specific antisera, provides an effective, rapid means of identifying abnormal proteins in serum and other fluids but does not provide quantitative information.

Once proteins are separated and fixed on supporting media, they can be identified with a variety of nonspecific dyes, all of which show relatively greater affinity for albumin than for globulin fractions.

Interpretation: Serum protein components as separated by electrophoresis represent a qualitative or semiquantitative approach, since albumin is often overestimated (due to the differential affinity of the dye) and densitometric determination of "minor" fractions—alpha, beta and gamma globulins—is relatively imprecise. Chronic renal disease produces a variety of qualitative alterations in electrophoretic patterns. In nephrotic syndrome, the serum shows a decrease in albumin with an increase in alpha–2-globulin.

4. Immunoglobulins

Specimen: Serum, urine or cerebrospinal fluid (CSF) may be used. Samples should be stored frozen at −15 °C if analyses will be delayed more than two to three days; repeated freeze-thaw cycles should be avoided, since protein degradation may occur. Most methods require approximately 100 to 150 μL of specimen for determining the major categories of immmunoglobulins.

Methods: All common quantitative methods are immunochemical, involving reaction of specific antisera and various classes of antisera. The simplest manual method is radial immunodiffusion (RID). Other manual techniques include counter current immunoelectrophoresis (CIE) and electroimmunoassay (EIA).

A major problem in interpreting the results of immunoglobulin quantitation is the lack of consensus regarding standardization of the methods.

Interpretation: Normal values for serum immunoglobulins vary considerably with age (see Appendix I).

5. Complement

Specimen: Serum or EDTA plasma may be used. EDTA is useful in blocking in vitro activation of complement. Prompt separation from cells, and storage at −70 °C is needed to preserve more labile complement components.

Methods: Immunoprecipitation methods involving RID or nephelometry have supplemented older techniques involving complement-mediated hemolysis in most clinical laboratories. Lack of reference materials and standardized procedures causes substantial variation among laboratories.

Interpretation: In clinical laboratories, C3 and C4 are the complement components most commonly requested for determination. One or both of these components may decrease in diseases that involve formation of immune complexes (e.g. SLE and poststreptococcal and membranoproliferative glomerulonephritis).

6. Specific Proteins in Renal Disease

a. Glomerular Proteinuria

Albuminuria is a sensitive marker for early alterations in glomerular permeability, and the ratio of the clearance of albumin to that of creatinine may have both theoretical and practical advantages over measurement of total protein in a 24-hour specimen (21):

$$\frac{CA}{C_{Cr}} = \frac{U_A/S_A}{U_{Cr}/S_{Cr}}$$

where C_A, U_A, S_A = clearance and urine and serum concentrations of albumin and C_{Cr}, U_{Cr}, S_{Cr} = clearance and urine and serum concentrations of creatinine.

Rapid assessment can also be made using urine albumin/creatinine ratio (see Chapter 8).

b. Tubular Proteinuria

Low molecular weight proteins serve as markers for tubular dysfunction. Lysozyme (MW 15,000 daltons) was one of the earliest marker proteins identified. Recently, immunochemical measurement of beta–2-microglobin (MW 11,800 daltons) has been used for this purpose, since normally less than 1% of beta–2-microglobulin is filtered at the glomerulus, the remaining fraction being reabsorbed or catabolized in the proximal tubules. Increased serum concentrations (>260 μg/dL) may be found in renal failure and increased urinary concentrations (>350 μg/L) in a variety of tubular disorders, and the test has been advocated as a way to monitor tubular function following renal transplantation (22).

References

1. Clayton BE, Jenkins P, Round JM (1980) Paediatric Chemical Pathology. Blackwell Scientific Publications, Oxford
2. Meites S (ed) (1981) Pediatric Clinical Chemistry. American Association for Clinical Chemistry, Washington DC
3. Hicks JM, Boeckxx RL (eds) (1984) Pediatric Clinical Chemistry. American Association for Clinical Chemistry, Washington DC
4. Tietz NW (ed) (1987) Textbook of Clinical Chemistry, 3rd edition, WB Saunders, Philadelphia
5. Chantler C, Barratt TM (1987) Laboratory evaluation. In: Holliday MA, Barrett TM, Vernier RL (eds) Pediatric Nephrology, 2nd edition. Williams and Wilkins, Baltimore, pp 282–299
6. Evans SE, Durbin GM (1983) Aspects of the physiological and pathological background to neonatal clinical chemistry. Ann Clin Biochem 20:193–207
7. Meites S, Glassco KM (1985) Studies on the quality of specimens obtained by skin-puncture of children. 2. An analysis of blood-collecting practices in a pediatric hospital. Clin Chem 31:1669–1672
8. Holzel WGE (1987) Intra-individual variation of some analytes in serum of patients with chronic renal failure. Clin Chem 33:670–673
9. Steffes MW, Freier EF (1976) A simple and precise method of determining sodium, potassium, and chloride concentrations in hyperlipemia. J Lab Clin Med 88:683–688
10. Narins RG, Jones ER, Stom MC, et al (1982) Diagnostic strategies in disorders of fluid, electrolyte and acid-base homeostasis. Am J Med 72:496–520

11. Harrington JT, Cohen JJ (1975) Measurement of urinary electrolytes—indications and limitations. N Engl J Med 293:1241–1243
12. Smithline N, Gardner KD (1976) Gaps–anionic and osmolal. JAMA 236:1594–1597
13. Dorwart WV, Chalmers L (1975) Comparison of methods for calculating serum osmolality from chemical concentrations, and the prognostic value of such calculations. Clin Chem 21:190–194
14. Beetham R (1982) A review of blood pH and blood-gas analysis. Ann Clin Biochem 19:198–213
15. Hicks JM (1985) In situ monitoring. Clin Chem 31:1931–1935
16. Graham G, Kenny MA (1980) Performance of a radiometer transcutaneous oxygen monitor in a neonatal-intensive-care unit. Clin Chem 26:629–633
17. Gosling P (1986) Analytical reviews in clinical biochemistry: calcium measurement. Ann Clin Biochem 23:146–156
18. Narayanan S, Appleton HD (1980) Creatinine: a review. Clin Chem 26:1119–1126
19. Spencer K (1986) Analytical reviews in clinical biochemistry: the estimation of creatinine. Ann Clin Biochem 23:1–25
20. Applegarth DA, Ross PM (1975) The unsuitability of creatinine excretion as a basis for assessing the excretion of other metabolites by infants and children. Clin Chim Acta 64:83–85
21. Barratt TM, McLaine PN, Soothill JF (1970) Albumin excretion as a measure of glomerular dysfunction in children. Arch Dis Child 45:496–501
22. Woo J, Floyd M, Cannon DC (1981) Albumin and β_2-microglobulin radioimmunoassays applied to monitoring of renal-allograft function and in differentiating glomerular and tubular diseases. Clin Chem 27:709–713

5
Clinical Testing and Evaluation of Glomerular Function

Pedro A. Jose and Robin A. Felder

I. Introduction

The kidney performs numerous functions, but only some can be evaluated indirectly in a clinical setting. In many instances, the function of both kidneys are evaluated; in others, the function of each kidney should be determined. The function of specific segments of the nephron can also be evaluated by indirect means. This chapter will deal mainly with clearance methods used to evaluate glomerular filtration rate (GFR), renal plasma flow (RPF) and water and solute excretion. Indirect methods to localize actions at specific nephron segments will also be discussed.

II. Definition of Clearance

The plasma clearance (C) of any substance (s) is defined as the volume of plasma required to supply the amount of substance appearing in the urine during any unit period of time (1). The amount of the substance excreted in the urine per unit time is equal to the concentration of the substance in the urine U_s times the urine flow (V). If the concentration of the substance in the plasma is (P), then the UV/P indicates the clearance of the substance. This ratio allows a quantitative assessment of the ability of the kidney to excrete a given substance in relation to its concentration in the plasma at any given time. Thus,

$$C_s = \frac{U_s\,(V)}{P_s}$$

where C_s is the clearance of any substance (e.g. inulin, creatinine, sodium, phosphate), U_s is the concentration of the substance in the urine (the clearance being measured) and P_s is the concentration of that substance in the serum or plasma.

In pediatrics, the clearance of a given substance is usually corrected to the body surface area (e.g. 1.73 m²) to allow comparison among patients of different body sizes. Thus,

$$(C_s \text{ mL/min/1.73 m}^2) = \frac{U_s\,(V)}{P_s} \times \frac{1.73}{SA}$$

where SA is body surface area in meters squared. For example, if the concentration of creatinine in the urine is 100 mg/dL, its concentration in plasma or serum is 1 mg/dL and the urine flow is 1 mL/minute, the creatinine clearance will be 100 ml/minute. If the body surfacde area is 1.2, then the creatinine clearance in mL/min/1.73 m² is 144.

The clearance of any substance is calculated in a similar fashion. For example,

$$\text{Osmolar clearance } (C_{osm}) = \frac{U_{osm}\,(V)}{P_{osm}}$$

where U_{osm} is the urine osmolarity, and P_{osm} is the plasma or serum osmolarity.

Clearance methods have also been used to determine sodium (Na) reabsorption in different segments of the nephron. Although these methods are limited, they are the only way to assess segmental Na reabsorption in a man with intact kidneys. Urine is diluted by the reabsorption of Na in the ascending limb of Henle and more distal segments. If one assumes that during water diuresis (water loading to decrease urine osmolarity close to the minimum value of 50), that the circulating antidiuretic hormone (ADH) level will be very low. If one also assumes that water does not back-diffuse at or beyond the diluting sites, then the rate of urine flow (V) must equal the rate at which fluid is delivered to the diluting sites. The urine becomes isosmotic at some point in the ascending limb of the loop of Henle. At that point, V is an index of fluid delivery to distal tubular sites (beyond the ascending limb of loop of Henle). $V \times P_{Na}$ would also be equal to the rate of distal Na delivery. Since the filtered Na is $GFR \times P_{Na}$, then the percentage of filtered Na or water delivered to the distal diluting segments will be expressed by the equation:

$$\text{Percent distal Na (or water) delivery} = \frac{V (P_{Na})}{GFR (P_{Na})} \times 100$$

$$= \frac{V}{GFR} \times 100$$

When Na is reabsorbed in the diluting segments, free water is formed, left in the tubular lumen and excreted (free water clearance, C_{H_2O}). If again one assumes that during maximal water diuresis, no free water diffuses back, then C_{H_2O} is an index of the amount of Na reabsorbed at these sites. Thus $C_{H_2O} \times P_{Na}$ is the amount of Na reabsorbed at distal diluting sites, C_{H_2O}/GFR is the fraction of filtered Na reabsorbed at these sites and C_{H_2O}/V is the fraction of Na delivered to the diluting segments that is reabsorbed. Note that P_{Na} cancels out.

The sum of C_{H_2O} (tubular fluid cleared of Na) and C_{Na} (tubular sodium remaining) also provides an estimate of distal Na delivery. The percent of distal Na reabsorption is expressed by the equation:

$$\text{Percent distal Na reabsorption} = \frac{C_{H_2O}}{C_{H_2O} + C_{Na}} \times 100$$

V is also the sum of C_{H_2O} and C_{osm}. Thus,

$$C_{H_2O} = V - C_{osm}$$

$$= V - \frac{(U_{osm} \times V)}{P_{osm}}$$

$$= V (1 - U/P_{osm})$$

When U/P_{osm} is 1, the urine is neither dilute nor concentrated compared to the plasma. When U/P_{osm} is less than 1 (urine osmolarity is less than plasma osmolarity), then free water is being made (C_{H_2O}). When U/P_{osm} is greater than 1 (urine osmolality greater than plasma), C_{H_2O} becomes a negative value; this negative C_{H_2O} is also known as $T^C_{H_2O}$. When solute excretion is high and medullary interstitial Na approaches plasma Na concentration, $T^C_{H_2O}$ can be used as an index of Na reabsorption in the medullary thick ascending limb of Henle. Using these clearance techniques, one can identify the nephron site being affected by drugs or conditions (Table 5-1). Agents decreasing proximal tubular reabsorption will increase C_{H_2O} (during maximal water diuresis), and $T^{C_{H_2O}}$ (during maximal antidiuresis) since distal reabsorption is enhanced as a consequence of increased distal load. Agents that decrease Na reabsorption at the diluting segments will decrease C_{H_2O}. $T^{C_{H_2O}}$ will be decreased if solute reabsorption in the medullary thick ascending limb is impaired but not when the cortical thick ascending limb is involved. This is due to the fact that Na reabsorbed in the medullary thick ascending limb of Henle increases medullary hypertonicity. This in turn results in increased water reabsorption in the collecting ducts (under the influence of ADH). When Na transport is decreased in the collecting ducts, C_{H_2O} is minimally affected (quantitatively, much less Na is reabsorbed at this site) but $T^{C_{H_2O}}$ will be decreased because water is reabsorbed at this site under the influence of ADH.

These calculations are approximations of what may occur in specific nephron segments. For example, micropuncture studies suggest that fluid delivery to the diluting segments is at least twice that estimated from C_{H_2O} calculations. However, clearance techniques are the only methods for quantitating kidney function as a whole, and for approximating transport at specific nephron sites. These techniques cannot distinguish variations among nephrons, cannot precisely localize function to specific nephron segments and may not distinguish reabsorption or secretion for substances that undergo both processes.

III. Clearance Methods to Determine Glomerular Filtration Rate

For the clearance rate of a substance to equal the GFR, the substance must be freely filtered, and neither reabsorbed nor secreted. In addition, the substance must be physiologically inert, nontoxic, not protein bound

TABLE 5-1. Localization of Site of Nephron Effects Using Clearance Techniques[a]

Nephron segment	C_{H_2O}[b]	$T^{C_{H_2O}}$[c]
Proximal tubule	+	+
Thick ascending limb		
Medullary segment	-	-
Cortical segment	-	0
Collecting duct	0	-

[a] +, increase; -, decrease; 0, minimal or no change.
[b] C_{H_2O} should be measured during maximum water diuresis.
[c] $T^{C_{H_2O}}$ should be measured during maximum antidiuresis.

and not subject to metabolism, synthesis or storage by the kidney. It must also have a clearance that is constant over a wide range of plasma concentrations (2).

Several substances have been suggested as markers for GFR including inulin, polyfructosan, urea, creatinine, vitamin B_{12}, chelating substances (EDTA, ethylenediaminetetraacetic acid; DTPA, diethylenetriamine pentaacetic acid), contrast media (iothalamate, diatrizoate) and mannitol, among others. Inulin, a fructose polymer with a molecular weight of 5,200 and molecular radius of 15 Å (Einstein-Stokes radius) meets all the criteria set by Smith (2) and is the standard substance used in the measurement of GFR. Polyfructosan is a synthetic fructose polymer with a molecular weight of 3,000. Its clearance does not differ significantly from inulin and its greater solubility may offer an advantage over inulin when high concentrations are required in urine and plasma.

Creatinine, derived entirely from muscle creatine and phosphocreatine, and routinely measured in clinical laboratories has been used as an index of GFR. About 1.6% of the total body creatine pool is converted to creatinine daily (3). Creatine turnover rate is relatively constant in normal subjects, but little is known about turnover rate in disease (4). The major determinants of the creatine pool are 1) the total muscle mass, which is influenced mainly by sex and age and 2) dietary (mainly meat) intake of creatine. About 1 g of urinary creatinine is excreted per 17.9 kg of muscle mass. There is a greater generation of creatinine in males than females, and in young adults than in the preadolescent and geriatric populations. Conditions associated with muscle wasting, such as malnutrition, hyperthyroidism, muscular dystrophy, muscular paralysis, dermatomyositis and other causes of negative nitrogen balance, are associated with reduced creatinine generation (4, 5). In the adult, creatine intake is about 500 to 800 mg/day; cooking converts creatine to creatinine (6) and can greatly influence endogenous creatinine clearance. The generation of creatinine is reduced in patients with renal disease and elevated serum creatinine. Adding to the problem in patients with renal disease and substantial reductions in GFR is the fact that up to 60% of the creatinine generated may be removed by extrarenal means (7).

The clearance of creatinine can be used as an index of GFR in those species in which creatinine is not secreted (e.g. dog, cat, turtle, rabbit). However, in man and primates, creatinine is secreted in the proximal tubule (1). In normal humans, about 10 to 40% of the excreted creatinine can be derived from tubular secretion; this increases to 50 to 60% in patients with renal disease (8,9). Moreover, certain substances (e.g. cimetidine, trimethoprim, probenecid) can interfere with creatinine secretion.

When urine flow is less than 0.5 mL/minute, significant amounts of creatinine may be reabsorbed within the kidney or from the lower urinary tract (1). Reabsorption of creatinine has also been demonstrated in congestive heart failure and uncontrolled diabetes mellitus (4). The presence of noncreatinine chromogens (e.g. protein, glucose, acetoacetate, pyruvate, uric acid, fructose, ascorbic acid, cephalosporins, bilirubin) in the plasma also makes the measurement of plasma creatinine imprecise. Schwartz and colleagues (5) have modified the Technicon procedure, allowing accurate measurements of creatinine especially at lower concentrations. These measurements are not affected by bilirubin.

The measurement of GFR using the ideal markers inulin and polyfructosan is not practical in the clinical setting. Very few laboratories are set up to measure inulin or polyfructosan routinely and radioactive markers may not be a well accepted alternative. Thus, the clearance of creatinine has been used in the clinical setting despite the uncertainties of using creatinine as a marker of glomerular filtration. The clearance of creatinine approximates inulin clearance, especially when the kidney function is within the normal range; the correlation coefficient between the clearance of inulin and clearance of creatinine from 3 to 192 mL/min/1.73 m² was 0.94 (5). When GFR was less than 20 mL/min/1.73 m², creatine clearance overestimated the clearance of inulin by 20%. Nonetheless, absolute reductions in creatinine clearance is a specific but not a sensitive indicator of reduced GFR (4). In general, a progressive decline in creatinine clearance indicates a decrease in GFR unless the patient is taking drugs that inhibit the tubular secretion of creatinine or the serum creatinine is falsely elevated.

IV. Technique of Measuring Glomerular Filtration Rate

The clearance of GFR markers such as inulin can be determined by several methods. The classic method involves the infusion of the marker substance until a steady-state concentration of the marker is attained in the plasma. Thereafter multiple samples of blood and urine are collected over a two- to four-hour period. The clearance of the marker substance is calculated as described above and the average of the determinations reported. The clearance of the marker is usually corrected for body surface area (e.g. mL/min/1.73 m²) to facilitate comparison among subjects of different sizes (10). Single injection and constant injection technique of inulin without urine collection can also be used to assess GFR (11). However, these latter methods may greatly overestimate the GFR in the early postnatal period (11).

Endogenous creatinine clearance is traditionally measured by collecting urine over 24 hours, obtaining serum creatinine at the middle or the end of the urine collection and calculating the clearance, as in any other clearance method. Inaccurate measurements of urine volume, whether the collection of urine is performed over 24 hours or shorter time intervals, can give erroneous results.

A. Isotope Methods of Determining Glomerular Filtration Rate

Sodium iothalamate, EDTA, sodium diatrizoate and DTPA among others can be radioisotopically labeled and can be used to measure GFR. The advantage of these methods is that the GFR of each kidney can be determined.

B. Serum Creatinine as an Estimate of Glomerular Filtration Rate

Serum creatinine has been used as an index of GFR to obviate the problems associated with urine collection. However, as indicated above, serum creatinine is not only influenced by GFR but also by other variables including age, meat intake, and muscle mass. Serum levels reflect not only renal excretion but also the generation, intake and metabolism of creatinine. Serum creatinine reflects only GFR under steady-state conditions. When GFR decreases or increases abruptly, steady state may not be achieved for several days. Serial measurements of serum creatinine may be the only reliable means of monitoring GFR. In the perinatal period, serum creatinine is also influenced by maternal creatinine. In term babies, serum creatinine increases by 0.09 ± 0.04 mg/dL within a few hours of birth, apparently due to a decrease in extracellular fluid volume, and decreases to about 0.4 mg/dL by the second week (5). Rudd and colleagues (12) have shown that the decrease in serum creatinine after birth is related to gestational age; it is fastest in full-term infants and slowest in the most premature infants (Figure 5-1). From two months to two years of age, serum creatinine remains stable, reflecting proportional increases in GFR and muscle mass (5). Beyond two years of age, serum creatinine increases in both sexes, but to a greater extent in males than females.

During maturation (1 to 20 years), serum creatinine can be calculated from the formula (13):

$$S_{cr} \text{ (males)} \quad = 0.35 + 0.025 \times \text{age (years)}$$

$$S_{cr} \text{ (females)} = 0.37 + 0.018 \times \text{age (years)}$$

In adult males (18 to 92 years), creatinine clearance (C_{cr}) can be calculated from the formula (14):

$$C_{cr} = (140 - \text{age in years})$$

$$\times \text{ weight (kg)/serum creatinine (mg/dL)} \times 72$$

In females, it is 85% of males.

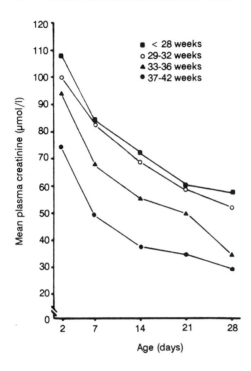

FIGURE 5-1. Plasma creatinine concentrations as a function of postnatal age in infants of different gestational ages. From Rudd PT, Hughes EA, Placzek MM, et al (1983) Reference ranges for plasma creatinine during the first month of life. Arch Dis Child 58:212–215, with permission.

This and other formulas overestimate creatinine clearance in obese and edematous patients. In children, Schwartz and colleagues (5) and others (15) have derived formulas that yield values of GFR that approximate those obtained from creatinine and inulin clearances:

$$GFR \ (mL/min/1.73 \ m^2) = k \ \text{body length (cm)}/S_{cr} \ (mg/dL)$$

where k is a constant that is a function of urinary creatinine per unit of body size. Table 5-2 gives the values and ranges of k in infants less than 1 year of age to subjects up to 21 years of age. The k values have to be adjusted downwards in patients with moderate to severe malnutrition, obesity and limb amputation, and in subjects with heart and renal failure (5). Body length may not be a true indicator of muscle mass in subjects with gross musculoskeletal deformities. For example, arm span rather than body length may be a better indicator of muscle mass in patients with myelomeningocele.

C. Serum Creatinine and Progression of Renal Failure

The reciprocal relationship between serum creatinine and creatinine clearance has led investigators to utilize the reciprocal of serum creatinine concentration to relate it to the decline in creatinine clearance. Although

TABLE 5-2. Mean and Ranges of k Used in Calculating GFR

Age group	k mean (range)
Low birth weight infants ($\leq$ 1 year)	0.33 (0.2–0.5)
Term infants ($\leq$ 1 year)	0.45 (0.3–0.7)
Children (2–12 years)	0.55 (0.4–0.7)
Females (13–21 years)	0.55 (0.4–0.7)
Males (13–21 years)	0.70 (0.5–0.9)

Adapted from Schwartz GJ, Brion LP, Spitzer A (1987) The use of plasma creatinine concentration for estimating glomerular filtration rate in infants, children and adolescents. Pediatr Clin North Am 34:571–590

the reciprocal of serum creatinine appears to decline at a constant rate in most patients with renal disease, the rate of decline may be influenced not only by GFR but also by tubular secretion, generation, intake and extrarenal elimination of creatinine. Some investigators suggest that determining the decline of renal function with time may be best studied by GFR measurements.

D. Glomerular Filtration Rate During Development (see renal functions, Appendix I)

After birth, GFR is variable but generally increases in the first two hours, followed by a decrease at four hours. In the first 24 hours of life, GFR may be as low as 2 mL/min/1.73 m^2 in infants of 25 weeks gestation and reaches term values of 25 mL/min/1.73 m^2 by 34 to 36 weeks. The GFR is the same in babies of similar conceptional ages, even if their postnatal ages are different. The rise in GFR after birth depends upon gestational age. In term babies, GFR may increase three- to fivefold within a week (16). The rise in GFR is less rapid in premature infants; the more premature the baby, the less will be the rise in GFR during the neonatal period. In preterm infants undergoing diuresis in the first few days of life, GFR may increase almost twofold by the second to the third postnatal day. In a minority of preterm infants who do not undergo diuresis after birth, the GFR does not change in the first week of life (17).

V. Clearance Method to Determine Renal Blood Flow

Until Doppler sonography is available to measure blood flow and blood flow distribution to specific organs, clearance techniques remain the most feasible way of measuring renal plasma flow (RPF). The most commonly used agent to measure RPF is *para*-aminohippurate (PAH). This agent is used because it is almost completely extracted by the kidney in a single pass. The use of clearance to measure RPF is based on the Fick principle and for PAH the equation is written as:

$$RPF = \frac{U_{PAH} \times V}{RA_{PAH} - RV_{PAH}}$$

where RPF is renal plasma flow in mL/min, U_{PAH} is the concentration of PAH in the urine, V is urine flow in milliliters per minute, RA_{PAH} is the concentration of PAH in the renal arterial blood and RV_{PAH} is the concentration of PAH in the renal venous blood. Determining the renal venous extraction of PAH is not usually necessary in the clinical setting in adults, since the renal venous extraction of PAH is almost 100%. In this situation, $RA_{PAH} - RV_{PAH}$ is the same as RA_{PAH}. Renal blood flow (RBF) can then be calculated from the formula:

$$RBF = \frac{RPF}{1 - \text{hematocrit}}$$

As in the case for GFR, for comparison of subjects of different sizes, the values can be corrected to 1.73 m^2 body surface area.

The Fick formula is not precisely applicable to measurement of RPF because renal venous outflow is less than the arterial inflow by an amount equal to urine flow and lymph flow. This problem increases with increasing urine flow, especially when the extraction of the marker substance is less than 50%. The extraction of PAH may reach this critical level in infants under three months of age.

The washout of radioactive gases such as Xenon-133 (^{133}Xe) from the kidney and single shot clearances of iodine-125 (^{125}I) PAH externally monitored have been used to determine renal plasma flow as well. Perfusion of each kidney can be determined with these methods.

VI. Renal Plasma Flow During Development

The clearance of PAH is not a true estimate of RPF in the newborn because the renal venous extraction of PAH may be as low as 60% compared to over 90% in older infants (>3 months). As with GFR, the most rapid increase in RPF occurs in the first three months of age (see Reference Intervals, in Appendix I). The filtration fraction (GFR/RPF) is similar in newborns and adults (0.2).

VII. Fractional Excretion

Under certain circumstances it may be necessary to determine the fractional excretion of different substance, i.e. amount excreted (U_s V) as a function of the filtered load ($GFR \times P_s$). This can be determined by the formula:

$$\text{Fractional excretion (\%)} = \frac{U_s(V)}{GFR \times P_s} \times 100$$

where U_s is the concentration of any substance in the urine, V is the urine flow and P_s is the plasma concentration of the substance in question. The formula can be rearranged so that fractional excretion of any substance can be measured without determining GFR or timing the urine collection:

$$\text{Fractional excretion (\%)} = \frac{U_s(V)}{U_{cr} \times V(P_s)/P_{cr}} \times 100$$

$$= \frac{U_s/P_s}{U_{cr}/P_{cr}}$$

Fractional excretion of a substance can be used to evaluate tubular function. Fractional excretion of Na is decreased in hypovolemia and Na depletion states and increased in acute tubular necrosis and Na repletion states. Fractional excretion of phosphate is increased in hypophosphatemic rickets and decreased in hypoparathyroidism. Fractional K excretion is low in hypoaldosteronism. Fractional excretion of Cl is decreased when the intake of Cl is low, and increased in Bartter's syndrome. Fractional reabsorption can also be used to assess renal tubular function:

$$\text{Fractional reabsorption} = 100 - \text{fractional excretion}$$

Renal function can also be evaluated, even when serum values are not available. The ratio of the concentration of a substance and creatinine in the urine (U_s/U_{cr}) has been used to assess renal function. For example, $U_{protein}/U_{cr} > 0.2$ indicates significant proteinuria and $U_{uric\ acid}/U_{cr} > 1$ indicates that hyperuricemia may be the cause of the renal failure; $U_{calcium}/U_{cr} > 0.2$ indicates hypercalciuria.

VIII. Serum Urea Nitrogen and Renal Function

A relationship between serum urea nitrogen (SUN) levels and renal function was noted before the concept of clearance evolved (18). Urea clearance is now rarely used as an index of GFR because of complex factors influencing the production and excretion of urea. Nonetheless, a SUN of 10 to 15 mg/dL almost always indicates a normal GFR. Low SUN is seen in overhydration, liver failure, malnutrition and inborn errors of urea metabolism. High SUN levels may be seen in hypovolemia, acute parenchymal renal failure, obstructive uropathy, inborn errors of urea excretion and states of increased urea production.

IX. Summary

Clearance techniques can be used to evaluate total and differential renal function as well as the function of specific nephron segments. Classic methods involve timed urine collections; however, formulas that require serum levels alone or "spot" urine samples without determinations of urine flows can be used with some degree of precision. In the pediatric age group, with changing renal function and body size, renal function is usually normalized to body surface area.

References

1. Levinsky NG, Levy M (1973) Clearance techniques. In: Orloff J, Berliner RW (eds) Renal Physiology. American Physiological Society, Washington, DC, pp 103–117
2. Smith HW (1951) The Kidney–Structure and Function in Health and Disease. Oxford University Press, New York
3. Heymsfield SB, Arteaga C, McManus C, et al (1983) Measurement of muscle mass in humans: validity of the 24-hour urinary creatinine method. Am J Clin Nutr 37:478–494
4. Levey AS, Perrone RD, Madias NE (1988) Serum creatinine and renal function. Ann Rev Med 39:465–490
5. Schwartz GJ, Brion LP, Spitzer A (1987) The use of plasma creatinine concentration for estimating glomerular filtration rate in infants, children, and adolescents. Pediatr Clin North Am 34:571–590
6. Macy RL, Jr, Naumann HD, Bailey ME (1970) Water soluble flavor and odor precursors of meat: 5. Influence of heating on acid-extractable non-nucleotide chemical constituents of beef, lamb and pork. J Food Sci 35:83–87
7. Hankins DA, Babb AL, Uvelli DA, et al (1981) Creatinine degradation I: The kinetics of creatinine removal in patients with chronic kidney disease. Int J Artif Organs 4:35–39
8. Shemesh 0, Golbetz H, Kriss JP, et al (1985) Limitations of creatinine as a filtration marker in glomerulopathic patients. Kidney Int 28:830–838
9. Bauer JH, Brooks CS, Burch R (1982) Clinical appraisal of creatinine clearance as a measurement of glomerular filtration rate. Am J Kidney Dis 2:337–346
10. McCrory WW (1972) Developmental Nephrology. Harvard University Press, Cambridge
11. Guignard JP, John EG (1986) Renal function in the tiny, premature infant. Clin Perinatol 13:377–401
12. Rudd PT, Hughes EA, Placzek MM, et al (1983) Reference ranges for plasma creatinine during the first month of life. Arch Dis Child 58:212–215
13. Schwartz GJ, Haycock GB, Spitzer A, et al (1976) Plasma creatinine and urea concentration in children: normal values for age and sex. J Pediatr 88:828–830
14. Cockroft DW, Gault MH (1976) Prediction of creatinine clearance from serum creatinine. Nephron 16: 31–41
15. Counahan R, Chantler C, Ghazali S, et al (1976) Estimation of glomerular filtration rate from plasma creatinine concentration in children. Arch Dis Child 51:875–878
16. Jose PA, Stewart CL, Tina LU, et al (1987) Renal disease. In: Avery GB (ed) Neonatology: Pathophysiology and Management of the Newborn. JB Lippincott Philadelphia, pp 795–849

17. Bidiwala KS, Lorenz JM, Kleinman LI (1988) Renal function correlates of postnatal diuresis in preterm infants. Pediatrics 82: 50–58
18. Kassirer JP, Gennari FJ (1979) Laboratory evaluation of renal function. In: Early LE, Gottschalk CW (eds) Strauss and Welt's Diseases of the Kidney. Little Brown and Co, Boston, pp 41–91

6
Imaging of the Kidney and Urinary Tract

Sharon M. Stein, Sandra G. Kirchner and
Richard M. Heller

I. Introduction

Imaging modalities available for the evaluation of the urinary tract in children have changed dramatically in the past several decades. Although the excretory urogram (EU) and voiding cystourethrogram (VCUG) are still important diagnostic tools, radionuclide imaging, ultrasonography

(US) and computed tomography (CT) have come to complement and even replace them in many clinical situations. Magnetic resonance imaging (MRI), an even newer technique, is still in the developmental stage but may also prove to be of value in urinary tract imaging.

Since a wide variety of techniques are available for assessing the urinary tract in pediatric patients, serious consideration must be given to using the proper technique in any given clinical situation so that the maximum amount of information can be obtained at a minimum risk, radiation exposure, trauma and cost to the patient. In this chapter, we will describe the most commonly used imaging modalities and discuss how they are currently employed in a variety of clinical situations. Preparation for radiological procedures is presented in Table 6-1.

II. Excretory Urography

Radiographic visualization of the kidneys, ureters and bladder by EU depends on the concentration and excretion by the kidneys of a radiopaque, iodinated organic compound that has been injected intravenously. The most commonly used agents are fully substituted tri-iodinated ben-

TABLE 6-1. Preparation for Radiological Procedures

Procedure	Preparation
Excretory urogram	1. Check history of allergy to iodinated contrast material 2. Inform radiologist if carbonated beverage is contraindicated 3. Hold last meal 4. One Dulcolax suppository 90 min prior to study; if no result, repeat in 45 min
Voiding cystourethrogram	No preparation
Ultrasound	No preparation
Radionuclide scintigraphy	No preparation
CT scan	Sedation[a]
MRI	Sedation[a]
Arteriography	1. Check history of allergy to iodinated contrast material 2. Sedation[a] or general anesthesia

[a]*Suggested sedation:*
<2 years: Chloral hydrate 50 mg/kg, oral or rectal (max 2 g)
>2 years: Meperidine (Demerol)   2 mg/kg, IM (max 100 mg)
          Promethazine (Phenergan)   1 mg/kg, IM (max   25 mg)
          Chlorpromazine (Thorazine) 1 mg/kg, IM (max   25 mg)
          or
          Demerol 2 mg/kg, IM (max 100 mg)
          Secobarbital (Seconal) 2 mg/kg, IM (max 100 mg)

zoic acid compounds, which are filtered by the glomeruli and are neither excreted nor absorbed by the renal tubule (1). Because the glomerular filtration rate (GFR) of the newborn and young infant is a fraction of that of the normal adult, EU in this group of patients can be suboptimal, and other imaging techniques are thus recommended (2).

The traditional high osmolar, ionic radiopaque contrast compounds are now being challenged by the low osmolar ionic and nonionic compounds (3). Current evidence suggests that the low osmolality is responsible for the reduced adverse effects seen with these compounds, and it has been shown that these radiopaque substances produce less in the way of vasodilation, hemodilution, vascular permeability and alteration of red blood cell (RBC) morphology than the older high osmolar agents (4). These materials, however, are more expensive than the high osmolar materials. In preparation for EU, oral intake is usually withheld for three to eight hours prior to the examination, depending on the age of the patient. When renal tomography is available, colonic cleansing is not required unless small renal calculi are being sought. On arrival of the patient in the radiology department, the examination is usually discussed with the parents. This allows an opportunity to acquire additional information and to explain the test, along with its potential risks. Although the risks may not be as great as in adults, minor reactions such as vomiting, sneezing, flushing and urticaria, and major life-threatening reactions such as laryngotracheal edema, asthma and cardiovascular shock can occur (5).

Prior to the intravenous injection of the contrast material, a plain scout radiograph of the abdomen is obtained. This radiograph serves the purpose of assuring that the technique is appropriate, gives the radiologist information as to how much gas and fecal material is present, provides the opportunity to assess for calcifications that might otherwise be obscured by radiopaque material and allows for evaluation of bony structures. After injection of the contrast material, filming is tailored to the patient's clinical problem and to the pathology revealed. A radiograph of the upper abdomen at one minute, during the nephrogram phase of the EU, usually provides the most optimal visualization of the renal outlines and renal substance (Figure 6-1A). If the kidneys are obscured by gas or fecal material, tomography is then performed. When tomography is not available, a radiograph with the X-ray beam angled slightly toward the head can be taken following the ingestion of a carbonated beverage. If the patient is to go from EU to surgery or is to take nothing by mouth for any other reason, this maneuver cannot be utilized. Oblique radiographs of the kidneys may also be helpful, especially if renal scarring is present. A radiograph of the entire abdomen at 10 to 15 minutes in most instances shows the renal collecting systems, ureters and bladder (Figure 6-1B). Delayed radiographs will be required if an obstruction is present.

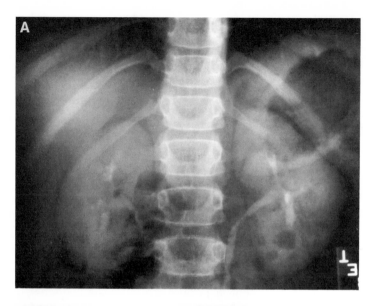

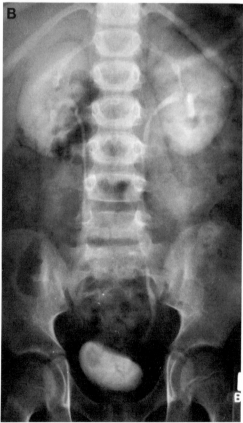

FIGURE 6-1. (A) Excretory urogram showing normal nephrograms bilaterally. (B) Abdominal film, at 15 minutes, from the same patient showing normal kidneys, collecting systems and ureters.

With the common use of US, CT and radionuclide scanning for imaging the urinary tract, the indications for EU have changed, but there are situations in which structural information concerning the upper urinary tract are required (6,7). Perhaps one of the most important of these situations is evaluation of the kidneys in children with urinary tract infection (UTI) and abnormal VCUG or US. Other indications for EU include suspected ectopic ureterocele (dribbling of urine in young girls), postsurgical assessment of the kidneys, abnormal renal US, hematuria and suspected urinary tract calculi. The EU is also performed in the initial examination of children with neurogenic bladder and when renal trauma is suspected and CT is otherwise not contemplated or available (6,7). Also, if the patient has a congenital anomaly associated with a high incidence of urinary tract disease, EU will be of use.

When a history of severe reaction to contrast material is obtained, other imaging modalities should be used to investigate the urinary tract. A history of allergy or a previous mild reaction to contrast material, however, are not absolute contraindications to EU.

III. Voiding Cystourethrography

Of all the techniques available for examination of the urinary tract, the VCUG gives the best anatomical detail of the lower urinary tract. It provides information concerning the bladder and urethral configuration, the presence or absence of vesicoureteral reflux and the size of the bladder (8). No advance preparation is required for the examination, although a full bladder is helpful to confirm that the catheter has been placed within the bladder. As with EU, the study is first discussed with the patient's parents and then a plain scout radiograph is obtained. The bladder is catheterized in a sterile technique with a #5 or #8 French catheter, and the bladder is emptied. The injection of a small amount of 9.5% aqueous lidocaine into the urethra of the male who is over the age of two years prior to catheterization reduces patient discomfort (8).

The contrast material, a 12.5 to 30% solution of conventional ionic contrast medium, is instilled into the bladder by gravity flow (8). The bladder is monitored intermittently with fluoroscopy throughout all phases of the examination for vesicoureteral reflux in particular but also for other dynamic abnormalities. Anteroposterior and oblique spot radiographs of the filled bladder are taken, followed by views of the bladder and urethra during voiding (Figure 6-2). If reflux occurs, its extent is also documented by fluoroscopic spot radiographs (Figure 6-3A,B). The catheter is removed during voiding and a postvoid radiograph completes the examination. Throughout the examination, care is taken to keep radiation dose to a minimum.

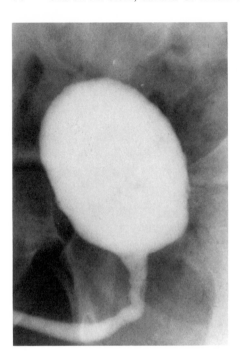

FIGURE 6-2. Normal voiding cystourethrogram in a male child. Note the normal bladder size and patent urethra.

The most common indication for the VCUG is the initial evaluation of a child with a UTI and suspected vesicoureteral reflux. Although there is some controversy on the subject (7), the VCUG is usually not performed until the child is infection free. The VCUG is also used to examine children with voiding abnormalities, the male infant with dribbling due to posterior urethral valves being a prime example of such a problem. Any infant or child in whom hydronephrosis is discovered should undergo VCUG to assess the possible role of vesicoureteral reflux in the process (7). The VCUG is also performed to evaluate the bladder in children with congenital anomalies, such as the prune belly syndrome, to assess the infant with anuria and to assess the previously continent child with recent-onset enuresis.

A. Urinary Tract Infection

The imaging evaluation of an infant or a child with the first appropriately documented and treated UTI will determine the the presence of vesicoureteral reflux, anatomical abnormalities and structural damage, all of which predispose to infection, and document base-line renal size to assess subsequent kidney growth (9).

Although the order of examinations may vary among centers, the VCUG is a useful test to start with (10). For the initial evaluation, a

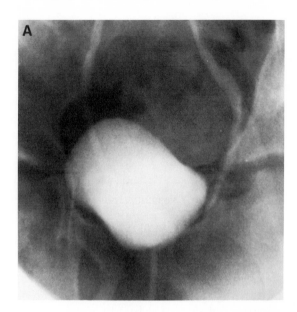

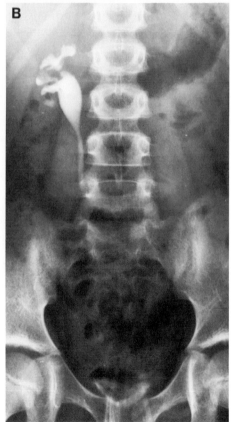

FIGURE 6-3. (A) A VCUG in a patient with urinary tract infection, showing a bilateral vesico-ureteral reflux. (B) Postvoid abdominal film in the same patient, showing retained contrast material in the right collecting system.

conventional fluoroscopic procedure is usually performed since this study provides better anatomical visualization of the bladder and urethra and, in the presence of vesicoureteral reflux, the ureters and collecting systems, than does the radionuclide cystogram. However, Bisset and colleagues contend that the conventional study provides little advantage over the radionuclide cystogram in girls (11). They now advocate a change in the traditional approach and recommend the use of the radionuclide cystogram instead of the conventional VCUG in the female child with the first UTI, since it delivers a significantly lower radiation dose to the ovaries and allows continuous monitoring for reflux. When the conventional VCUG is performed, the bladder is assessed for abnormalities such as diverticula, and if vesicoureteral reflux is observed, its severity is documented as is the degree of drainage.

In boys, abnormalities of the urethra can be detected during the voiding phase. For follow-up of children with known vesicoureteral reflux, the radionuclide cystogram is suggested because of its reduced radiation dose as compared to the fluoroscopic study.

Following the VCUG, an EU is performed to provide anatomical visualization of the kidneys and collecting systems if vesicoureteral reflux or any other significant abnormality is observed (Figure 6-4). In the absence of significant reflux, a US may be performed; however, minor renal

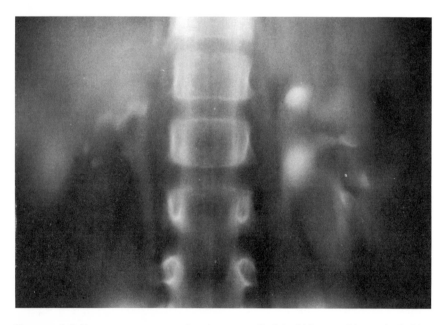

FIGURE 6-4. Excretory urogram showing a small right kidney, with cortical thinning secondary to chronic pyelonephritis.

scars and duplicated collecting systems can be missed with this method (12,13). If an abnormality is detected with US, it is advisable to perform an EU. Recently, renal scintigraphy has been advocated as a substitute for EU and US to evaluate renal structure and function in children with UTI (9). An approach to the radiographic study of patients with UTI is shown in Figure 9-1.

IV. Ultrasound

The development of high resolution, real-time sector scanners has greatly expanded the use of urinary tract ultrasound (US) in the pediatric patient because of the superior quality of the images obtained. The examination is short and painless, does not require sedation and does not expose the child to ionizing radiation. Ultrasonography does not, however, provide information about renal function; radionuclide scintigraphy is therefore used as a complementary modality if this information is required.

Sonographic evaluation of the kidneys begins with the determination of location, size, shape and echogenicity. The kidneys are then examined for abnormalities such as cysts, masses, calculi and hydronephrosis. Multiple views are obtained in the sagittal and transverse planes. A complete study will include examination of the bladder, although it is not always possible to obtain views of a full bladder in the young child.

Renal size varies with age, weight and height. Normal ranges are available from several sources (14–18) (see Appendix III). Renal cortical echogenicity is compared to that of the liver. In the neonate, and in infants up to three or four months of age, the renal cortex can be as echogenic as the liver (19); the renal cortex of premature infants may be more echogenic than the liver (20,21) (Figure 6-5). Above four months of age, the renal cortex is normally less echogenic than the liver and the renal sinus is very echogenic (Figure 6-6). This is due to the different types of tissues located therein, such as fat, infundibula, blood vessels and lymphatics.

A. Indications

The echogenicity of the renal parenchyma is increased in any form of *renal parenchymal disease* in childhood. This is a nonspecific finding in terms of disease entities, but the degree of echogenicity correlates significantly with the degree of parenchymal abnormality (19). The increased echogenicity is due to changes such as edema, sclerosis, infiltrate, fibrosis or calcium deposition. In older children, it is most frequently due to acute glomerulonephritis or nephrosis, whereas in the neonate and young infant it is more often due to renal vein or artery thrombosis and renal cortical necrosis.

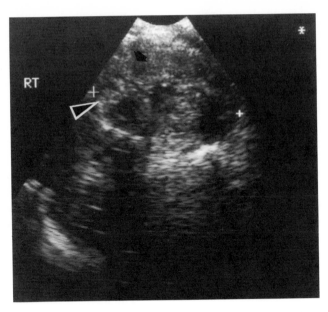

FIGURE 6-5. Renal ultrasound in a premature infant. Note that the renal cortex (triangle) is more echogenic than the adjacent liver (arrow).

Improved resolution has made US the primary imaging modality in the evaluation of *renal cystic disease.*

In infantile (autosomal recessive) polycystic disease, the kidneys are enlarged and echogenic with a sonolucent rim due to compressed renal cortex, as well as central sonolucency due to the prominent renal pelvis and calyces (22). The diffusely increased echogenicity is due to echoes reflected off the multiple interfaces caused by the ectatic tubules.

The findings in adult (autosomal dominant) polycystic kidney disease (APKD) are those of renal enlargement with multiple cysts; however, normal parenchymal thickness is usually preserved between the cysts. In infancy, the findings of APKD are similar to those with infantile polycystic disease but without the sonolucent rim, the larger cysts developing with increasing age. The cysts in APKD may be diagnosed as early as 12 weeks gestation, but may be seen for the first time as late as 30 years of age.

In the classic form of *multicystic dysplastic kidney* caused by complete ureteral obstruction before 10 weeks gestation, the kidney is enlarged and contains multiple noncommunicating cysts (23). There is no demonstrable parenchyma or pelvis. The hydronephrotic form, caused by obstruction after the 10th week, shows a central cyst with peripheral cysts budding off (24). The distinction between this condition and hydronephrosis on US may be difficult.

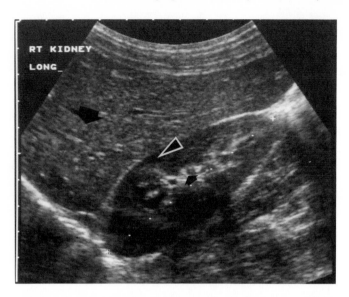

FIGURE 6-6. Normal renal ultrasound in an eight-year old male. The renal cortex (triangle) is less echogenic than the adjacent liver (large arrow), and the renal sinus (small arrow) is very echogenic.

In *multilocular cystic disease*, the normal kidney is compressed by a mass of multiple cysts separated by echogenic septa.

Medullary sponge kidneys are rarely diagnosed in children. They generally appear normal sonographically, although renal calculi may be seen.

Sonographic evaluation of *hydronephrosis* includes a complete examination of the ureters, bladder and bladder outlet in order to determine a cause for the hydronephrosis. It is important to demonstrate continuity between the dilated calyces and the renal pelvis in order to differentiate hydronephrosis from renal cystic disease.

In hydronephrosis caused by ureteropelvic junction obstruction, the ureter is not dilated, whereas in conditions such as ureterovesical junction obstruction, vesicoureteral reflux, primary megaureter, neurogenic bladder and bladder outlet obstruction, a dilated ureter may be demonstrated. Bilateral ureteral dilation suggests a neurogenic bladder or an obstruction distal to the bladder. Simple and ectopic ureteroceles are readily identified sonographically but differentiation between the two may be difficult, and correlation with VCUG or EU is required.

Fetal hydronephrosis detected on antenatal US should be followed up in all cases. With the normal dehydration that occurs in the early neonatal period, the renal appearance may revert to normal in milder cases. It is, therefore, important to reevaluate these babies once rehydration has occurred. Prenatal diagnosis of obstructive uropathy is discussed in Chapter 21.

Renal tumors of childhood include Wilms' tumor, renal cell carcinoma, mesoblastic nephroma and the conditions related to Wilms' tumor (renal blastoma, nephroblastomatosis and epithelial nephromablastoma).

Sonographically, these lesions may be difficult to distinguish from one another, since they may vary in echogenicity from one patient to another. Indeed, there may be areas of varying echogenicity within the same tumor, including anechoic areas representing hemorrhage or necrosis. It is extremely important to evaluate the contralateral kidney very carefully, since a significant proportion of Wilms' tumors are bilateral.

The greatest usefulness of US in renal tumors to the surgeon is its accuracy in the evaluation of the renal vein, inferior vena cava (IVC) and right atrium for tumor extension. Wilms' tumor can obstruct the IVC by compression without actual invasion, and the ease with which the sonographer can visualize the IVC in multiple different planes makes this an important modality in the preoperative workup of the child with a renal tumor.

V. Radionuclide Scintigraphy

Radionuclide scintigraphy includes methods for the evaluation of renal structure and function with a low patient radiation dose. It is frequently used in conjunction with ultrasound and the combination of these two modalities provides a relatively noninvasive, low radiation dose method of evaluating many renal problems. No patient preparation is required. A pharmaceutical is labeled with a radioisotope such as technetium-99m or iodine-131. The resulting radiopharmaceutical is then injected intravenously. The dose is calculated according to the child's weight. Imaging is subsequently performed with a scintillation camera interfaced to a computer.

Radiopharmaceuticals used for renal imaging fall into two broad groups. The first group contains those agents used for cortical imaging, providing information of an anatomical nature as well as evaluating renal cortical function. Technetium-99m dimercaptosuccinic acid (^{99m}Tc-DMSA) is an example of this type of radiopharmaceutical. The second group of agents assesses renal function. These agents include iodine-131 hippuran and technetium-99m diethylene triamine pentaacetic acid (^{99m}Tc-DTPA). Technetium-99m glucoheptonate (^{99m}Tc-GH) possesses features of both groups (Table 6-2).

A. Cortical Imaging

99mTc-DMSA is bound to plasma proteins and is taken up by the cells of the proximal and distal tubules, where it is retained for approximately

TABLE 6-2. Agents Used in Radionuclide Scintigraphy

Radiopharmaceutical	Excretory pathway (%)	Uses
^{99m}Tc-DTPA	Glomerular filtration (100)	GFR; vascular flow; collecting system/obstruction
^{131}I-Hippuran	Glomerular filtration (20) Tubular secretion (80)	Renal function
^{99m}Tc-DMSA	Tubular secretion (100)	Parenchymal anatomy
^{99m}Tc-GH	Glomerular filtration ($>$50) Tubular secretion ($<$50)	Renal function Parenchymal anatomy; collecting system/obstruction; vascular flow

24 hours. Imaging is performed 2 to 4 hours after injection with the cameras in the posterior position. This technique is used to determine whether a renal mass is functioning. It can detect renal scarring and differentiate a column of Bertin from a neoplasm.

B. Functional Imaging

The GFR is calculated using ^{99m}Tc-DTPA, since this agent is excreted by glomerular filtration only. The ^{99m}Tc-DTPA is also used for flow studies, in which images are obtained over the abdominal aorta, renal arteries and kidneys every 1.5 seconds immediately following an intravenous bolus of the radiopharmaceutical.

Iodine-131 hippuran is the most commonly used agent for assessing renal function. It is excreted by glomerular filtration (20%) and tubular secretion (80%). After intravenous injection, posterior, five-minute images are obtained for 30 minutes and a computer generated time activity curve is obtained for the region of interest drawn around each kidney. A normal kidney shows peak activity in three to five minutes; the activity will sharply decline thereafter.

If ureteric obstruction is identified, with increasing activity in the collecting systems and renal pelvis, a diuretic renogram is then performed. Furosemide is injected intravenously and five-minute images are obtained for another 30 minutes. If obstruction is partial, activity in the collecting systems will decrease, whereas if it is high grade or complete, there will be no significant reduction in activity (Figures 6-7A,B and 6-8A,B).

Split renal functions are also calculated from the renogram by computer analysis. The number of counts in each region of interest in the first five-minute image indicates the percentage of total renal function contributed by each kidney.

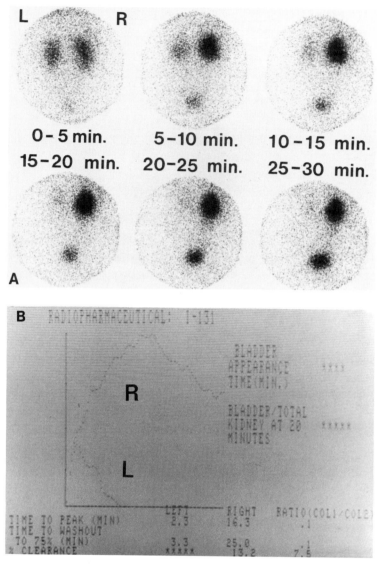

FIGURE 6-7. (A) ¹³¹I-hippuran renogram in a four-year-old child with partial right ureteropelvic junction obstruction. Sequential five-minute images show normal function on the left, with increasing activity in the right renal pelvis. (B) Computer generated time activity curves from the same patient, showing a normal curve for the left kidney, and increasing activity in the right kidney to 16.3 minutes, followed by a minimal decrease in activity.

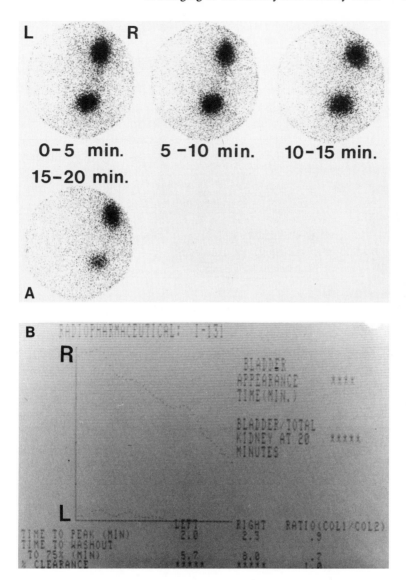

FIGURE 6-8. (A) Renogram obtained after the same patient was injected with furosemide shows a minimal decrease in right renal pelvic activity. (B) Computer-generated curve shows some decrease in activity in the right renal pelvis.

C. Radionuclide Cystography

Cystography may be used for follow-up of the vesicoureteral reflux, previously documented by VCUG. It is not as good as the initial investigation because resolution is not high enough for accurate documentation of anatomical abnormalities of the ureters, bladder or urethra, or detection of minimal reflux. However, it is the ideal method for follow-up because of the much lower radiation dose to the bladder and gonads. With radionuclide cystography, gonadal exposure is approximately one hundredth that of standard radiographic VCUG (25).

No preparation is required for this examination. The child is placed supine on the scanning table with the scintillation camera in the posterior position. Catheterization is performed using sterile technique, with an infant feeding tube or a #8 French catheter. The bladder is emptied and the catheter connected to a bag of normal saline with a three-way stopcock through which 500 μCi to 1 mCi ^{99m}Tc-DTPA is instilled into the bladder. Saline is then allowed to run into the bladder, and an image is taken after every 50 cc. Most children tolerate up to 200 cc, but occasionally 300cc will be required in the older child. If possible, voiding and postvoiding images are obtained (Figure 6-9).

VI. X-Ray Computed Tomography

A new dimension to kidney evaluation became available in the mid–1970s when X-ray computed tomography (CT) instrumentation became commonplace. Prior to that time, EU, tomography, VCUG, renal scans and US constituted the tools available to study the urinary tract. Both US and CT have allowed the radiologist to evaluate the kidneys independent of renal function. Additionally, these techniques have decreased the indications for angiography in children.

X-ray computed tomography is the method of choice in the evaluation of the child suspected of having a renal tumor. It can be used to determine whether a lesion is intrarenal or extrarenal, or single or multiple, and when the lesion is malignant, to establish if metastasis to the lungs has occurred. It may also be helpful in the evaluation of the traumatized child suspected of having a renal laceration or fracture, and in the recognition of nephrocalcinosis (26,27).

A. Technique

Almost all our CT scans are performed one hour after oral administration of dilute contrast material for opacification of the bowel; 2 cc/kg body weight of ionic or non-ionic contrast material are also injected as a rapid intravenous bolus into one of the larger, upper extremity veins. Two sets of cross-sectional images, one before and one after the intravenous injection of contrast material, are obtained. In the trauma patient, we perform only contrasted studies. Scans, 8 mm thick are then obtained, and in every study of the abdomen we include the lung bases and the entire

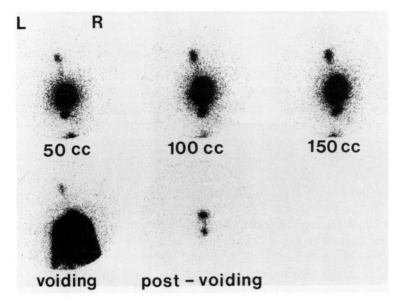

L   R

50 cc   100 cc   150 cc

voiding   post – voiding

FIGURE 6-9. Radionuclide cystogram showing left sided reflux during filling. The postvoiding image shows bladder and urethra and no activity in the left collecting system or ureter.

pelvis. These images are most valuable because they demonstrate the vascular anatomy and relationships of soft tissue masses to normal structures, permitting the extraction of optimal information from the study (28–30). The lack of intraabdominal fat planes in the young child is a limitation to CT as compared to adults, in whom perivisceral fat provides good radiographic contrast.

B. In Wilms' Tumor

X-ray computed tomography is the most accurate way to demonstrate the extent of the primary tumor (whether it is unilateral or bilateral and whether metastases have developed), and to evaluate renal function. Sonography is the method of choice for demonstration of tumor in the renal vein and the IVC.

The appearance of Wilms' tumor, as shown by CT, has been well described in the literature (31,32). Most tumors are quite large and distort the calyces. Small, centrally placed tumors are less common and do not distort the renal outline. Occasionally, an exophytic Wilms' tumor will develop at the periphery of the kidney and leave the calyceal pattern intact.

The initial, pre-contrast scans of a Wilms' tumor will demonstrate that the mass lacks homogeneity. After intravenous contrast material administration, this lack of homogeneity is exaggerated. Areas of necrosis and hemorrhage within the mass, and occasionally calcification, are easily seen (Figure 6-10).

Growth of the tumor into the renal vein and IVC may be documented on the contrast-enhanced study, and the extent of the tumor thrombus determined. The presence of multiple lesions in one kidney, bilateral tumors and nephroblastomatosis can be documented by CT (33).

At the time of initial diagnosis of Wilms' tumor, the retroperitoneum must be evaluated for nodal disease. Large nodes immediately adjacent to the mass may well contain tumor, whereas smaller, remote nodes are usually reactive in nature.

Liver involvement at the time of presentation is uncommon unless lung disease is also present. Even in the presence of a normal chest radiograph, chest CT must be performed to identify metastases not visible on conventional studies.

Follow-up evaluation of the abdomen of children treated for Wilms' tumor is usually performed by sonography. There are occasional cases, however, when evaluation of the renal bed by US is equivocal. In this setting, CT may prove very helpful.

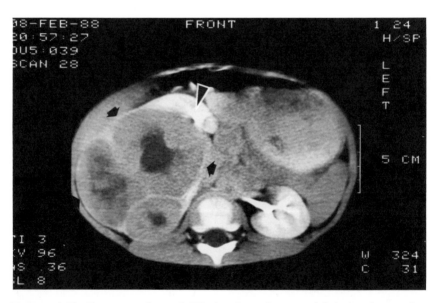

FIGURE 6-10. Contrast-enhanced CT showing a large multilobulated mass (between arrows) with areas of necrosis intrinsically distorting the calyces of the right kidney (triangle) and compressing and displacing the normal renal parenchyma anteriorly (Wilms' tumor)

C. In Trauma

X-ray computed tomography is the imaging modality of choice in the child injured by blunt abdominal trauma in which kidney injury is suspected. This modality permits early recognition of kidney laceration or contusion and the formation of perirenal hematoma formation and urinoma. There is a wide range of renal injury, from a small area of contusion to disruption and fragmentation of the kidney. In addition to providing anatomical information, CT will provide functional data.

VII. Magnetic Resonance Imaging

Magnetic resonance imaging (MRI) of the kidneys and retroperitoneum offers the following advantages at the present time:

1. Superlative tissue contrast capability
2. Generation of images in multiple planes
3. Capability to demonstrate vascular anatomy without intravenous or arterial injections of contrast material
4. No ionizing radiation

The major limitations of MRI at the present time include inability to image calcifications, and image degradation by respiratory motion. The future challenges for scientists applying MRI techniques to the study of the genitourinary systems include 1) the study of metabolic and physiological derangements utilizing magnetic resonance spectroscopy and 2) the application of MRI technology to recognize early signs of kidney rejection in the transplant patient (34–36).

The latest imaging modality to be applied to the study of the genitourinary system, MRI should not be thought of as competing with CT or US but rather as offering the unique advantages listed above. There are, however, certain advantages to MRI, and limitations to CT and US. A CT of the kidneys in children is occasionally limited by a paucity of perirenal fat; the superlative tissue contrast resolution capability of MRI is not so impaired. Imaging by CT usually requires intravenous contrast material injection for optimal resolution, but it may not be prudent to subject some children to toxic contrast material. In these patients, MRI is ideal because no contrast material is needed or used. Ultrasound is an operator-dependent modality, whereas MRI requires much less skill to generate images (37–39).

A. Normal Anatomy

Magnetic resonance imaging clearly depicts the normal anatomy of the kidneys and retroperitoneum in coronal, sagittal or axial projections, unlike CT in which the images are displayed in an axial or a transverse format.

The fat that surrounds the kidney on spin-echo images will be very bright due to the short T1 relaxation time. Although the renal capsule is not commonly visualized, the renal cortex is easily separated from the medulla on spin-echo images because the renal cortex has a shorter T1 relaxation time than the medulla. The renal sinus has a bright signal because of the fat content. Blood vessels appearing at the renal hilus have no signal because moving blood does not generate a signal. Recently, techniques have been developed whereby cine MRI technology permits study of magnetized blood in motion in the heart and vessels. Conceptually, the blood flow in the renal artery may be evaluated with this technique.

In spin-echo techniques, the pelvicalyceal system will appear dark because of the low signal intensity due to the long T2 relaxation time of urine. In this regard, the bladder is easily identified (40).

B. Techniques

Both axial (transverse) and coronal MRI images are generated for the initial studies of a child with suspected kidney pathology. Multiplanar images in other projections can be made to evaluate further the relationship between an abdominal mass and the surrounding tissues.

We utilize axial spin-echo images with short TE or TR parameters that are relatively T1 weighted. We next utilize a long TE and long TR pulse sequence (SE 60/2000 or SE 120/2000). These sequences are especially useful in differentiating a tumor thrombus from a blood clot (41).

C. Indications for Use

The differentiation between cystic and solid *renal masses* is within the capability of MRI, as well as the capability to demonstrate hemorrhagic cysts. With a short TR interval (SE 30/500), simple renal cysts will appear as low-level areas of homogeneous intensity, clearly separated from the remainder of the kidney. If there has been a recent hemorrhage into a cyst, there will be a high signal intensity on pulse sequences with short TE and TR intervals. In general, the degree of brightness of the signal correlates with the age of the hemorrhage and the degree of resolution (41).

D. In Wilms' Tumor

Many imaging modalities and strategies have been devised to assist in the rapid diagnosis of an *abdominal mass* including Wilms' tumor, neuroblastoma, hydronephrosis, hepatosplenomegaly, duplication cysts and the like (42). It has been documented that plain radiographs rarely permit a confident diagnosis, although the type, distribution and character of calcification may be very helpful. An EU or renogram may show lack of function of one kidney or may not permit clear-cut differentiation of an intrarenal mass from an extrarenal mass that distorts and displaces the kidney (43).

Real-time US has the disadvantage of not being able to image the entire mass. If the mass is large, it is sometimes a problem determining its origin and how it relates to other organs (44). Again, CT is limited by the axial plane depiction of the anatomy and pathology, and may not differentiate between intrarenal or extrarenal tumors (42).

However, MRI permits imaging in oblique planes as well as the standard axial, sagittal and coronal planes. The entire abdomen can be visualized on one image, and there is excellent tissue contrast differentiation (45). It is tempting to say that one can dispense entirely with contrast studies; however, it is important to know the function of the "uninvolved" kidney, so that at some point in the preoperative workup of a child suspected of having a Wilms' tumor, a contrast study of the patient can be implemented to be certain that the "uninvolved" kidney functions.

Current MRI technique routinely includes two pulse sequences, the first employing a moderately T1-weighted spin-echo technique, and the second employing a moderately T2-weighted technique with a slice thickness of 5 mm. Sedation with chloral hydrate may be required.

Magnetic resonance imaging demonstrates the renal origin of the suspected mass. However, capsular penetration may be difficult to detect. The technology is extremely useful in recognition of tumor in the IVC as well as metastases in the liver. In this regard, MRI has the potential for replacing studies that offer similar information such as CT, US and liver and spleen scanning (46,47) (Table 6-3, Figures 6-11A,B and 6-12A,B).

Abdominal *neuroblastoma* is a common pediatric tumor. Thus, it is important to differentiate it from other masses such as Wilms' tumor.

TABLE 6-3. Use of MRI in the Diagnosis of Wilms' Tumor

Parameter	MRI
Ability to identify kidney as site of abdominal mass	Accurate
Capsule penetration	May not show the renal capsule; local invasion may be missed
Enlarged lymph nodes	Can demonstrate enlarged nodes but cannot reliably indicate their histology
Wilms' tumor invasion of renal vein and IVC	Accurate, although experience is not extensive (46)
Hepatic metastases	Accurate; accuracy exceeds that of contrast-enhanced CT when gadolinium-DTPA is used as a paramagnetic contrast-enhancement agent

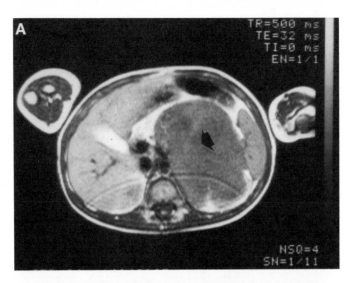

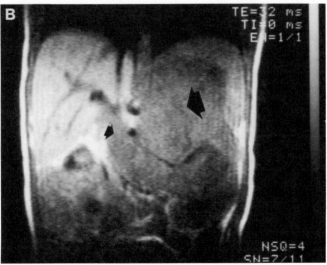

FIGURE 6-11. MRI: (A) Axial T1 weighted image through upper abdomen. Note the huge left-sided mass (arrow). (B) Coronal T1 weighted image. The tumor is seen in the left renal vein (small arrow) and a mass lesion (large arrow) is again seen.

An MRI study of the abdomen, especially in the coronal plane, facilitates recognition of lesions arising in the adrenal gland, and the coronal plane study helps to differentiate a mass arising in the adrenal gland from one arising in the liver or kidney (48).

An important contribution of MRI to the management of selected cases of neuroblastoma is the identification of spinal involvement by tumor.

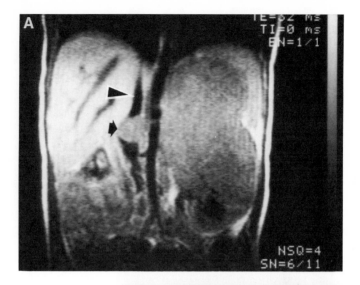

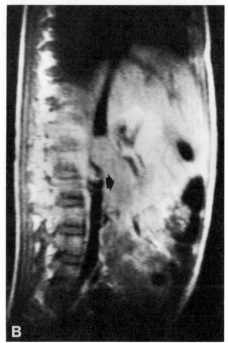

FIGURE 6-12. MRI: (A) Coronal T1 weighted image through the inferior vena cava and aorta. Tumor thrombus (arrow) is present in the inferior vena cava (triangle). (B) Sagittal T1 weighted image confirms the coronal image. Note the tumor thrombus (arrow) in the renal vein and the inferior vena cava.

In the past, myelography, or metrizamide-enhanced CT scanning, was performed to evaluate intraspinal extension of the tumor (49). Now MRI can provide a noninvasive way to determine the intraspinal extent of the tumor (50) (Table 6-4).

TABLE 6-4. Use of MRI in the Diagnosis of Abdominal Neuroblastoma

Parameter	MRI
Ability to identify correctly adrenal gland as site of origin of abdominal mass	Accurate
Ability to identify characteristic calcification seen in a high percent of neuroblastomas	No signal emanates from calcification
Ability to identify extent of lesion including intraspinal and vascular involvement	Accurate

The pulse sequences employed to study a child suspected of having an abdominal neuroblastoma are the same as those employed to study a Wilms' tumor. One major limitation of MRI is its inability to image the calcification that is characteristic of this lesion, but not infrequently a signal void can be recognized in what is shown by another imaging modality to be an area of calcification.

In some cases, MRI can replace myelography and CT in the study of abdominal neuroblastoma especially in those children who show neurological findings or abnormalities of the spine or paraspinal regions on conventional radiographs of the abdomen.

VIII. Renal Arteriography

Renal arteriography, although safe in experienced hands, is an invasive procedure and should only be performed when the result will influence the clinical management of the patient and the diagnosis cannot be made by other imaging modalities. Close interaction between the referring physician and radiologist is therefore of paramount importance.

Contraindications to arteriography are bleeding tendencies, severe anemia and a history of previous severe reaction to iodinated contrast material. If the arteriogram is essential and such a history of severe allergy is present, the patient should be premedicated with steroids (prednisone 2 mg/kg daily) for three days, and diphenhydramine (Benadryl) given immediately prior to the study. Most children can undergo the procedure under sedation (see Table 6-1); however, general anesthesia is recommended if the sedated child is incooperative.

An informed consent should be obtained and the potential risks of the procedure (infection, hematoma, femoral arterial thrombosis and allergy to the contrast material) should be outlined. An intravenous line is started the evening before study, and nothing by mouth is allowed after midnight (children under two years are allowed clear fluids). Sedation is administered 30 minutes before the study.

Arteriography is generally performed via the right femoral artery. An aortic injection at the level of the renal arteries is usually performed, followed by selective renal artery injection if necessary. At the end of the procedure, the catheter is removed and pressure is applied over the puncture site for 10 to 15 minutes, or until bleeding has stopped. Frequent inspections of the groin area, strict bed rest and no bending of the leg should be enforced for eight hours.

Three phases are seen on the normal renal arteriogram—the arterial phase lasting three seconds; the nephrogram phase, three to eight seconds; and the venous phase, eight to ten seconds after injection.

Renal arteriography in children is primarily indicated in the diagnosis of masses, trauma, renal artery thrombosis and suspected renovascular hypertension (Figure 6-13).

A. Masses

The multiple, noninvasive imaging modalities discussed earlier in this chapter have reduced the need for arteriography in the diagnosis of renal masses; however, the procedure is of value in suspected large tumors and

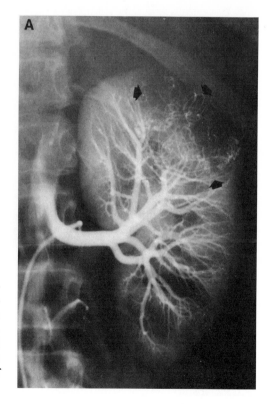

FIGURE 6-13. (A) Renal arteriogram from an 11-year-old female who presented with blurred vision, malignant hypertension, proteinuria and pyuria. She was found to have a reninoma in the upper pole of the left kidney (arrows).

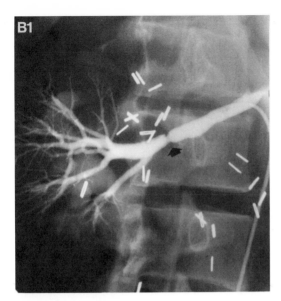

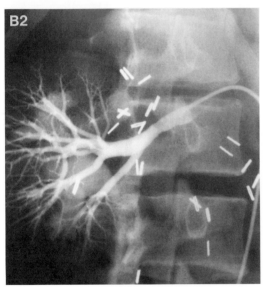

FIGURE 6-13. (B1) A renal arteriogram from a 13-year-old boy with a restenosed renal artery following surgical correction of renal artery stenosis (arrow). (B2) Renal arteriogram of the same patient showing the renal artery following balloon angioplasty.

bilateral Wilms' tumor, and in embolization of vascular tumors. Arteriography may be the only modality to pick up a small Wilms' tumor in the contralateral kidney. Children who are prone to develop bilateral disease are those with sporadic aniridia (51) and hemihypertrophy (52,53). Renal arteriography may be required also to differentiate between benign ipsilateral nephromegaly and Wilms' tumor in patients with hemihypertrophy. The vascular pattern is also useful in differentiating the type of a tumor (angiomyolipoma, renal cell carcinoma and lymphoma), which may also be bilateral. The procedure may be used also to embolize very vascular tumors with gelfoam prior to surgery in order to decrease the intraoperative blood loss. A protocol for imaging neonates with an abdominal mass is presented in Figure 6-14.

B. Trauma

Generally, EU and CT will provide sufficient information about renal damage and function in most cases of renal trauma. Indications for angiography in such cases include 1) unilateral nonvisualization of a kidney on EU, suggesting pedicle damage, and 2) EU or CT findings suggesting preexisting renal disease. Abnormal kidneys are more susceptible to damage in a trauma situation; here indications for arteriography include 1) persistent hematuria with normal EU, CT and cystourethrogram, 2) suspicion of an intrarenal arteriovenous fistula, and 3) onset of hypertension.

C. Renovascular Hypertension

Arteriography confirms the presence of renovascular disease, and transluminal angioplasty can offer the patient a relatively safe, effective alternative to surgery in selected cases of focal renal artery stenosis. It is

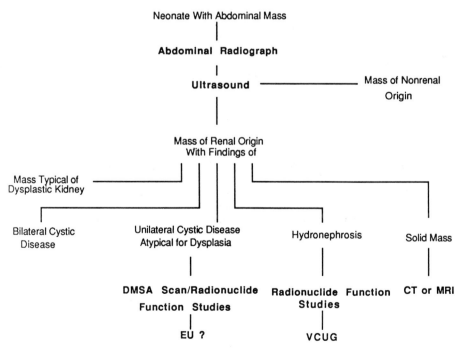

FIGURE 6-14. Suggested imaging protocol for a neonate with an abdominal mass.

also useful in following patients who have deteriorated following successful surgery. Medial fibrodysplasia is the commonest cause of renovascular hypertension in children, the middle and distal thirds of the renal artery being predominantly affected. Angiographically, this lesion appears as alternating areas of constriction and dilation. Aneurysms may be also present. Neurofibromatosis, which is usually proximal and often bilateral, is the next most common cause of renovascular hypertension. Renal artery narrowing may also follow umbilical artery catheterization or irradiation. A protocol for imaging a child with hypertension is presented in Figure 6-15.

X. Renal Venography

The technique of venography is identical to arteriography, but here the femoral vein is catheterized and the catheter advanced into the IVC with possible renal vein selection. Indications for this procedure include venous sampling in hypertensive patients, suspected renal vein thrombosis, possible tumor invasion (a cavagram is first performed in this instance) and evaluation of splenorenal shunts.

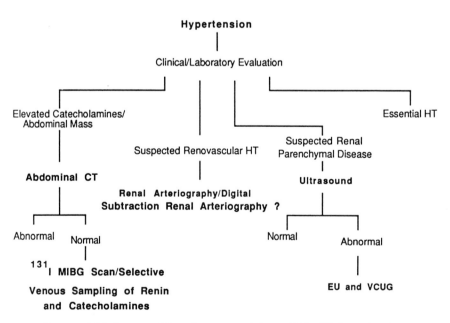

FIGURE 6-15. Suggested imaging protocol for a child with hypertension.

References

1. Denneberg T (1965) Clinical studies of kidney function with radioactive sodium diatrizoate (Hypaque®). Acta Med Scand 179 (Suppl 442) 442:1–134
2. Martin DJ, Gilday DL, Reilly BJ (1975) Evaluation of the urinary tract in the neonatal period. Radiol Clin North Am 13:359–368
3. McClennan BL (1987) Low osmolality contrast media: Premises and promises. Radiology 162:1–8
4. Dawson P (1984) New contrast agents. Chemistry and pharmacology. Invest Radiol 19:S294–S300
5. Gooding CA, Berdon WE, Brodeur AE, et al (1975) Adverse reactions to intravenous pyelography in children. AJR 123:802–804
6. Lebowitz RL, Ben-Ami T (1983) Trends in pediatric uroradiology. Urol Radiol 5:135–147
7. Lebowitz RL (1985) Pediatric uroradiology. Pediatr Clin North Am 32:1353–1362
8. Hilton SvW, Edwards DK, Hilton JW (1984) Practical Pediatric Radiology. WB Saunders, Philadelphia.
9. Liebowitz RL, Mandell J (1987) Urinary tract infection in children: Putting radiology in its place. Radiology 165:1–9
10. Blickman JG, Taylor GA, Lebowitz RL (1985) Voiding cystourethrography: The initial radiographic study in children with urinary tract infection. Radiology 156:659–662
11. Bisset GS III, Strife JL, Dunbar JS (1987) Urography and voiding cystourethrography: findings in girls with urinary tract infection. AJR 148:479–482
12. Leonidas JC, McCauley RGK, Klauber GC, et al (1985) Sonography as a substitute for excretory urography in children with urinary tract infection. AJR 144:815–819
13. Kangerloo H, Gold RH, Fine RN, et al (1985) Urinary tract infection in infants and children evaluated by ultrasound. Radiology 154:367–373
14. Blane CE, Bookstein FL, DiPietro MA, et al (1985) Sonographic standards of normal infant kidney length. AJR 145:1289–1291
15. Han BK, Babcock DS (1985) Sonographic measurements and appearance of normal kidneys in children. AJR 145:611–616
16. Holloway H, Jones TB, Robinson AE, et al (1983) Sonographic determination of renal volumes in normal neonates. Pediatr Radiol 13:212–214
17. DeVries L, Levene MI (1983) Measurement of renal size in preterm and term infants by real-time ultrasound. Arch Dis Child 58:145–147
18. Rosenbaum DM, Korngold E, Teele RL (1984) Sonographic assessment of renal length in normal children. AJR 142:467–469
19. Hayden CK Jr, Santa-Cruz FR, Amparo EG, et al (1984) Ultrasonographic evaluation of the renal parenchyma in infancy and childhood. Radiology 152:413–417
20. Cramer BC, Jequier S (1984) Factors associated with renal parenchymal echogenicity in the newborn. Presented at the 70th Scientific Assembly of the RSNA, Washington, DC
21. Erwin BC, Carroll BA, Muller H (1985) A sonographic assessment of neonatal renal parameters. J Ultrasound Med 4:217–220

22. Hayden CK Jr, Swischuk LE, Smith TH, et al (1986) Renal cystic disease in childhood. Radiographics 6:97–116
23. Beck AD (1971) The effect of intrauterine urinary obstruction upon the development of fetal kidney. J Urol 105:784–789
24. Felson B, Cussen LJ (1975) The hydronephrotic type of unilateral congenital multicystic disease of the kidney. Semin Roentgenol 10:113–123
25. Majd M, Belman AB (1979) Nuclear cystography in infants and children. Urol Clin North Am 6:395–407
26. Kuhn JP, Berger PE (1981) Computed tomography of the kidney in infancy and childhood. Radiol Clin North Am 19:445–461
27. Berger PE, Munschauer RW, Kuhn JP (1980) Computed tomography and ultrasound of renal and perirenal diseases in infants and children. Relationship to excretory urography in renal cystic disease, trauma and neoplasm. Pediatr Radiol 9:91–99
28. Damgaard-Pedersen K, Yssing M (1982) The clinical value of CT whole body scanning in pediatric tumour investigation. Pediatr Radiol 12:191–195
29. Damgaard-Pedersen K, Yssing M (1982) CT in the surveillance and current control of children with extracranial malignant tumours. Pediatr Radiol 12:197–200
30. Kirks DR, Rosenberg ER, Johnson DG, et al (1985) Integrated imaging of neonatal renal masses. Pediatr Radiol 15:147–156
31. Fishman EK, Hartman DS, Goldman SM, et al (1983) The CT appearance of Wilms' tumor. J Comput Assist Tomogr 7:659–665
32. Miller JH, Lang WE (1984) Urinary tract. In: Miller JH (ed) Imaging in Pediatric Oncology, Williams and Wilkins, London, pp 252–258
33. Montgomery P, Kuhn JP, Berger PE, et al (1985) Multifocal nephroblastomatosis: Clinical significance and imaging. Pediatr Radiol 14:392–395
34. James AE Jr, Partain CL, Holland GN, et al (1981) Nuclear magnetic resonance imaging: the current state. AJR 138:201–210
35. Wolfson BJ, Gainey MA, Faerber EN, et al (1985) Renal masses in children. An integral imaging approach to diagnosis. Urol Clin North Am 12:755–769
36. Dietrich RB, Kangarloo H (1986) Kidneys in infants and children: evaluation with MR. Radiology 159:215–221
37. Buonocore E, Borkowski GP, Pavlicek W, et al (1983) NMR imaging of the abdomen: technical considerations. AJR 141:1171–1178
38. Kulkarni MV, Partain CL, Tishler JM, et al (1985) Magnetic resonance imaging of the abdomen. In: Peterson SB, Muller RN, Rinck PA (eds) An Introduction to Biomedical Nuclear Magnetic Resonance. Georg Thieme Verlag, Stuttgart, pp 146–154
39. Leung AW-L, Bydder GM, Steiner RE, et al (1984) Magnetic resonance imaging of the kidneys. AJR 143:1215–1227
40. LiPuma JP (1984) Magnetic resonance imaging of the kidney. Radiol Clin North Am 22:925–941
41. Hricak H, Moon KL Jr (1983) Kidneys and adrenal glands. In: Margulis AR et al (eds) Clinical Magnetic Resonance Imaging. Radiology Research and Educational Foundation, San Francisco, pp 209–228
42. Currarino G (1985) The genitourinary tract. In: Silverman FN (ed) Caffey's Pediatric X-Ray Diagnosis: An Integrated Imaging Approach, 8th edition. Year Book Medical Publishers, Chicago, pp 1587–1743

43. Canty TG, Nagaraj HS, Shearer LS (1979) Nonvisualization of the intravenous pyelogram: a poor prognostic sign in Wilms' tumor? J Pediatr Surg 14:825–830
44. Jaffe MH, White SJ, Silver TM, et al (1981) Wilms' tumor: ultrasonic features, pathologic correlation, and diagnostic pitfalls. Radiology 140:147–152
45. Kangarloo H, Dietrich RB, Ehrlich RM, et al (1986) Magnetic resonance imaging of Wilms' tumor. Urology 28:203–207
46. Belt TG, Cohen MD, Smith JA, et al (1986) MRI of Wilms' tumor: promise as the primary imaging method. AJR 146: 955–961
47. Kulkarni MV, Shaff MI, Sandler MP, et al (1984) Evaluation of renal masses by MR imaging. J Comput Assist Tomogr 8:861–865
48. Dietrich RB, Kangarloo H, Lenarsky C, et al (1987) Neuroblastoma: The role of MR imaging. AJR 148: 937–942
49. Armstrong EA, Harwood-Nash DCF, Ritz CR, et al (1982) CT neuroblastomas and ganglioneuromas in children. AJR 139:571–576
50. Kagan AR, Steckel RJ (1986) Retroperitoneal mass with intradural extension: value of magnetic resonance imaging in neuroblastoma. AJR 146:251–254
51. Pilling GP,IV (1975) Wilms' tumor in seven children with congenital aniridia. J Pediatr Surg 10:87–96
52. Janik JS, Seeler RA (1976) Delayed onset of hemihypertrophy in Wilms' tumor. J Pediatr Surg 11:581–582
53. Kirks DR, Shackleford GD (1975) Idiopathic congenital hemihypertrophy with associated ipsilateral benign nephromegaly. Radiology 115:145–148

7
The Kidney Biopsy

JEAN-PIERRE DE CHADARÉVIAN and
BERNARD S. KAPLAN

I. Introduction

The use of percutaneous biopsy to obtain and study renal tissue by light, immunofluorescent and electron microscopy has advanced our understanding of renal disease. As a result, useful clinicopathological correlations were developed and it has become possible to diagnose diseases more precisely, to predict prognosis and to offer treatment based on an understanding of the underlying pathological abnormalities rather than on clinical and laboratory findings alone. Two recent advances, the development of the disposable biopsy needle (Tru-cut needle, Travenol Laboratories, Inc. Deerfield, IL) and the use of renal ultrasonography, have made percutaneous renal biopsy safer and easier to perform. Percutaneous renal biopsy has been performed on thousands of children over the past 30 years and is now an established, safe and practical procedure.

II. The Biopsy: A Clinicopathological Consultation

The indications for kidney biopsy are variable, and experience shows that the more pertinent and precise the question asked, and the better known the limitations of what a biopsy can assess, the more rewarding the results. Disappointment with results is often caused by "fishing expeditions" and poor judgment of the indications. Therefore, it is strongly suggested to do the biopsy in conjunction with the pathologist who can best judge the usefulness of the procedure in a given case, and set the priorities and methods of handling the specimen once obtained. When the amount of tissue is very limited, a decision has to be made as to what should be done with it. The study of one glomerulus may establish by light microscopy alone the diagnosis of membranous nephropathy, whereas the diagnosis of focal sclerosis requires 5 to 10 deep glomeruli. In IgA nephropathy, immunofluorescence is a must. In Alport's syndrome, electron microscopy is crucial. This means that for a biopsy to indicate, for example, the cause of recurrent hematuria of glomerular origin, a sampling for all techniques is required. Predicting in advance which technique will provide the answer requires knowing the diagnosis, or an unusually lucky intuition.

A technician should be available on site, with all the necessary instruments, media and fixatives once the biopsy specimen is obtained. The technician will make sure that glomeruli are present in all samples, that the fragment for electron microscopy is minced properly without crushing and placed in fresh chilled fixative (glutaraldehyde, paraformaldehyde, etc.) and that the sample for immunofluorescence is transported in the medium of choice of the laboratory for rapid freezing and processing. Furthermore, planning and timing of the biopsy in conjunction with the laboratory is also necessary for proper handling soon after procurement: A specimen in glutaraldehyde needs to be taken out of the fixative and rinsed in buffer one to three hours later; the specimen for immunofluorescence needs to be frozen as soon as it reaches the laboratory. Therefore, performing a biopsy toward the end of the day creates superfluous problems, which may jeopardize the results.

III. Limitations Due to Sampling

Familiarity with what a needle renal biopsy can assess is of great help when deciding whether to biopsy. Therefore, it is worth remembering that when one looks at the slide, one is scanning an area measuring about 1 cm × 1 mm. Changes that are extremely patchy or limited to a particular area, such as embolic infarcts, abscesses, segmental hypoplasia or a cyst, will not be picked-up unless biopsied under some means of very precise visualization. Such lesions seldom need to be biopsied, but in the case of glomerular lesions, the limitations of the method may be serious. One of the better illustrations of this problem is seen in nephrotic syndrome, when the possibility of early focal sclerosis is feared. Sampling in these cases is essential, since sclerosis may have affected only a few glomeruli and, therefore, a large number of glomeruli is needed. Also glomeruli have to be obtained from the corticomedullary junction where early changes develop. Adequate sampling is also necessary for proper evaluation of the severity of focal and segmental lesions and conditions in which crescents may be seen.

Table 7-1 lists the most commonly biopsied renal conditions in which there could be discrepancy between the biopsy findings and the actual state of the kidney because of insufficient sampling.

IV. Nondiagnostic Lesions

It is important to be aware of the fact that many renal changes observed in a biopsy are nondiagnostic. Such changes indicate the presence of an abnormality and may even point out the level and degree of involvement, but they fail to establish the exact diagnosis. Under such circumstances, the pathologist will give a descriptive diagnosis. In the case of electron microscopic study in particular, many observations with presently unknown significance may be made. However, they are recorded for the

TABLE 7-1. Renal Conditions with Focal, Localized or Patchy Lesions for Which an Ample Biopsy Sampling Is Crucial

Focal and segmental sclerosis and minimal change nephrotic syndrome
Glomerulonephritis with crescents (percentage of crescentic glomeruli)
Henoch-Schönlein purpura nephritis
Embolic nephritis (purulent, bacterial endocarditis, shunt nephritis, intravenous drug abuse)
Polyarteritis nodosa
Wegener's granulomatosis
Tubulointerstitial disease
Renal cortical necrosis
Systemic lupus erythematosus

sake of completeness and may have to await further progress of our knowledge before they are fully understood.

Several conditions may show nondiagnostic lesions on biopsy. The value of the biopsy in such instances may be debated; however, it helps to rule out other possibilities or to assess the degree of renal involvement. Examples of these conditions are minimal change nephrotic syndrome (MCNS), some advanced disease states and various hereditary and congenital disorders, such as oligomeganephronia, segmental renal dysplasia (Ask-Upmark kidney) and juvenile nephronophthisis. In MCNS, the only change observed is effacement of foot processes (also called fusion of podocytes), a nonspecific ultrastructural change also seen in many other glomerular diseases. Yet, in the proper context, its documentation in the absence of other lesions is essential to the diagnosis. Similarly, in several hereditary and/or congenital, nonprimarily renal syndromes in which there is associated renal involvement, the lesions themselves may not be diagnostic. This is the case for example with the cortical cysts that may be seen in Meckel's syndrome, Zellweger's syndrome, tuberous sclerosis, Hippel-Lindau disease, oral-facial-digital syndrome, Lejeune's asphyxiating thoracic dystrophy and some trisomies, to mention only a few. Cortical cysts may be isolated also, and their significance remains unclear.

V. Indications for Renal Biopsy in Children

In the more mundane practice, the pediatric nephrologist resorts to the biopsy after gathering a detailed personal and family history and performing a complete physical examination and laboratory workup. Although it is usually prudent to await the results of the noninvasive studies before doing the biopsy, it is becoming apparent that in certain circumstances, such as in Goodpasture's syndrome or in patients with a necrotizing vasculitis, a biopsy should be done as soon as possible in order to institute appropriate treatment. The common indications of renal biopsy in children are presented in Table 7-2.

VI. Special Considerations

1. Nephrotic Syndrome

Since over three-quarters of children with nephrotic syndrome have the minimal change variety, a renal biopsy is not recommended in the newly diagnosed nephrotic child unless there are features in the clinical history, physical examination or laboratory findings that point to a structural glomerular lesion (see Chapter 8). Indications for a renal biopsy in the child with nephrotic syndrome are presented in Table 8-11. A family history of renal disease associated with deafness (Alport's syndrome),

TABLE 7-2. Common Indications for Renal Biopsy in Children

Persistent and recurrent hematuria of unknown cause
Atypical or severe acute glomerulonephritis
Rapidly progressive glomerulonephritis
Nephrotic syndrome resistant to steroids or with features not typical of MCNS
Persistent nonorthostatic proteinuria
Suspected familial or hereditary nephritis
Acute intrinsic renal failure of unknown cause
Chronic renal failure of unknown cause
Evaluation of renal involvement in systemic disease (anaphylactoid purpura, SLE)
Evaluation of renal allograft
Other forms of renal disease (Bartter's syndrome, some tubular disorders)
Monitoring course of glomerular disease in response to treatment

clinical features of the nail-patella syndrome, and clinical findings of ambiguous genitalia (suggestive of the syndrome of abnormal gonadal differentiation, nephropathy and Wilms' tumor) are other indications for biopsy. Before performing a biopsy on patients with unexplained proteinuria, it is imperative that orthostatic proteinuria be excluded (see Chapter 8).

2. Acute Nephritic Syndrome

A biopsy is not indicated in a patient in whom there is an unequivocal diagnosis of acute poststreptococcal glomerulonephritis. In primary acute nephritic syndromes with atypical presentation, persistant hypocomplementemia and no evidence of a prior streptococcal infection, and in acute nephritis secondary to systemic disease, the biopsy will establish diagnosis and type and degree of damage and will help in planning therapy and making a prognosis.

Some of these patients may have IgA nephropathy or hereditary nephritis. Patients with membranoproliferative glomerulonephritis may present with acute nephritis and massive proteinuria, the so-called nephritic-nephrotic picture. A suspicion of necrotizing or crescentic glomerulonephritis is an indication for an urgent biopsy (see Chapters 10 and 19).

3. Hematuria

A biopsy is advisable in a patient with hematuria if there is a family history suggestive of Alport's syndrome. Patients who have microscopic hematuria unaccompanied by gross hematuria and/or substantial proteinuria (>1 g/1.73 m^2 daily) are not usually biopsied. Table 7-3 illustrates the logic prompting a biopsy in the case of recurrent hematuria of glomerular origin; Table 7-4, in the case of acute renal failure.

TABLE 7-3. Differential Diagnosis of Recurrent Glomerular Hematuria in Children

Clinical entity	Diagnostic clue on biopsy	Usual pathology
Berger's disease (IgA-IgG nephropathy)	Intramesangial IgA	Near normal by light microscopy or moderate to severe segmental mesangioproliferative change ± tubulointerstitial involvement
Alport's syndrome	No deposits, thickening, splitting and fragmentation of lamina densa by electron microscopy	Near normal by light microscopy or segmental mild to severe glomerulosclerosis ± tubulointerstitial change
Benign (familial or not) recurrent hematuria	Very attenuated glomerular basement membrane by electron microscopy; no deposits	Near normal histology

TABLE 7-4. Differential Diagnosis of Acute Renal Failure

Clinical entity	Diagnostic clues on biopsy
Hemolytic uremic syndrome	Microangiopathy; subendothelial involvement of glomerular capillaries by electron microscopy
Cortical necrosis	Diffuse glomerular, tubular and interstitial ischemic damage
Postinfectious glomerulonephritis	Subepithelial deposits without spiking
Membranoproliferative glomerulonephritis, Type II	Band-like, intramembranous dense deposits
Renal vein thrombosis	Zones of hemorrhagic infarction, often unilateral
Acute tubular injury (toxic, shock, dehydration, etc.)	Tubulointerstitial injury with relative sparing of glomeruli; no deposits
Hyperuricemia	Uric acid crystals (sometimes associated with leukemic or lymphomatous infiltrates)

4. Henoch-Schönlein Nephritis

The use of biopsy in patients with Henoch-Schönlein nephritis should be restricted to those excreting more than 1 g/m^2 of protein daily (>1 g in those over 1 m^2), to those who have hypertension and to those with decreased renal function.

5. *Lupus Nephritis*

A biopsy should be done in all patients who have systemic lupus ery-thematosis (SLE) associated with clinical or laboratory evidence of renal disease. More debatable, however, is the question of whether to biopsy all cases of SLE irrespective of whether there is evidence of renal in-volvement. Many nephrologists believe that the latter course of action should be taken because of the finding of substantial renal involvement in some patients in whom clinical and laboratory findings were trivial or even nonexistent. The biopsy findings may also be invaluable in terms of monitoring the effects of treatment in some conditions such as SLE and membranoproliferative glomerulonephritis (see Chapter 19).

6. *Hemolytic Uremic Syndrome*

In the past, biopsies were done routinely on patients with the hemolytic uremic syndrome once the platelet count had returned to normal. Al-though not all nephrologists are in agreement, there are some who believe that a biopsy should be done in every case to determine the extent of renal damage and to see whether renal involvement is primarily glo-merular, arteriolar or both.

7. *Other Conditions*

Renal biopsy may be performed also in patients with suspected nephro-calcinosis, and in some patients with sickle cell disease to ascertain the severity and extent of the renal damage. A biopsy may be done also in neonates suspected of having acute cortical necrosis. The procedure is safe in neonates. We have performed percutaneous renal biopsies suc-cessfully and without complications in 1-kg babies. We have also biopsied patients with pyelonephritis to ascertain whether or not there was still evidence of ongoing infection. The biopsy is also commonly used in monitoring renal graft rejection, efficacy of immunosuppressive therapy and recurrence of the original disease in the allograft.

VII. Contraindications and Complications of Kidney Biopsy

The procedure is very safe when performed by experienced hands and when good judgment has been exercised in weighing the risk and eval-uating the indications and contraindications. Absolute contraindications of percutaneous needle kidney biopsy include a solitary kidney, an ab-normal vascular supply to the kidney, the presence of intrarenal tumor and noncorrectable bleeding diathesis. Markedly obese and uncooperative patients are difficult candidates. Those who cannot stand surgery represent a high risk in case it is required after the procedure. The biopsy is relatively contraindicated when there is a risk of dissemination of pus or tumor or of significant bleeding (bleeding diathesis and uncontrolled hypertension). Hydronephrosis, cystic kidneys, end-stage renal disease and bilateral contracted kidneys are not usually biopsied.

In the absence of contraindications, and when all precautionary measures have been taken, morbidity is minimal. The main complication of the procedure is hematuria. Macroscopic hematuria occurs in about 5% of biopsies; it is usually self-limited. Only 0.5 to 2% of biopsies will bleed to the extent of the patient needing a blood transfusion. Colic secondary to the passage of clots may occur. Perirenal hematomas are not infrequent and usually require observation and reassurance only. An arteriovenous fistula is suspected if a bruit is heard over the biopsy site. Affected patients may also develop systolic hypertension with very wide pulse pressure. A pseudoaneurysm of the small renal vessels has been rarely observed, but the majority of vascular abnormalities resolve spontaneously. Other complications are presented in Table 7-5.

VIII. Preparation of the Patient

The patient can be hospitalized one day before, or on the morning of the biopsy. A physical examination and an accurate blood pressure measurement should be done, and laboratory studies performed. The procedure should be explained to the parents and the child, indicating that during the procedure the child will be lightly sedated and lying on the table with a roll under the abdomen, that the skin will be anesthetized so that there will be very little discomfort and that the child will be asked to take a deep breath and hold it a number of times during the procedure. An ultrasound examination of the kidneys must be done the day before, or immediately before the biopsy to establish the presence of two kidneys and the absence of structural anomalies or localized lesions. A prebiopsy checklist is presented in Table 7-6.

TABLE 7-5. Complications of Kidney Biopsy

Hematuria requiring transfusion (0.5–2%)
Macroscopic hematuria, usually self-limited (5%)
Perirenal hematoma (0.5–1.5%)
Arteriovenous fistula (0.5%)
Exceptional complications (puncture of viscera or
    major renal vessels, renal infection, sepsis)
Death (less than 0.1%)

TABLE 7-6. Pre-biopsy Check List

Laboratory studies:
   Complete blood cell count, platelet count, prothrombin time,
      partial thromboplastin time, bleeding time, fibrinogen
   Type and hold one unit of blood
   Other studies as indicated
Consent form signed
Make arrangements with pathology department
Make arrangements with ultrasound department
Day of biopsy
   Nothing by mouth for 6 hours
   Insert a blood line
   Premedicate 1 hour before biopsy with:
      Meperidine (Demerol)   2 mg/kg (max. 50–100 mg)
      Promethazine (Phenergan)   1 mg/kg (max. 25 mg)
      Chlorpromazine (Thorazine) 1 mg/kg (max. 25 mg)
   Send patient to ultrasound on stretcher

IX. Localization of the Kidney

The patient is placed in a prone position on the biopsy table, with the head lying comfortably on a pillow and the face turned to one side. A rolled sheet is placed under the abdomen at the level of the biopsy site. The left kidney is usually preferred, but either kidney can be biopsied without difficulty. The site of biopsy should be about 1 cm above the border of the lower pole, midway between the medial and lateral aspects of the kidney. A number of techniques are available for localizing the kidney for biopsy, including intravenous urography, fluoroscopy, radionuclides and ultrasound; the latter is usually preferred. The lower pole is identified and an indelible mark is made on the patient's back with a pen.

X. Biopsy Procedure

Blood pressure and pulse should be monitored prior to biopsy and during the procedure at regular intervals. The operator and the assistant wear sterile surgical gloves. An area of the skin 20 to 25 cm in diameter is disinfected. A sterile spinal sheet is draped over the biopsy site with the site centered in the middle of the hole in the sheet. The skin is infiltrated with the local anesthetic, using a #25 disposable needle. The subcutaneous tissue and deeper layers are then anesthetized using a #22 1½-in. needle. If resistance is encountered in the attempt to inject the local anesthetic, the possibility that the needle has penetrated the kidney should be considered and the needle should be withdrawn slightly. In most prepubertal children, the kidney is 2.5 to 4 cm deep; in infants, it is usually not deeper than 2 cm. A small longitudinal incision about 0.5 cm in length is now made in the skin at the bipsy site using the # 11 scalpel blade. The purpose of the incision is to allow free oscillation of the scout needle and to allow the biopsy needle to pass unimpeded through the skin. The stylet of the lumbar puncture needle is used as a scout needle to determine the depth of the kidney. The patient is asked to hold his or her breath in mid-inspiration. The needle is then passed directly or placed in the biopsy needle guide (Needle Guide for 720 Scanheads, Amedic USA, Phoenix, AZ) and inserted slowly in a slight (10 to 20°) cephalad direction through the skin and subcutaneous tissue. As the stylet penetrates the kidney capsule, a definite give, or loss of resistance, can be felt by the operator. The child should be asked to breathe and if the stylet is inside the kidney capsule, there will be a definite swing in a cephalocaudal direction with respiration. Furthermore, arterial pulsations are often transmitted to the stylet when the kidney has been penetrated and this can be also used to indicate that the kidney has been reached. The stylet is now withdrawn very slowly until the respiratory swing and arterial pulsation stop. At this depth, the stylet is just at the surface of the kidney. The position of the stylet is checked by ultrasound and then withdrawn, and the depth noted. The patient should be asked to hold his or her breath in mid-inspiration every time a needle is inserted in or withdrawn from the kidney. In infants and younger children, this of course cannot be achieved and the biopsy should be performed as quickly as possible. The biopsy needle is now inserted directly, or through the biopsy guide attached to the tranducer of the ultrasound machine, which is held steady by the ultrasonographer.

The biopsy is performed by advancing the specimen notch unsheathed into the kidney for the desired distance. Once the specimen notch is in the kidney, the cannula is advanced over it to cut off the piece of tissue that is lying in the notch. This must be done without, at the same time, advancing the specimen notch. With practice and the use of ultrasound guidance, it is possible to obtain tissue with almost every attempt. After one or two cores of tissue have been obtained, the renal ultrasound is repeated to determine whether or not bleeding into or around the capsule has occurred. If success is not encountered after several tries, however, it is best to desist and to try again on another day, preferably using the same side to limit the risk of injury to one kidney. A simple, firm dressing is applied. An assessment is made of the patient's condition, and if it is satisfactory, he or she is returned to bed by rolling him or her gently onto it from the biopsy table.

XI. Postbiopsy Care

The child should remain in bed for 24 hours, and the blood pressure and vital signs determined frequently. It is advisable to have cross-matched blood ready in the blood bank for possible transfusion, although the chance of needing a transfusion is only 0.5 to 2%.

Abdominal pain, colic or mass may suggest hemorrhage and a renal ultrasound should be performed. The child is usually discharged home 24 hours after the procedure if no complications appear; however, harsh play and trauma to the biopsy site should be avoided for at least one month. The postbiopsy orders are presented in Table 7-7.

XII. Reading the Biopsy

The information obtained from the biopsy has to be integrated into the total picture. This is best done by going over the biopsy slides and micrographs with the pathologist. This is not only a learning exercise, but it also allows better understanding of the wording of the biopsy report, provides a visual picture of the disease process and its severity and often gives useful leads for further investigation of the patient.

Reading the biopsy requires a minimum of familiarity with the histological, ultrastructural and immunopathological appearance of the normal and abnormal kidney, as well as with the terminology used to describe it, and some understanding of the purpose of the various stains used (1-4).

XIII. Terminology and Basic Lesions

Reading the biopsy involves a systematic evaluation of the glomeruli, tubules, interstitium and extraglomerular blood vessels. Tubular, interstitial and vascular lesions are usually straightforward but may be non-specific and secondary to glomerular disease.

TABLE 7-7. Postbiopsy Orders

Apply a firm dressing to biopsy site

Keep patient flat in bed for 24 hours; first 4 hours on back with a rolled sheet under the biopsy site

Check blood pressure and vital signs every 15 minutes for 2 hours, every 30 minutes for 2 hours, every 1 hour for 8 hours, and every 2 hours for 12 hours

Perform urinalysis and hematocrit 4 and 24 hours after the procedure, and as indicated thereafter

Observe all samples of urine for gross hematuria and clots

Resume previous diet and medication. If fluid is not restricted, force fluids

Inform house officer if blood pressure >140/90 or <90/50, and about any change in vital signs

Inform house officer if patient does not void by 12 hours following biopsy

Discharge home next morning, if no complications appear. Before discharge, change dressing to a small one and check for a bruit over the biopsy site with the bell of the stethoscope.

There are four basic parameters in the evaluation of glomerular disease. The pattern of distribution of the lesions, the nature of the lesion, its severity (or degree of activity) and its chronicity. When describing the distribution of the glomerular lesions, the following four terms are generally used: *focal, diffuse, segmental* and *global*. They all refer to the histological pattern in a given section, and not to patterns obtained with electron microscopy or histological examination of a serially sectioned block of tissue. The term *diffuse* means that all glomeruli appear abnormal as opposed to *focal,* in which some glomeruli seem to be spared. The term *segmental* implies that, in a given glomerulus, only segments of the tufts are affected, whereas *global* lesions imply total involvement of a tuft. Therefore, theoretically, four combinations are possible: diffuse and global, focal and global, focal and segmental and diffuse and segmental. Description of the lesion itself is also complicated by a profuse and variable terminology. However, it is essential to be familiar with the basic types observed; most of these changes are best demonstrated by electron microscopy (Figure 7-1 and Table 7-8).

XIV. Histological Stains

In all laboratories, the parafin-embedded tissue is serially sectioned. Some levels are stained with routine nonselective stains such as hematoxylin-eosin (H&E) or hematoxylin-phloxin-saffron (HPS). The purpose of these stains is to give a general view of the tissue, and the level and pattern of the disease. They should not be used to evaluate specific components such as mesangial matrix increases, basement membrane thickening or deposits. Other stains are used to complement the study (special stains). They may vary from one laboratory to another. The following special stains are almost universally employed. The periodic acid-Schiff (PAS) stains all polysaccharides and in particular the glomerular and tubular basement membrane as well as the mesangial matrix. The role of the periodic acid-silver methenamine stain (PASM) and related silver-impregnation stains is similar. They sharply outline basement membranes; mesangial deposits (immune) within these structures do not pick up the silver and thus are easily visualized. Splitting and spiking of basement membranes as well as diffuse segmental mesangial matrix increase are demonstrated with these stains. Masson's trichrome stains cytoplasms and collagen blue-green, and deposits appear red-orange. The Congo-red stain demonstrates amyloid (apple-green birefringence under polarized light). The Giemsa stain may be used for identification of cells present in an inflammatory infiltrate. Alizarin-red stains calcification. Demonstration of granules in the juxtaglomerular apparatus requires special fixation prior to exposure to Bowie's stain. Demonstration of crystals (urates, cystine, oxalate) often require fresh frozen tissue, and examination under polarized light.

XV. Immunopathological Studies

These ordinarily complement the histological and ultrastructural evaluation of glomerular diseases. They are also useful in demonstrating antitubular basement membrane activity. They are usually performed to detect the presence of immunoglobulins (IgG, IgM, IgA, IgE), complement and fibrinogen, and can be used to detect various antigens such as thyroglobulin, and nucleic acids, and in particular those associated with infectious agents such as *Treponema pallidulm, Candida, Plasmodium malariae, Mycoplasma pneumoniae,* hepatitis B virus, *Streptococcus, Staphylococcus,* and measles and rubella viruses. However, antigen detection is seldom performed in the course of a routine biopsy.

The most widely used technique of immunopathological study is immunofluorescence. However, other nonfluorescent techniques are available (immunoperoxidase, immune-gold technique for light and electron microscopy). The distribution pattern may be diffuse, focal, segmental or global. Within a given glomerulus, the pattern of involvement may be confined to the periphery of the glomerular loops (membranous), be purely mesangial or be mesangial and peripheral. The character of the immunofluorescence also varies. It may be linear (Goodpasture's syndrome), granular or pseudolinear (resulting from coalescence of granular deposits). Although the demonstration of an antigen serves a very specific purpose, demonstration of immunoglobins, complement and fibrinogen require interpretation in the light of clinical, histological and ultrastructural findings. With a few exceptions (Masugi-type nephritis, Berger's disease, membranous nephropathy), the immunopathological findings are usually nondiagnostic. There are many circumstances in which "staining" is nonspecific and there are no diagnostic combinations of positivity.

XVI. Open Surgical Biopsy

This is another method of obtaining renal tissue for study. It has limited indications and the major disadvantage of requiring general anesthesia. Some use it in very young children, although trained hands can successfully biopsy kidneys of very small infants. Marked obesity, risk of uncontrollable bleeding, a solitary kidney and abnormal renal vascular supply are also situations in which it may be considered. When a surgical biopsy is performed, the surgeon should be made aware of the tremendous artifacts the forceps and even the scalpel can cause. Therefore, when the

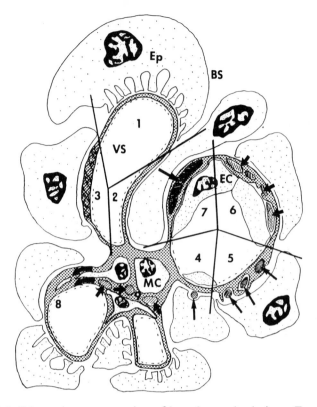

FIGURE 7-1. Schematic representation of key glomerular lesions. Four capillary loops are represented. The glomerular basement membrane and mesangial matrix are shaded. *Zone 1:* Normal appearance. VS: vascular space; BS: Bowman's or urinary space; Ep: visceral epithelial cell with its arcade forming major foot processes, along the glomerular basement membrane. The dotted line on the vascular side of the basement membrane represents the fenestrated epithelium (membrana fenestrata). *Zone 2:* Effacement of the major foot processes, as seen in the minimal change nephrotic syndrome. *Zone 3:* "Basket-weaving" of the membrane as seen in Alport's syndrome. *Zone 4:* An arrow indicates a sub-epithelial deposit as seen in post-infectious glomerulonephritis. *Zone 5:* Membranous nephropathy. Arrows, subepithelial deposits. There is an associated basement membrane reaction forming spikes that tend to engulf and eventually surround the deposits, in the advanced stages of the process. This leads to marked peripheral and diffuse thickening of the glomerular capillary wall. *Zone 6:* Subendothelial deposits, gradually incorporated within the membrane, leading to a "tram-track" appearance or duplication of the membrane. EC: endothelial cell. Note the marked endothelial prominence (endocapillary process). This is seen in membranoproliferative glomerulopathy, Type I. *Zone 7:* Type II membranoproliferative GN, with mid-membranous dense deposits having a "ribbon-like" appearance. *Zone 8:* Mesangial proliferation and basement membrane duplication secondary to mesangial cell interposition (curved arrows) within the thickened basement membrane of the paramesangial region. *Zone 9:* The mesangium, which is the area located between the capillary loops (*mes:* in the middle, in between: *angio:* vessel). It is made up of mesangial matrix (shaded area) and mesangial cells (MC). The arrows indicate intramesangial deposits, which are seen in many conditions. In Berger's disease, the IgA and IgG deposits are confined to this area.

TABLE 7-8. Summery of Findings in Major Glomerulopathies

Acute postinfectious GN
Diffuse increase in cellularity. Polymorphs. Subepithelial deposits without spikes.
Granular C_3 along GBM

Membranous GN
Diffuse thickening of glomerular capillary walls. No mesangial reaction. Subepithelial
deposit with spiking. Uniform granular subepithelial IgG and C_3.

Membranoproliferative GN
Diffuse increase in mesangial cells and matrix. Lobulated appearance. Thickening of
capillary walls due to subendothelial deposits. GBM duplication. Mesangial cell
interposition. Granular C_3 deposits at periphery of lobules and mesangium with IgG
and IgM being less constant, and no IgA. In Type II (dense deposit disease) very dense
ribbon-like deposits within GBM and linear C3 along capillary walls

Anti-GBM antibodies associated GN
Segmental, often crescentic with fibrinoid necrosis. Sometimes intraglomerular
multinucleated giant cells. Linear IgG along GBM, but no deposits by EM

Systemic lupus erythematosus
Variable: Focal and segmental proliferative, diffuse proliferative or membranous.
Combinations may be observed. All forms show mesangial proliferation with
intramesangial deposits (usually IgG and C_3). Occasional linear IgG without
complement along GBM. Hematoxyphil bodies, wire loops, polymorphs, segmental
fibrinoid necrosis and crescents may be seen. Tubuloreticular structures in
endothelium by EM

IgA nephropathy
Normal or mesangioproliferative change + tubulointerstitial changes by LM.
Mesangial IgA deposits by IF

Henoch-Schönlein purpura
Similar to IgA nephropathy but may be crescentic with fibrinoid necrosis. May show
subepithelial, subendothelial and mesangial deposits. No specific IF but positivity for
mesangial IgA a prerequisite

Minimal change nephrotic syndrome
Normal appearance by LM. Effacement of major process of podocytes by EM.
Negative IF

Focal glomerulosclerosis
Segmental nonproliferative mesangial sclerosis. IF consistant only for mesangial IgM
and C_3

GN: glomerulonephritis; GBM: glomerular basement membrane; LM: light microscopy;
EM: electron microscopy; IF: immunofluorescence.

purpose of the open biopsy is not primarily to obtain a large sample, it
is preferable that, after exposing the kidney, a needle biopsy be performed.

References

1. Zollingger HU, Mihatsch MJ (1978) Renal Pathology in Biopsy. Springer-Verlag, New York
2. Striker GE, Quadracci LJ, Cutler RE (1978) Use and Interpretation of Renal Biopsy. Major Problems in Pathology, Volume 8. WB Saunders, Philadelphia

3. Churg J, et al. Volume 1 (1982), Volume 2 (1985), Volume 3 (1987) Classification and Atlas of Renal Diseases. Igaku-Shoin, New York
4. Tisher CG, Brenner BM (1989) Renal Pathology with Clinical and Functional Correlations. JB Lippincott, Philadelphia

8
Hematuria and Proteinuria

LETICIA U. TINA and ROBERT D. FILDES

I. Introduction

Hematuria and proteinuria are the most important laboratory signs of renal disease. Clinical investigation of these findings in children must be both logical and orderly, taking into consideration the clinical presentation, natural history and judicious testing of a patient-tailored differential diagnosis (1–3). Accurate prognostication and management may depend more on a well-structured clinical evaluation than on the availability of sophisticated and invasive studies such as renal biopsy.

II. Hematuria

A. Definition

Small numbers of red blood cells (RBC) are normally excreted in the urine. With careful examination of a freshly voided, clean-catch concentrated urine, hematuria may be defined as the excretion of more than three RBCs in a high power field (hpf) in two or more urine samples. Measurement of RBC excretion in children by a timed urine collection is estimated to be 240,000 RBC in 12 hours (4,5).

B. Tests for Hematuria

The dipstick uses an orthotoluidine-impregnated paper strip; the peroxidase-like activity of hemoglobin and myoglobin catalyze the oxidation of orthotoluidine to a blue product. The test, which is more sensitive in detecting free hemoglobin and myoglobin than intact RBCs, can detect a hemoglobin concentration of 0.015 to 0.062 mg/dL, equivalent to about 5 to 20 intact RBC/hpf (see Chapter 3).

C. Hemoglobinuria and Myoglobinuria

Not all red urine is hematuria. Several substances may color the urine red (Table 8-1). Hemoglobin and myoglobin alter the normal color of urine to reddish-brown (6). These pigments, both of which may produce

TABLE 8-1. Causes of Red or Dark Urine

Acetophenetidin	Lead
Antipyrine	Myoglobin
Azathioprine	Phenolphthalein
Beets	Phenothiazines
Benzene	Pyridium
Bile pigments	Rifampicin
Blackberries	Rhodamine B
Desferroxamine mesylate	*Serratia marcescens* infection
Diphenylhydantoin	(red diaper syndrome)
Hemoglobin	Urates

TABLE 8-2. Agents Causing Hemo-globinuria

Aniline dyes	Oxalic acid
Arsine	Phenacetin
Carbon monoxide	Phenol
Chloroform	Phosphorus
Fava beans	Quinine
Mushrooms	Sulfonamides
Naphthalene	

acute renal failure, give a positive orthotoluidine test in the absence of RBCs. Methods to differentiate hemoglobin from myoglobin include cellulose acetate electrophoresis and immunoassays (see Chapter 3). A presumptive test is based on the principle that myoglobin is soluble in 80% saturated ammonium sulfate solution, whereas hemoglobin is not. The test is performed as follows:

1. Centrifuge a sample of fresh urine
2. Add 2.8 g of ammonium sulfate to 5 mL of urine, making an 80% saturated solution, allow to stand for five minutes and then filter. Myoglobin in the urine will remain in solution, whereas hemoglobin will precipitate and will be detected on the filter paper.

1. Hemoglobinuria with Hematuria

This occurs following hemolysis when the urine is highly alkaline or when it has a very low specific gravity.

2. Hemoglobinuria Without Hematuria

This results from hemoglobinemia in conditions associated with intravascular hemolysis. Plasma haptoglobin levels fall, the plasma acquires a pinkish color and the spun urine remains red. Agents causing hemoglobinuria are presented in Table 8-2.

3. Myoglobinuria

This is relatively uncommon in pediatrics. Acute renal failure may follow such precipitating events as increased muscle exertion (physical exercise, grand mal seizures, status asthmaticus, inflammatory muscle disease, toxins, trauma, burns and heat stroke). Unlike hemoglobinuria, the serum here is clear. The creatine phosphokinase level is usually elevated.

D. Red Blood Cell Morphology

A simple method to localize the source of hematuria consists of the examination of urinary RBC morphology by phase-contrast microscopy (7–9). A 10-ml sample of fresh urine is centrifuged for 10 minutes at 1500 rpm, and 9.5 mL of the supernatant is discarded. The sediment is resuspended in the remaining 0.5 mL of urine and examined under high power with a phase microscope. At least 50 to 100 cells are examined; a glomerular basis for hematuria is suspected when at least 10% of the total RBCs examined are dysmorphic or distorted and pitted with irregular outlines. Small blebs of cytoplasm are also seen to extrude from the cell membrane (Figure 8-1A). In contrast, nonglomerular urinary RBCs are uniform in size and have normal morphology (Figure 8-1B). A Wright stain of the centrifuged sediment examined by conventional light microscopy also differentiates normal and abnormal RBCs very effectively and is well suited in an outpatient setting. Although the method has certain limitations, familiarity with this technique provides a simple and practical approach to localize the source of hematuria. This allows the physician to make a more intelligent differential diagnosis and direct the workup accordingly, avoiding expensive and unnecessary investigations. An algorithm for the diagnostic approach to children with isolated hematuria is shown in Figure 8-2.

E. Clinical Approach to Isolated Hematuria

1. History and Physical Examination

A complete history and physical examination should be performed, with emphasis on diseases that affect the kidney. Height, weight and blood pressure should be measured accurately and plotted on standard charts.

Family history should be detailed, stressing renal failure in a parent or sibling, hematuria with or without hearing loss and ocular abnormalities, sickle cell disease, bleeding disorders, IgA nephropathy, polycystic and medullary cystic disease, congenital abnormalities of the kidney and urinary tract, nephrolithiasis and others (see Chapter 2).

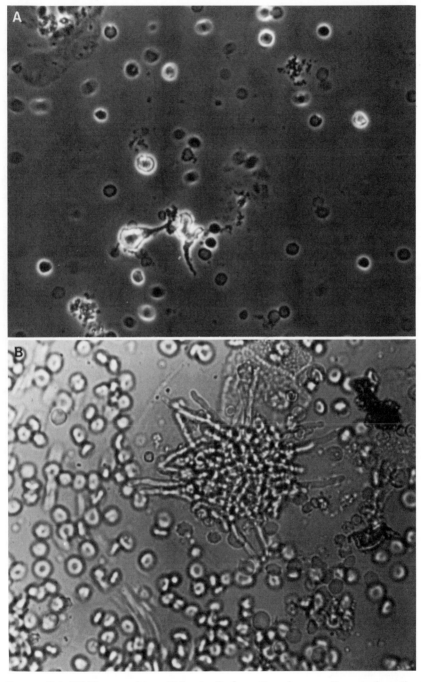

FIGURE 8-1. (A) Dysmorphic red blood cells from the urinary sediment of a patient with glomerular hematuria (phase-contrast microscopy, × 40). (B) Normal red blood cells from the urinary sediment of a patient with nonglomerular hematuria (phase-contrast microscopy, × 40).

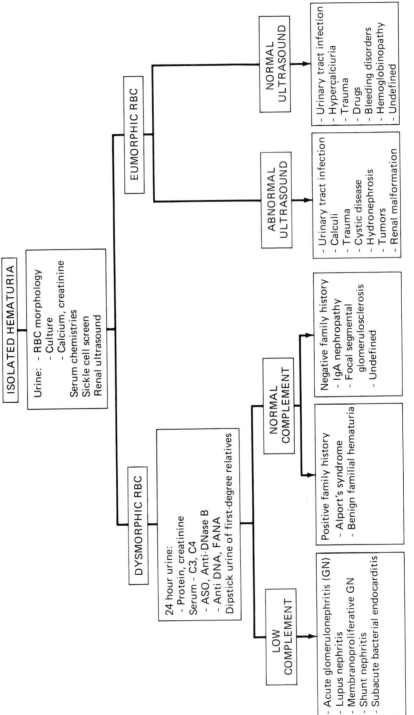

FIGURE 8-2. Diagnostic approach to isolated hematuria in children.

2. Differential Diagnosis of Isolated Hematuria (10–12)

a. Isolated Hematuria with Dysmorphic Red Blood Cells
(see Chapters 10 and 19)

Poststreptococcal glomerulonephritis is characterized by antecedent history of a recognizable Group A beta hemolytic streptococcal infection. Typical clinical features include microscopic or gross hematuria, oliguria, edema, and hypertension. There is also a depressed level of serum complement which normalizes after four to eight weeks. Prognosis is favorable.

IgA nephropathy is accompanied by recurrent episodes of gross hematuria that occur during or shortly after an upper respiratory tract infection or excessive exercise, normal serum C_3 complement and diffuse IgA-IgG deposits in glomerular mesangium on immunofluorescence that do not resolve (13).

Henoch-Schönlein purpura is associated with recurrent episodes of gross hematuria with skin, joint and gastrointestinal manifestations (bleeding, abdominal pain); normal serum C_3 complement; and diffuse IgG, IgA, C_3 and fibrin deposits in glomerular mesangium and skin and gastrointestinal vessel wall that may resolve.

Systemic lupus erythematosus (SLE) is a multisystem disease involving the renal, cutaneous, central nervous, pulmonary and cardiovascular systems. Photosensitivity, anemia, specific serological and hematological abnormalities, decreased serum complement (C_3, C_4, CH_{50}) and normal to varying degrees of glomerular involvement classified as mesangial, diffuse, proliferative and membranous may be also present.

Focal segmental glomerulosclerosis characterized initially by persistent microscopic and recurrent episodes of gross hematuria, normal serum C_3 complement and segmental or global sclerosis with extensive interstitial fibrosis and tubular atrophy on renal biopsy. Immunofluorescent microscopy shows deposits of IgM and C_3.

Shunt nephritis occurs in patients with infected ventriculoatrial shunt. The affected child appears ill with fever, weight loss, lethargy, lymphadenopathy, hematuria and hypertension. Serum complement is decreased. The renal histology is similar to membranoproliferative glomerulonephritis and is associated with the presence of granular deposits of immunoglobulins and complement.

Membranoproliferative glomerulonephritis occurs in about 7% of children with the nephrotic syndrome. Edema and hematuria are the predominant presenting symptoms. Hypocomplementemia is present in 75% of cases, persistently low in some patients. Renal biopsy may reveal three different types of histologic lesions:

Type I: Mesangial and subendothelial deposits containing IgG, IgM, IgA, C_3, and properdin

Type II: Intramembranous dense deposits within basement membranes of glomerular capillaries, Bowman's capsule and convoluted tubules with heavy deposition of C_3.

Type III: Isolated epimembranous deposits associated with changes similar to Type I.

Hereditary nephritis or *Alport's syndrome* is associated with a family history of hematuria, with or without hearing loss or ocular deformities, and recurrent macroscopic hematuria (14). Affected males have severe renal disease with or without sensory neural hearing loss, and glomerular basement membrane lesions characterized by thickening, splitting and fragmentation of the lamina densa by electron microscopy. Immunofluorescent microscopic studies are negative.

Familial benign hematuria is characterized by a family history of hematuria without hearing or ocular abnormalities, normal renal function and ultrastructural demonstration of uniform thinning of the glomerular basement membrane. Immunofluorescent microscopic studies are negative.

Recurrent benign hematuria is associated with episodic gross hematuria in the absence of other abnormalities. Diagnosis is usually made by exclusion.

Bacterial endocarditis associated with glomerulonephritis can occur with congenital heart disease with or without previous cardiac surgery, with placement of prosthetic heart valves, rheumatic fever, abuse of parenteral illicit drugs. Clinical features include high fever, new or changing murmurs, splenomegaly, anemia, and positive blood cultures. Serum complement is usually depressed. Hematuria which may be persistent or intermittent, microscopic or gross occurs in 11 to 93% of affected individuals (15). The hematuria is secondary to small renal infarcts, focal or diffuse glomerulonephritis. Granular deposits of immunoglobulins and complement are described by immunofluorescent microscopy.

Interstitial nephritis is usually due to exposure to drugs or toxins. Skin rash and eosinophilia may suggest the disease (see Chapter 10).

b. Isolated Hematuria with Normal RBC Morphology

This may be due to various conditions:

Urinary tract infection (see Chapter 9)

Idiopathic hypercalciuria is characterized by a positive family history of renal calculi, recurrent episodes of macroscopic hematuria, nephrocalcinosis, calculi and increased urinary calcium excretion (>4 mg/kg daily or a urine Ca/Cr ratio >0.2) (16).

Renal calculi (see Chapter 18)

Congenital renal anomalies and obstructive uropathy are accompanied by a positive family history, associated chromosomal and other organ system abnormalities, recurrent urinary tract infection (UTI), palpable enlarged kidneys, poor urinary stream and gross hematuria following trauma.

Tumors of the kidney usually present with an abdominal mass and sometimes hematuria. Aniridia and hemihypertrophy may be associated with Wilms' tumor; tuberous sclerosis with angiomyolipoma. Renal cell carcinoma is rare in children.

Drug-induced hematuria is suggested by the presence of fever, a morbilliform rash and a history of antecedent exposure to such drugs as methicillin and other antibiotics (see Table 8-3).

Sickle cell anemia is characterized by hematuria, gross or microscopic, in about 20% of sickle cell patients and to a lesser extent in sickle cell trait.

Schistosoma hematobium as a cause of hematuria should be suspected in patients who have recently traveled to endemic areas.

Traumatic hematuria is suspected in children with a history of trauma or instrumentation or the presence of bruises or evidence of a foreign body or child abuse.

Exercise may be followed by a transient hematuria. Other causes of hematuria should be excluded before this diagnosis is made.

F. Workup of Isolated Hematuria

Any child presenting with red urine should be studied systematically, and the following questions should be answered (3,12):

1. Is the red urine due to true hematuria? Hemoglobinuria, myoglobinuria and various other factors producing a red urine should be excluded (Table 8-1 and 8-2), and the presence of RBCs should be documented by microscopy.
2. Is the bleeding renal or extrarenal? The presence of RBC casts, significant proteinuria, decreased renal function and evidence of associated systemic disease indicate renal bleeding. The demonstration of dysmorphic RBCs suggests glomerular hematuria (section II.D).
3. How far should a child with hematuria be studied? A systematic intelligent workup should avoid unnecessary invasive procedures, unless

TABLE 8-3. Agents Causing Hematuria

Ampicillin	Cyclophosphamide
Amphotericin	Indomethacin
Anticoagulants	Lead
Aspirin	Methicillin
Carbon tetrachloride	Penicillin
Chlorpromazine	Phenacetin
Chlorthiazide	Phenol
Colchicine	Phenylbutazone
Corticosteroids	Sulfonamides

indicated. A renal biopsy should be performed, for example, when there is evidence of persistent glomerular hematuria and when the information obtained will help the physician determine the prognosis and treatment. Extrarenal hematuria may be studied by imaging methods and cystoscopy.

A diagnostic approach to children with isolated hematuria is presented in Figure 8-2. Common causes of hematuria at different ages are presented in Table 8-4. Work-ups for different entities are discussed in other chapters. Renal trauma may be diagnosed by a CT scan or renal arteriogram; tumors with ultrasound, CT scan or MRI and undefined hematuria, particularly gross hematuria, may require cystoscopy (see Chapter 17). Children with documented persistent hematuria should be referred to a pediatric nephrologist for a systematic workup.

G. Hematuria and Proteinuria

The association of hematuria and proteinuria suggest conditions that are of renal origin (3). These conditions, along with guidelines for their evaluation, are described under the section on proteinuria. A renal biopsy may be necessary to establish the nature of the renal disease, thus providing the physician with useful information in establishing the prognosis and planning the treatment.

III. Proteinuria

"Bubbles on the surface of the urine are a sign of disease of the kidneys . . ." Hippocrates.

TABLE 8-4. Common Causes of Hematuria at Different Ages

Newborn	*Late childhood*
Congenital abnormalities of the kidney and urinary tract	Menstruation
Renal vascular disorders	Trauma
Renal cortical necrosis	Glomerulonephritis
	Acute glomerulonephritis
Infancy	Henoch-Schönlein purpura
Renal vein thrombosis	Systemic lupus erythematosus
Hemolytic uremic syndrome	Recurrent benign hematuria
Acute infections	IgA nephropathy
Wilms' tumor	Hypercalciuria
Early childhood	
Acute glomerulonephritis	
Hemorrhagic cystitis	
Trauma	
Henoch-Schönlein purpura	

A. Definitions

1. Proteinuria

Normal daily urinary protein excretion in an afebrile individual at rest is around 100 mg/m^2. There are age and sex differences, in addition to diurnal variation in physiological proteinuria (Table 8-5 and 8-6) (17–19). Significant proteinuria may be conveniently defined for clinical purposes as shown in Table 8-7. The composition of excreted urinary protein varies with age. In the newborn, there is increased excretion of albumin, β_2-microglobulin and alpha-amino nitrogen. Two-thirds of the physiological (normal) urinary protein in children is albumin, and one-third represents a mixture of Tamm-Horsfall protein (a large glycoprotein secreted primarily in the thick ascending limb of the loop of Henle as well as more distal sites) and globulins. This ratio is reversed in adults.

Normal protein excretion is dependent on the interaction of glomerular and tubular mechanisms. Disease processes affecting either the glomeruli or the proximal tubules can result in an increased urinary excretion of protein.

TABLE 8-5. Age-Dependency of Normal Urinary Protein Excretion in Children (mean values and 95% confidence limits)

Age		Daily urinary protein excretion (mg/m^2)	
		Daily (range)	Hourly mean
Preterm	(5–30 days)	182 (88–377)	7.6
Term	(7–30 days)	145 (68–309)	6.0
Infants	(2–12 months)	109 (48–244)	4.5
Children	(2–4 years)	91 (37–223)	3.8
Children	(4–10 years)	85 (31–234)	3.5
Children	(10–16 years)	63 (22–181)	2.6

From Miltenyi M (1979) Urinary protein excretion in healthy children. Clin Nephrol 12:216–221

TABLE 8-6. Effects of Sex and Time of Collection on Urinary Albumin Excretion Rate in Children Aged 4–16 Years (geometric mean values in mg/m^2 an hour)

Sex	24-hour period	Day	Night
Male	0.16	0.19	0.10
Female	0.20	0.27	0.10

From Davies AG, et al (1984) Urinary albumin excretion in school children. Arch Dis Child 59:625–630

TABLE 8-7. Clinical Definition of Significant Proteinuria

Semi-quantitative methods

Dipstick: If sp gr $\leq$1.015, 1+ (30 mg/dL). If sp sg $\geq$1.015, 2+ (100 mg/dL) for two of
  three random urines collected at one-week intervals

Sulfosalicylic acid: If sp gr $\leq$1.015, 1+ (turbidity only, 15–30 mg/dL).
  If sp gr $\geq$1.015, 2+ (white cloud, no precipitate, 40–100 mg/dL) for two of three
  random urines

Urine protein/creatinine ratio $\geq$0.2 for urines obtained randomly during normal
  daytime activity.

Quantitative methods[a] (timed urine collections; 24 hours recommended)

Normal: $\leq$ 4 mg/m^2 an hour
Abnormal: 4–40 mg/m^2 an hour
Nephrotic: $\geq$ 40 mg/m^2 an hour

[a]For children over 1 year of age.

2. Glomerular Proteinuria

Abnormal glomerular proteinuria may be the result of an increased filtered load of protein from an increased glomerular filtration rate or an
increased plasma concentration or an altered glomerular permeability.
Such events as glomerular endothelial or epithelial cell injury (mediated
by immunological, toxic or ischemic insults), structural damage to the
glomerular basement membrane or loss of the characteristic charge barrier
from an alteration in the distribution of key glycoproteins/proteoglycans
(which impart a negative charge to the basement membrane) may readily
affect the filtered load of protein. Normal tubular reabsorptive mechanisms may be overwhelmed, and albumin, as well as some larger ma-
cromolecules, will appear in increased amounts in the urine. Glomerular
diseases are the commonest cause of proteinuria associated with serious
manifestations such as the nephrotic and nephritic syndromes, hypertension or progressive renal failure (20).

3. Tubular Proteinuria

Direct micropuncture studies have demonstrated that albumin and other
small molecular weight proteins are present in Bowman's space in very
small concentrations. The proximal tubule largely reabsorbs these proteins, primarily by endocytosis, and subsequently merges the formed en-
dosomes with lysosomes that break down proteins to their constituent
amino acids, which are transported across the basolateral membrane into
the circulation. Tubulointerstitial disorders (metallic poisons, chronic
pyelonephritis, inflammation, etc.) can cause excess loss of proteins
through impaired reabsorption. In these disorders, the urine contains
largely low molecular weight proteins such as lysozyme and β_2-microg-
lobulin, in addition to Tamm-Horsfall protein. Tubular proteinuria does

not usually exceed 2 g/1.73 m² a day. Albumin may be present in such low concentrations that no or trace amounts are found with the dipstick method.

4. Overload Proteinuria

Conditions associated with overproduction of low molecular weight plasma proteins that filter through the glomeruli in large amounts overload the tubular reabsorptive capacity, and protein appears in the urine. Increased protein excretion produced by this mechanism is called overload (overflow) proteinuria. The amount of protein lost daily may vary from 100 mg to 10 g/1.73 m² in a given patient. The most common example of such proteinuria is seen in multiple myeloma patients who excrete immunoglobulin light chains (Bence Jones proteins). Similarly, amyloidosis and Waldenstrom's macroglobulinemia may be associated with this type of proteinuria. Lysozymuria in patients with monocytic and monomyelocytic leukemias, as well as myoglobinuria due to rhabdomyolysis, are other examples. Occasionally, albuminuria may follow repeated albumin or blood transfusions. Once again, overload proteinuria, like tubular proteinuria, may register a disproportionately low concentration for protein if the dipstick method is used alone, compared with turbidometric methods (sulfosalicylic acid precipitation). Urine electrophoresis will show a monoclonal peak of the specific protein.

5. Microalbuminuria

Reportedly, 40% of insulin-dependent diabetics have albumin excretion rates that are above the upper limit of normal detectability by radioimmunoassay techniques (2.0–25 mg/day), but still well below excretion rates conventionally accepted as clinical proteinuria. This subclinical increase in albumin excretion, called microalbuminuria, has been shown in long-term prospective studies to be strongly predictive of persistent proteinuria and to identify more than 80% of the patients who will progress to diabetic nephropathy (21). The levels of albuminuria reported are 15 to 70 μg/minute, depending on the method of urine collection and the period of follow-up. This particular glomerular proteinuria has not yet found general clinical applicability outside diabetes research.

B. *Methods of Detection* (see Chapter 3)

The dipstick and turbidometric methods and protein/creatinine ratios are semiquantitative tests for proteinuria. True quantitation of the urine protein is usually performed on a 24-hour timed collection. The availability of the dipstick (Labstix, Multistix, Albustix, etc.) has simplified office screening of urine for protein. These methods have several important limitations (see Table 3-2). Interobserver variability may be high, and both urine pH and concentration must be accounted for in interpreting the results. As a screening tool on random urine specimens, significant proteinuria may be considered when the dipstick reads 1+ (30–99 mg/dL) for a specific gravity (sp gr) of <1.015, or, 2+ (100–299 mg/dL) for a sp gr >1.015. Turbidometric methods (acid precipitation or heating) detect all types of proteins.

A high correlation between the urine protein/creatinine ratio (Up/Ucr) and quantitative protein excretion (timed urine collections) has been documented for both normal children and adults as well as patients with renal disease over a wide range of protein excretion (22). The interest in this observation lies in the fact that random, single voided specimens are used to assess the protein excretion thus, obviating the cumbersome 24-hour urine collection. However, some nephrologists have observed misleading elevations of the Up/Ucr ratio in some patients with orthostatic proteinuria. Using the 95th percentile as a cut-off point for normalcy, children under two years of age should have a Up/Ucr <0.5, whereas children over two years should have a ratio <0.20. We have found this ratio to be reliable for screening and monitoring proteinuria, but we do not rely on it in the initial evaluation of proteinuric children. Quantitative assessment of urinary protein excretion is usually performed on a 24-hour collection; however, split timed collections are useful when orthostatic proteinuria is suspected (see below). Some information as to the adequacy of the collection may be obtained by determining the creatinine excretion in the specimen and comparing this value with the accepted excretion rates based on the child's weight and sex.

1. Protein Selectivity Index

This is calculated by measuring the clearance ratio of a single large protein (usually IgG) to that of a smaller protein (either albumin or transferrin). When it is greater than 0.2, proteinuria is termed nonselective; when it is less than 0.1 it is selective (23). Selectivity usually indicates a minimal change nephrotic syndrome responsive to steroids, whereas nonselectivity denotes a glomerulonephritis resistant to steroids. This test is not infallible and should not be a substitute for renal biopsy, when indicated.

C. Etiologies of Proteinuria

Classification of proteinuria in children is presented in Table 8-8. In effect, the constancy of proteinuria is the most important sign of renal disease.

1. Intermittent Proteinuria

Proteinuria, detectable in some but not all of a patient's urine specimens is the most common form of proteinuria in children and is usually not associated with serious renal disease. Having excluded such confounding

TABLE 8-8. Etiology of Proteinuria in Children

Intermittent proteinuria

Non-postural
  Urinary contamination (vaginal discharge)
  False positive result (Table 3-2)
  Random finding (may be physiological in young)
  Functional, nonrenal: fever, strenuous exercise, exposure to cold, emotional stress,
    congestive heart failure, seizures, abdominal surgery, infusion of epinephrine
  Urological abnormalities: obstruction
  Glomerular lesions: IgA nephropathy, focal gomererulonephritis
Orthostatic (postural) proteinuria

Persistent proteinura

Glomerular disorders
  Reduction/loss of glomerular polyanion and charge selectivity: congenital nephrosis,
    MCNS
  Hemodynamic: hyperfiltration in disorders like early diabetes mellitus, residual
    nephrons in chronic renal insufficiency or following unilateral nephrectomy
  Inflammatory diseases of the glomeruli: postinfectious glomerulonephritis (GN),
    mesangiocapillary GN, SLE, HSP, SBE, "shunt nephritis," other immune-complex
    diseases
  Late diabetes mellitus; hereditary nephritis
  Idiopathic: isolated asymptomatic proteinuria
Nonglomerular disorders
  Overload proteinuria
  Tubular proteinura: tubulointestinal disease secondary to pyelonephritis, acute tubular
    necrosis, heavy metal poisoning, analgesic abuse, hypercalcemia, postrenal
    transplantation; tubular disorders such as Fanconi's and Lowe's syndromes,
    galactosemia, hereditary fructose intolerance, etc.
  Secretory proteinura: with pyelonephritis and in neonates (Tamm-Horsfall protein);
    diseases of the prostate

GN: glomerulonephritis; SLE: systemic lupus erythematosus; HSP: Henoch-Schönlein
purpura; SBE: subacute bacterial endocarditis

conditions as urinary contamination (e.g. vaginal secretions) and drugs
(false positive tests), intermittent proteinuria is either the manifestation
of some transient/hemodynamic condition, the expression of urological
disease (obstruction, etc.), or an early sign of glomerular disease, or it is
a random occurrence without an identifiable cause (idiopathic transient
proteinuria).

2. Functional or Hemodynamic Proteinuria

This transient proteinuria is occasionally seen with high fever, strenuous
exercise, exposure to cold, seizures, emotional stress, congestive heart
failure or essential hypertension. Urine protein returns to normal after
recovery from the precipitating event. Renal disease has not been seen
in these patients.

3. Postural or Orthostatic Proteinuria

This type of proteinuria appears only when the child is upright (24, 25). This may be found in some (transient) or all (persistent) urine specimens collected in the upright position. Total protein excretion rarely exceeds 1.5 g/1.73 m² daily. Some studies suggest that orthostatic·proteinuria accounts for nearly 60% of all childhood and perhaps even a greater percentage of adolescent proteinuria. It occurs more commonly in girls than boys until the age of 16, when boys and young men have a higher incidence. Although the exact pathophysiology of this condition is unknown, some effect of altered renal hemodynamics (renal blood flow, filtration fraction, renin-angiotensin) on glomerular protein handling is generally accepted as the most probable mechanism. This pattern of proteinuria may occur with a variety of relatively minor glomerular lesions. In spite of this, several studies in both adults and children have underlined the benign clinical course and good long-term prognosis for these patients. It is important to note that most patients with glomerular disease will also have an orthostatic component to their proteinuria. Therefore, the diagnosis of orthostatic proteinuria must be reserved for patients who have normal urinary protein excretion rates at rest (<100 mg/m² daily).

4. Persistent (Fixed) Proteinuria

This pattern of proteinuria, by definition, means that protein is found in every urine specimen. Although the actual amount of protein may vary from one specimen to another in a given patient, the proteinuria persists for a recognizable length of time and may continue indefinitely, or resolve, depending on the underlying renal disorder. Persistent proteinuria is one of the most important signs of renal parenchymal disease. Its presence, with or without other renal symptoms or signs, indicates the necessity for a detailed diagnostic evaluation.

In children, this pattern of proteinuria is of glomerular etiology; however, nonglomerular causes may also result in significant proteinuria. Table 8.8, although not meant to be exhaustive, provides a useful clinical frame of reference. Clearly, the differential diagnosis is sufficiently broad as to require careful organization of the diagnostic workup. The clinical course may be quite benign, although renal biopsy may be the only way to arrive at this reassuring conclusion in a timely fashion.

D. Diagnosis of Proteinuria

An appropriately structured plan for the evaluation of proteinuria in children must avoid unnecessary extended testing of patients with isolated benign proteinuria and permit adequate identification of that small group of children in whom proteinuria is a sign of potentially serious renal disease. An essential point to establish early in the evaluation is whether the increased urinary excretion of protein is asymptomatic or whether it is accompanied by such clinical manifestations as hematuria, edema, hypertension, change in urine protein excretion rates, abdominal pain and decrease in renal function. Symptomatic proteinuria may occur in the context of the nephrotic syndrome, acute/chronic glomerulonephritis, pyelonephritis, congenital/hereditary renal disorders and other conditions.

Prior to initiating a probing history and physical examination, it is worthwhile to exclude false positive results (see Table 3-2). In addition, nonrenal etiologies of proteinuria should be considered according to the clinical observations present at the time the proteinuria was noted.

A complete history and physical examination should be performed, with special consideration of symptoms and signs suggestive of either an underlying renal disease or a systemic illness potentially affecting the kidney. Edema and skin rash and genitourinary and systemic symptoms should be looked for and an accurate physical examination including blood pressure determination should be performed (see Chapter 2).

The assistance of laboratory and imaging modalities may be judiciously organized according to the clinical data, further documentation of proteinuria, and the presence or absence of orthostatic proteinuria. Renal biopsy should be reserved for children presenting with persistent, non-orthostatic type proteinuria (>1 g/1.73 m^2).

E. Clinical Approach to Proteinuria

Following the initial discovery of proteinuria, at least two additional, first-morning voided urine specimens should be examined. If only the initial sample is positive, the child probably has transient (random) proteinuria and the family may be reassured; however, a repeat urinalysis should be performed in three to six months. Obtaining samples with a pH <6.0, and a sp gr >1.018 (first morning void) will enhance the value of these urinalyses.

The presence of signs or symptoms or both of renal disease accelerates the process of evaluation, and the presence of an abnormal urinary sediment (hematuria, etc.) changes the general prognosis of the patient. Such children should be thoroughly evaluated in order to make authoritative recommendations to the family and provide informed reassurance when indicated. Our approach to the patient with proteinuria is outlined in Figure 8-3.

If the child's confirmed proteinuria is truly asymptomatic, further characterization of the proteinuria to determine the effect of posture or activity or both on this finding is essential. The collection method presented in Table 8-9 provides both the total daily urinary protein excretion and documents the effect of posture on protein excretion rates. Patients with confirmed orthostatic proteinuria who excrete less than 1.5 g/1.73 m^2

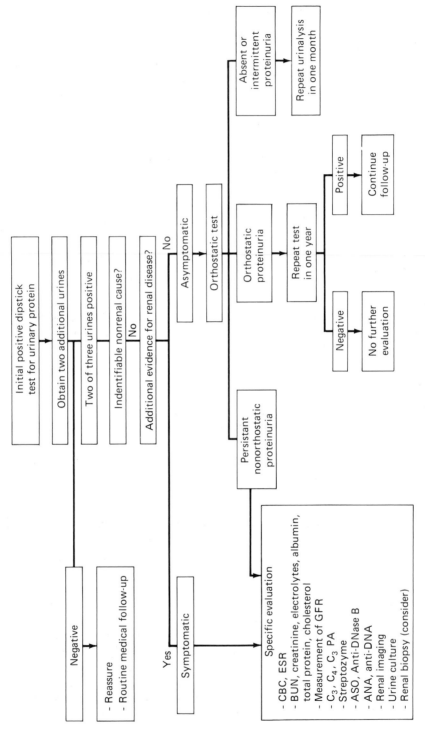

FIGURE 8-3. Diagnostic approach to isolated proteinuria in children.

TABLE 8-9. Orthostatic Test for Proteinuria

1. Collection period begins with the patient voiding prior to going to bed. This urine is discarded, and the time/date noted. Following this void, the patient must stay in bed throughout the night
2. Collect all urines during the night including the first urine in the morning prior to beginning morning activity. Patient records the time of this first-morning void. Label this sample #1
3. Patient walks about for two hours and voids into a separate container and notes time. Label this sample #2
4. Thereafter, collect all urines in a third container until bedtime at which point the patient must void and save this last urine in the same container #3. Write down the time/date
5. Keep urine samples refrigerated until they are taken to the laboratory

daily and who are clearly in good health may be reassured, and seen at yearly intervals. Serum chemistries, creatinine clearance and urine protein quantitation may be performed during these visits. Patients excreting more than 1.5 g protein/1.73 m^2 daily, with a clear orthostatic pattern, and children with persistent nonorthostatic proteinuria, should be evaluated completely as shown in Figure 8-3.

If all the ancillary and imaging studies performed during this extensive evaluation are normal, and if the proteinuria is mild to moderate (<0.5 g/m^2 daily), serious renal disease is unlikely, and reassurance may be given. Such children may have isolated asymptomatic proteinuria or a resolving mild renal disorder. Generally, the proteinuria will either disappear with time, or it may persist for a long period without any evidence of progressive renal insufficiency. These children should be seen again in three months for physical examination, urinalysis, creatinine clearance and Up/Ucr, and depending on the results, subsequent follow-up should be performed at six- to twelve-month intervals.

F. Nephrotic Syndrome

The hallmark of the nephrotic syndrome is massive proteinuria (defined by some as more than 40 mg/m^2 an hour and by others as 50 mg/kg a day) and hypoalbuminemia (serum albumin <2.5 g/dL). Edema and hyperlipidemia are generally present, although variable in degree. Table 8-10 presents an abbreviated classification of disease states associated with the nephrotic syndrome in children. Although many glomerular diseases may present clinically as nephrosis, in children the primary (idiopathic) nephrotic syndrome predominates, accounting for about 90% of all cases.

1. Primary Nephrotic Syndrome

These primary glomerular diseases, with no identifiable etiology or evidence of systemic disease, have certain distinguishing clinical features, in addition to well-characterized morphological differences. These permit

TABLE 8-10. Causes of Nephrotic Syndrome in Children

Primary glomerular disease (see Table 10-3)

Secondary nephrotic syndrome associated with specific disorders/diseases that result in glomerular lesions

Multisystem disease
  SLE (rash, serositis, arthritis, CNS disease, ANA, anti-DNA, low serum complement, active urinary sediment, etc.)
  Henoch-Schönlein purpura (purpura, arthritis/arthralgia, abdominal pain, hematuria, etc.)
  Goodpasture's syndrome (pulmonary hemorrhage, hematuria, anti-GBM antibody)
  Vasculitides (Kawasaki's, PAN, Wegener's, etc.)
  Others: essential cryoglobulinemia, ulcerative colitis, partial lipodystrophy, amylordosis

Heredofamilial and metabolic disease
  Alport's syndrome (hematuria, sensorineural deafness, keratoconus/cataracts)
  Infantile microcystic disease (Finnish type congenital nephrotic syndrome): placentomegaly, hematuria, glycosuria, aminoaciduria
  Nail-patella syndrome (malformed nails, absent or hypoplastic patella, abnormal radial head)
  Sickle cell disease
  Alpha–1-antitrypsin deficiency (cirrhosis, emphysema)

Allergens/immunization
  Bee sting, pollens, poision ivy, poison oak, DPT immunization, etc.

Medications/drugs (captopril, organic gold, D-penicillamine, mesantoin, probenecid, all forms of mercury, heroin)

Infections
  Bacterial: poststreptococcal GN, SBE, "shunt nephritis," congenital syphilis, tuberculosis, chronic vesicoureteral reflux with pyelonephritis
  Viral: hepatitis B, CMV, EBV (infectous mononucleosis), AIDS
  Protozoal: Toxoplasmosis, malaria

Neoplastic: Leukemias, lymphomas, carcinomas

Miscellaneous
  Chronic renal allograft rejection
  Renal vein thombosis
  Congenital heart disease
  Papillary necrosis

SLE: systemic lupus erythemetosus; CNS: central nervous system; ANA: antinuclear antibody; anti-DNA: anti-deoxyribonucleic acid; anti-GBM: anti-glomerular basement membrane; PAN: periarteritis nodosa; GN: glomerulonephritis; SBE: subacute bacaterial endocarditis; CMV: cytomegalo virus; EBV: Epstein-Barr virus; AIDS: acquired immune deficiency syndrome

their classification when adequate biopsy specimens are processed for light, immunofluorescent, and electron microscopy (see Table 10.3). Minimal change nephrotic syndrome (MCNS), is the most common primary nephrosis of childhood, accounts for over 80% of cases (see Chapter 10) (26,27).

2. Secondary Nephrotic Syndrome (see Chapter 10)

3. Diagnostic Approach to the Child with Nephrotic Syndrome

Since over 80% of nephrotic children have MCNS as their underlying lesion, a particular orientation is observed and a management strategy different from that structured for adult patients with nephrosis is followed. Indeed, the initial evaluation is performed to confirm the diagnosis of nephrosis, rule out common secondary forms, and identify those children with probable MCNS quickly so that corticosteroid therapy may be given and steroid responsiveness ascertained. We recommend that the initial evaluation be performed during hospitalization, particularly in children under 10 years of age and also in older children and adolescents unless the patient is nearly asymptomatic, and special circumstances prevail. During the evaluation useful ancillary studies include:

Urine:	Urinalysis and urine culture
	24-hour urine for protein and creatinine
	Protein selectivity index
Blood:	Serum electrolytes, calcium, phosphorus, urea nitrogen, creatinine, total protein/albumin
	Complete blood cell count, platelet count (the erythrocyte sedimentation rate is rarely useful, since it is generally increased in nephrosis)
	Lipid profile (cholesterol, triglycerides)
	Serum complement (C_3, C_4, C_3PA)
	FANA and anti-DNA, as indicated
	Streptozyme if glomerulonephritis is identified
	Hepatitis screen, Epstein-Barr virus serology and drug screen, as indicated
Imaging:	Chest x-ray, renal ultrasound, renal scan or intravenous pyelogram (IVP) when indicated

PPD 5 Tuberculin units prior to use of corticosteroids

Following the above assessment, it is often possible to exclude secondary forms of childhood nephrosis and to make a reasonable clinical differentiation of the common primary nephroses in children (see Table 10-3). Classically, the characteristics supportive of the diagnosis of MCNS include age over one year but less than ten years; male:female ratio, 2:1, absence of hematuria, hypertension, hypocomplementemia, azotemia and protein selectivity. However, as shown in Table 10-3, many patients with MCNS have one or more findings that suggest other nephrotic lesions. Clinical differentiation is most successful in children under 10 years of age. In older children, renal biopsy appears to be the best means of differentiation. The exact role of the renal biopsy remains controversial; however, we present our indications for its use in nephrotic children in Table 8-11.

TABLE 8-11. Indications for Renal Biopsy in Children with Nephrotic Syndrome (NS)

Initial evaluation

Presenting in the first year of life (congenital or infantile NS)
Presenting in older children/adolescents
Evidence to support a diagnosis of either a secondary NS or non-MCNS (hematuria, hypertension, and decreased renal function may suggest the presence of a structural glomerular lesion)

Following prednisone therapy

Initial nonresponse to a six-week course of steroids
Frequently relapsing NS
Steroid-dependent NS
Altered clinical course in a child with presumed MCNS

Once the diagnosis of MCNS has been made, the empirical use of oral prednisone is recommended to assess responsiveness of the nephrosis to steroids, as an integral part of the diagnosis. One regimen that has been accepted among nephrologists worldwide is the use of prednisone (60 mg/m^2 a day in three divided doses for three to four weeks, followed by 60 mg/m^2 given as a single dose in the morning on alternate days for an additional four weeks. The prednisone is then abruptly discontinued. A positive response is the disappearance of proteinuria for three consecutive days. Early nonresponse, subsequent nonresponse, and frequent relapses are patterns associated with many non-MCNS disorders, which usually signal the need to perform a renal biopsy, if it has not already been performed.

In addition to the differential diagnosis of nephrosis, as outlined above, an affected child must be carefully assessed for the presence of any of the known complications of this disorder. Hypovolemia with orthostasis/shock, infection (peritonitis, pneumonia, etc.) related to low levels of Factor B and IgG, and hypercoagulability with secondary thrombosis (inferior vena cava, renal veins, hepatic veins, pulmonary arteries/veins, femoral veins, deep leg veins and the saggittal sinus) must be anticipated and diagnosed as soon as they occur, so as to avoid further morbidity and mortality.

References

1. Dodge WF, West EF, Smith EH, et al (1976) Proteinuria and hematuria in school children: Epidemiology and early natural history. J Pediatr 88:327–347
2. Kitagawa T (1988) Lessons learned from the Japanese nephritis screening study. Pediatr Nephrol 2:256–263
3. West CD (1976) Asymptomatic hematuria and proteinuria in children: Causes and appropriate diagnostic studies. J Pediatr 89:173–182

4. Lyttle JD (1933) The Addis sediment count in normal children. J Clin Invest 12:87–93
5. Snoke AW (1938) The normal Addis sediment count in children. J Pediatr 12:473–478
6. Glassock RJ (1983) Hematuria and pigmenturia. In: Massry SG, Glassock RJ (eds) Textbook of Nephrology. William and Wilkins, Baltimore, pp 4.14–4.24
7. Fairley KF, Birch DF (1982) Hematuria: A simple method for identifying glomerular bleeding. Kidney Int 21:105–108
8. Rizzoni G, Braggion F, Zacchello G (1983) Evaluation of glomerular and non-glomerular hematuria by phase-contrast microscopy. J Pediatr 103:370–374
9. Stapleton FB (1987) Morphology of urinary red blood cells: A simple guide in localizing the site of hematuria. Pediatr Clin North Am 34:561–569
10. Ingelfinger JR, Davis AE, Grupe WE (1977) Frequency and etiology of gross hematuria in a general pediatric setting. Pediatrics 59:557–561
11. Northway JD (1971) Hematuria in children. J Pediatr 78:381–396
12. Leiberman E (1976) Work-up of the child with hematuria. In: Leiberman E (ed) Work-up of the Child with Hematuria. JB Lippincott, Philadelphia, pp 12–25
13. Emancipator SN, Gallo GR, Lamm ME (1985) IgA nephropathy: perspectives on pathogenesis and classification. Clin Nephrol 24:161–179
14. Grünfield J-P (1985) The clinical spectrum of hereditary nephritis. Kidney Int 27:83–92
15. Barakat AY, Dakessian B (1986) The kidney in heart disease. Int J Pediatr Nephrol 7:153–160
16. Moore ES (1981) Hypercalciuria in children. In: Berlyne GM (ed) Contributions to Nephrology. Karger, New York, pp 20–32
17. Davies AG, Postlethwaite RJ, Price DA, et al (1984) Urinary albumin excretion in school children. Arch Dis Child 59:625–630
18. Houser M (1984) Assessment of proteinuria using random urine samples. J Pediatr 104:845–848
19. Miltenyi M (1979) Urinary protein excretion in healthy children. Clin Nephrol 12:216–221
20. Kaysen GA, Meyers, BD, Couser WG, et al (1986) Mechanism and consequences of proteinuria. Lab Invest 54:479–498
21. Mogensen CE, Christensen CK, Christiansen JS, et al (1986) On predicting and preventing diabetic nephropathy. In: Friedman EA, L'Esperance FA, Jr (eds) Diabetic Renal Retinal Syndrome, volume 3. Grune & Stratton, Orlando, FL, pp 81–109
22. Ginsberg JM, Chang BS, Matarese RA, et al (1983) Use of single voided urine samples to estimate quantitative proteinuria. New Engl J Med 309:1543–1546
23. Cameron JS, Blandford G (1966) The simple assessment of selectivity in heavy proteinuria. Lancet 2:242–247
24. Houser MT (1987) Characterization of recumbent, ambulatory, and postexercise proteinuria in the adolescent. Pediatr Res 21:442–446
25. Rytand DA, Spreiter S (1981) Prognosis in postural (orthostatic) proteinura: forty to fifty year follow-up of six patients after diagnosis by Thomas Addis. N Engl J Med 305:618–621
26. Vehaskari VM, Robson AM (1981) The nephrotic syndrome in children. Pediatr Ann 10:42–64
27. Wynn SR, Stickler GB, Burke EC (1988) Long-term prognosis for children with nephrotic syndrome. Clin Pediatr 27:63–68

9
Urinary Tract Infection

Ziad M. Shehab

I. Introduction

Urinary tract infection (UTI), a common infection in children, is characterized by the presence of significant numbers of bacteria in the urine. In the study of Kunin, the cumulative incidence of infection in school girls followed over a 10-year span was 5% (1). In addition, 10 to 20% of affected children developed pyelonephritic scars even after the first uncomplicated UTI, and 20 to 35% had radiographic evidence of vesicoureteral reflux (2). Accurate identification of the child with UTI is of paramount importance in order to reduce the morbidity and sequelae associated with these infections. Confirmation of the diagnosis will dictate therapy and further workup of the child with UTI. To be effective, the method used for diagnosis should be sensitive and specific, since overdiagnosis of UTI may lead to missing the basic disease responsible for the urinary symptoms, in addition to the cost, invasiveness and radiation exposure resulting from the diagnostic studies. Furthermore, this may lead to unnecessary therapy. On the other hand, underdiagnosis of UTI will lead to persistence of annoying symptoms and, more importantly, to progression of renal scarring and loss of renal function.

In this chapter, we will assess the relative value of the different methods used for collection of urine specimens submitted for culture and review the criteria for diagnosis of UTI based on the findings of the urine culture. We will also review adjunctive laboratory methods to identify a UTI and discuss the methods available to localize the site of infection in children. Finally, we will present an approach to the workup of the child with UTI.

II. Definitions

Significant bacteriuria is thought to result from the multiplication of bacteria within the urinary tract, i.e. bladder or renal parenchyma. Bacteriuria may be symptomatic or asymptomatic. A *contaminated urine*, on the other hand, is one in which the bacteria are thought to originate and multiply outside of the urinary tract. In *upper UTI* the infection is localized in the renal parenchyma (*acute pyelonephritis*), whereas in *lower UTI* the renal parenchyma is spared and only the bladder is involved. *Chronic pyelonephritis* is a confusing term, but is usually considered to be the histological sequelae of bacterial infection of the kidney.

III. Epidemiology

The prevalence of asymptomatic bacteriuria has been estimated to be less than 1% among healthy, full-term neonates during the first three days of life. The incidence is thought to be 1 to 1.4% at the end of the first week and during the second week. The incidence declines to 0.2% of boys and 0.8% of girls of preschool age and to 1.2% of school girls and 0.03% of school boys. Young women 15 to 24 years of age have an incidence of asymptomatic bacteriuria of 2%. The frequency of symptomatic infections is more difficult to define and is estimated at 0.14% during the neonatal period and at 0.7% for boys and 2.8% for girls aged one month to eleven years (2–5).

IV. Clinical presentation

The clinical presentation of UTI in children is variable and depends to a large extent on the age of the child . Often, symptoms are nonspecific or lacking. Therefore, in order to make a prompt diagnosis a high index of suspicion of UTI should be maintained at all times. In neonates, the symptoms are nonspecific. In this age group, UTI is more common in males and may present with weight loss, loss of appetite, vomiting, diarrhea, jaundice and failure to thrive. In addition, lethargy, irritability and seizures can be the presenting symptoms. More importantly, sepsis with hypo- or hyperthermia is a common accompaniment of UTI in the neonate, and 21 to 33% of these infants will have a concomitant bacteremia (6,7). Urinary tract infection should be considered in any neonate with unexplained fever.

In toddlers, symptoms of UTI may be nonspecific or may refer to the urinary tract. Children may have urinary frequency, fever and abdominal pain; however, eating problems, failure to thrive, diarrhea and vomiting are also quite common. In older children, the presentation is more similar to that seen in adults. Children with cystitis usually present with dysuria, frequency and urgency; fever, flank pain, malaise and chills are more suggestive of pyelonephritis. The clinician should be aware of the significant amount of overlap of these clinical symptoms particularly in children with pyelonephritis (3,4,7–9).

V. The Specimen for Urine Culture

Urine culture remains the mainstay of diagnosis of UTI. The significance of microbial growth in a urine culture is heavily dependent on the method of collection of the urine sample, the temperature at which it is stored and the rapidity with which it is processed. Midstream, early-morning voided urine is adequate in most children. In small infants, a bag with adhesive may be used but it should be removed immediately after the urine is voided to avoid contamination. Since the urethra, perineum and vagina are usually contaminated with bacteria, the urethral meatus of girls and the preputial fold in boys should be cleansed with water. Antiseptics may reduce the number of bacteria in the urine and should be avoided. In the absence of gross fecal contamination, contamination rates after collection of specimens without cleansing are acceptably low (10–13). In midstream and in bag urine specimens, the important contributor to colony counts is time to refrigerating or plating the specimen (14). The presence of multiple organisms in low counts probably represents contamination and does not warrant further workup or follow-up cultures.

A suprapubic, or catheterized, urine specimen is necessary when the collection of a clean specimen is impossible or when a therapeutic decision is necessary because of the patient's clinical status or because of confusion resulting from the interpretation of a clean-catch specimen culture. Indications for obtaining suprapubic or catherized urine sample are 1) extensive dermatitis of the perineum, which increases the chances of contamination of a voided or bag specimen; 2) a child in whom antimicrobial therapy is being started and in whom a UTI is a reasonable suspicion, 3) indeterminate colony counts on a clean-catch urine, which may have resulted from dilution of the specimen or the presence of low colony counts in a child prone to the development of pyelonephritis and 4) isolation of multiple species of bacteria on one or more clean catch urine specimens.

Suprapubic urine is obtained by puncturing the full bladder about 1.5 cm above the symphysis pubis. Local anesthesia is not essential. Bladder cathererization may introduce infection and its routine use should be discouraged; however, when indicated, it may be performed gently using a soft, thin catheter.

Many studies have illustrated the superiority of a suprapubic bladder aspiration compared to a bag urine culture in infants (15–17). Aronson compared these two collection methods in 86 infants. Bag urine culture yielded misleading information when compared to a suprapubic urine specimen in 31 infants. In twenty-seven infants, the bag urine yielded a false positive result; in four infants it yielded a false negative result. Thus, a bag urine culture should not be relied upon if the child is to be started on antibiotic therapy, since further clarification of the diagnosis may not be possible. In children some of the same problems are encountered with clean-catch urines. The clean-catch specimen yielded a false positive result compared to a suprapubic urine specimen in 20% of children with a UTI, whereas a false negative result was obtained in 28% of those with evidence of a UTI.

The urine obtained by any of these studies should be sent to the laboratory immediately or stored at 4 °C to avoid multiplication of bacteria. The doubling time of organisms in urine at room temperature is 20 minutes.

In general, the diagnostic accuracy can be significantly improved by the collection of more than one specimen: the specificity of a single clean-catch specimen is 80%; it is improved to 90% with the collection of two specimens and to over 95% with three specimens (2).

In the classic study of Kass, a colony count on a catheter urine of more than 10^5 colony-forming units (cfu) per milliliter in women generally correlated with pyelonephritis or lower tract disease (18,19). This concept is well accepted in children and forms the basis of our interpretation of urine cultures (2,8). Counts of 10^5 or greater, if confirmed, are diagnostic of a UTI in continent girls. Counts between 10^4 and 10^5 are suspicious. In boys, in whom contamination is less likely, counts over 10^4 represent a UTI. In the incontinent child, these determinations are fraught with error and a suprapubic or catheterized specimen should be considered. Catheterized specimens with counts over 10^3 and suprapubic urines with any colony growth are considered representative of UTI. In Slosky and Todd's study, one-third of the children with a confirmed UTI had counts of 10^4 to 10^5 (20).

VI. Urinalysis

Although the definitive diagnosis of UTI is based on a quantitative urine culture, urinalysis can be of great help, especially when the patient presents with symptoms and signs of UTI. The presence of pyuria correlates poorly with bacteriuria, since only 43% of children with UTI will have more than five white blood cell in a high power field, and only 75% of children with pyuria have significant bacteriuria (14). Pyuria is a sign of inflammation and in children, along with bacterial and nonbacterial infection, it may be seen in association with a number of conditions including dehydration, trauma, chemical irritation, renal tuberculosis and acute glomerulonephritis, and following polio virus immunization, respiratory infections and appendicitis. One should keep in mind that only 10% of children with dysuria, frequency or burning on urination will have a bacterial UTI, as compared to 50% of adults (14). Thus, the presence of pyuria in association with urinary symptoms does not establish the diagnosis of UTI. Additionally, a normal white blood cell count in the urine does not exclude UTI in children, particularly in patients with recurrent UTI.

Demonstration of bacteria on an unspun urine specimen correlates with the presence of more than 10^5 colonies/mL (21). The criteria used for the microscopic evaluation of a urine specimen for bacteria are imperfect and a consensus on any one set of criteria by which to evaluate the urine is lacking. Recently, urine microscopy has been reviewed for its accuracy in the prediction of bacteriuria (22). The best sensitivity and specificity are achieved with the use of a Gram-stained, uncentrifuged urine specimen. This method has a sensitivity of 95% and a specificity of 89% when more than 1 organism in an oil immersion field (oif) is seen. The observation of more than 5 organisms per field improves the specificity to 95% for bacteriuria at a level of $>10^5$ cfu/mL with a resultant sensitivity of 87%. Thus, the use of the Gram-stained centrifuged urine specimen may offer the clinician the most sensitive and specific nonculture method to detect significant bacteriuria.

VII. Microbiology of Urinary Tract Infections

Kunin, in his decade-long study of bacteriuria in 501 school girls, identified *Escherichia coli* as the most common pathogen involved in UTI (72%) (1). The *Klebsiella-Enterobacter* group accounted for 16.5% of the infections, *Proteus sp.* 5%, *Staphylococcus* 5% and *Pseudomonas sp.* and other organisms 1.5%. The distribution of organisms responsible for UTI in the neonate is similar. *Proteus sp.* and coagulase-negative *Staphylococcus* have a relatively greater role in infections of pubertal girls and boys, although *E.coli* remains the main pathogen in this population. In complicated UTI, the most common pathogen remains *E.coli,* although unusual organisms such as *Proteus sp., Pseudomonas sp., Kebsiella sp., Enterobacter sp.,* enterococcus and *Candida* assume a greater role.

VIII. Urine Culture

The standard setup for the urine culture is the use of two plates: sheep blood agar (BAP) and MacConkey or EMB (eosin-methylene blue) plates (23). These allow for the isolation of the common Gram-positive and -negative organisms often found in urine specimens as well as the isolation of yeast. The MacConkey plate, in addition to being a selective medium for Gram-negative organisms, will allow rapid recognition of the lactose reaction of the organism isolated.

The use of a quantitative technique is essential in the interpretation of urine cultures. For this purpose, a calibrated loop is used for inoculation of the urine specimen. The loop, delivering either 0.01 mL of urine (suprapubic or catheterized urine) or 0.001 mL (clean catch), is heated, allowed to cool and immersed in the urine specimen, which has been agitated. The loop is streaked down the center of the plate. Without flaming the loop, it is then streaked across the entire plate in a pattern perpendicular to the original streak. The plate is then rotated 90° and the streaking is repeated. The same process should be repeated after flaming the loop for the MacConkey or EMB plate. An effective and less costly procedure is to use bi-plates; here, half the plate consists of BAP and the other half of MacConkey or EMB agar. To ensure even distribution of the specimen, inoculating each half of the bi-plate separately is recommended.

A number of commercially available culture kits may be used by the clinician. The most reliable is the dipslide kit, which allows the isolation and subculture of urinary pathogens. By comparison with supplied standards, a semiquantitative assessment of the number of bacteria is obtained. Its results correlate fairly well with those of standard pour plates or of plates cultured by calibrated loop methods (8).

A rapid assessment of the type of organism growing on the culture plate allows for a preliminary identification of the organism. Gram-negative organisms will grow on both the BAP and MacConkey plates with roughly equivalent colony counts. Gram-positive bacteria and yeast will grow only on the BAP. When discrepancies in colony counts are noted between the BAP and MacConkey plates, a careful search for colonies of different morphology, which would indicate that different organisms are present, should be undertaken. The lactose reaction will allow for further presumptive identification. On the MacConkey plate, *E.coli, Klebsiella* and *Enterobacter* will appear as pink colonies, since they ferment lactose. *Klebsiella-Enterobacter* will appear as a mucoid or "wet"-looking colony, whereas *E.coli* is dry. *Pseudomonas* and *Proteus* will appear as clear colonies, since they do not ferment lactose. In addition, *Proteus* colonies will swarm on the BAP plate. The Gram-negative organisms mentioned above will usually give a relatively large gray colony on the BAP. The BAP and MacConkey plates should be carefully scrutinized for colonies of different morphology, which may indicate the presence of more than one species of organism in the urine specimen.

The colony count is obtained from the BAP, since Gram-positive organisms may not grow on MacConkey agar and Gram-negative organisms may be stunted in their growth on this selective medium. Coagulase-negative *Staphylococcus* usually appears as small white colonies and should not be confused with enterococcus, which is an important cause of UTI and will appear as small gray colonies on the BAP. *Staphylococcus* can also be confused with yeast, which produces colonies of similar morphology but with a somewhat duller appearance.

From the practical standpoint, the clinician is interested in the number of colonies in the specimen. If the colony counts are suggestive of a UTI, the organism should be sent to a reference laboratory for confirmation and complete identification. Antimicrobial susceptibility testing may be determined by the tube dilution method or diffusion test. If intermediate counts are obtained or if a mixture of organisms is isolated, another specimen should be collected and the initial findings confirmed prior to embarking on further studies or therapy.

IX. Localization of the Site of Urinary Tract Infection

A child with UTI associated with systemic symptoms, fever, tenderness over the kidney and significant bacteriuria probably has pyelonephritis and little needs to be done to determine the site of infection. However, about 20% of girls with asymptomatic bacteriuria or with clinical cystitis have been shown by direct localization studies to have upper urinary tract disease (24).

It is generally widely assumed that parenchymal damage to the kidney in the course of a UTI is the result of bacterial invasion. Thus, some effort has been made to localize the site of infection in order to better target the treatment. Localization of infection may be achieved by direct or indirect methods, none of which is reliable enough to identify the site of infection accurately.

A. Direct Methods

The direct methods are invasive and time consuming. These include kidney biopsy, ureteral catheterization and bladder washout studies. The renal biopsy is usually of limited value, given the invasiveness of the procedure and the limitations of an erratic sampling method.

The ureteral catheterization method of Stamey (25) is the optimal method but has had limited use in children because of the requirement for general anesthesia in this population. In this method, the bladder is sterilized and washed out and the ureters catheterized, with urine cultures obtained from each ureter.

The bladder washout technique described by Fairley (26) determines the level of infection without the need for ureteral catheterization. In this method, the bladder is catheterized, sterilized and washed out, and urine specimens are then immediately obtained from fresh urine in the bladder and cultured. Hellerstein and colleagues have developed criteria based on research on 100 children to interpret bladder washout technique results (27). Upper UTI is usually characterized by an abrupt increase in the concentration of bacteria following sterilization of the bladder, whereas lower UTI is characterized by scant or nonexistent growth after the bladder is sterilized. However, if renal bacteriuria is slight or intermittent, misinterpretation as lower tract disease is possible.

B. Indirect Methods

Indirect methods to localize the site of UTI have been disappointing. They tend to discriminate poorly between upper and lower tract disease. Loss of urine concentrating ability during an episode of upper UTI, which is restored in eight to twelve weeks, is met by the problems of strictly controlling fluid intake in an outpatient setting and determining the relative contribution of each kidney to the total concentrating ability (24). However, if the concentration defect does not correct itself, persistent infection, renal scarring or urinary tract obstruction should be suspected. An increase in serum creatinine suggests marked parenchymal damage or bilateral hydronephrosis. A scarred kidney has a decreased ability to excrete a sodium load and a reduced renal threshold to bicarbonate.

Serological tests assessing the antibody responses to the patient's infecting organism or to pools of urinary pathogens have been contradictory but have in general lacked sensitivity (24). Autoantibodies to the Tamm-Horsfall protein, a renal epithelial glycoprotein produced in the ascending loop of Henle, may be a good indicator of upper tract disease and deserves further evaluation (24).

In patients with fever and symptoms of upper urinary tract disease, acute phase reactants, such as the C-reactive protein, erythrocyte sedimentation rate, increased white blood cell count and increased number of polymorphonuclear leukocytes or immature cell forms, have correlated with the presence of upper UTI. However, these tests detect the presence of upper UTI in girls when there is fever and when the symptoms of upper tract disease are clinically evident (28–30).

A number of enzyme preparations have been proposed to distinguish upper tract disease from lower tract disease. Isoenzyme 5 of urinary lactic dehydrogenase has yielded mixed results; β-glucuronidase has not been useful (24).

A test using antibody-coated bacteria was initially reported to correlate well with the site of infection in adults with UTI (31,32). This test is based on the assumption that only bacteria infecting the renal parenchyma are coated with antibody. Unfortunately, the studies in children were disappointing. The positive predictive value of the test in children has been calculated as 35%, but its negative predictive value was 69% (24,33).

Bacteria embedded in a cellular cast in a urinary sediment are reliable evidence of upper tract disease, since these bacteria could have only been incorporated in the cast in the renal parenchyma. Unfortunately, the usefulness of this test is severely limited by the rarity of these findings in children with upper tract disease (24).

X. Approach to the Child with Suspected Urinary Tract Infection

Because the child with symptoms and signs suggestive of upper UTI (fever, toxicity, flank pain) needs to be attended to immediately, a specimen collected by suprapubic bladder aspiration or by bladder catheterization is necessary. This avoids the higher risk of contamination of the urine obtained by clean-catch or bag collection, since accurate diagnosis and therapy are essential. Colony counts of less than 10^5 cfu/mL and cultures yielding more than one type of organism may be significant here. Urinalysis is not a substitute for urine culture, but it may be helpful in suggesting a UTI or possibly other etiologies of the child's symptoms, such as appendicitis in the child with pyuria and no bacteria on the Gram stain.

We approach the mildly symptomatic child or the child needing a follow-up because of a previous UTI with a modification of the approach proposed by Todd (23). A nitrite test is performed on the first-morning specimen. This test relies on the conversion of nitrate to nitrite by bacteria incubating in the bladder for a prolonged period of time, such as may occur in concentrated urine specimens (e.g. first-morning specimen). The presence of nitrite is detectable by a change of color of the indicator strip on most urine dipsticks. If the urine is tested immediately after voiding, this method avoids conversion to nitrite by organisms collected from the urethra or the perineum. It should be noted, however, that some organisms such as *Streptococcus* and *Pseudomonas* do not convert nitrate to nitrite. If there are no other pigments in the urine, such as hemoglobin, rifampin or pyridium, this is very sensitive and specific in detecting UTI at home by parents of children with suspected UTI or for follow-up of UTI (23,34,35). If the nitrite test is positive, a UTI is presumed and the urine is cultured; if it is negative, a urine microscopic examination is performed. If a Gram stain of the urine reveals more than 1 organism/oif, another specimen is obtained by a clean-catch collection or catheter. The specimen is cultured and another urine microscopic examination is performed. A presumptive diagnosis of UTI is made if the examination again reveals more than 1 organism/oif pending results of the urine culture.

For children being monitored for recurrence of a UTI, the nitrite test can be very convenient. An early morning specimen is obtained and arrangements are made for a urine culture if the specimen is nitrite positive or if the child is symptomatic. It should be stressed that urine culture is the only reliable way to rule out a UTI.

Once the diagnosis of UTI is documented, adequate therapy should be instituted and the child evaluated. In addition to a thorough history and physical examination, a urinalysis, complete blood cell count, quantitative protein determination or a urine protein/creatinine ratio, creatinine clearance and imaging studies should be performed. Imaging studies should be performed, preferably following the first documented UTI particularly in males, in patients with unusual organisms in the urine and in patients resistant to antimicrobial treatment. Females may be studied after the second infection. A palpable bladder or loin mass, hypertension, acidosis, electrolyte disturbances, azotemia and failure to respond to the proper antimicrobial agent suggest urinary tract obstruction.

The upper urinary tract can be studied with renal ultrasound or intravenous pyelogram (IVP), and the lower tract with a voiding cystourethrogram (VCUG). The VCUG should be performed after adequate antimicrobial therapy to prevent seeding of bacteria in the kidney, in case vesicoureteral reflux is present. Although VCUG radiography is recommended for the initial study, radionuclide VCUG is preferred for follow-up of patients with reflux because of the substantial reduction in radiation. Kidneys, ureters and the bladder may be visualized by TcDTPA scan, which may also serve to test the renal function. The DMSA scan is superior in detecting parenchymal damage and renal scarring (see Chapter 6). The radiologic workup of the child with UTI is shown in Figure 9-1.

XI. Summary

Urinary tract infection is common in children. Its diagnosis requires a high degree of suspicion because of the nonspecific nature of the symptoms, particularly in infants and young children. Proper diagnosis is important, since UTI is frequently associated with congenital abnormalities of the urinary tract and may be complicated by renal scarring. The diagnosis is established only by a urine quantitative culture. No finding on urinalysis (pyuria, bacteria on microscopy) is diagnostic of UTI. Addi-

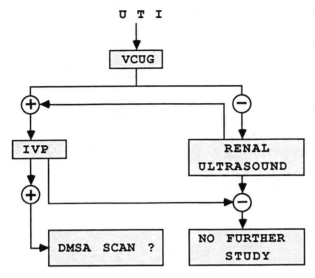

FIGURE 9-1. A radiological workup of the child with a urinary tract infection.

tionally, a normal urinalysis does not exclude the diagnosis of UTI. Children with UTI should be promptly and adequately treated so that renal scarring can be avoided. They should also have a radiological workup and a close follow-up, with periodic urine cultures and sensitivity tests on isolated microorganisms to determine the correct therapy.

References

1. Kunin CM (1970) A ten-year study of bacteriuria in school girls: Final report of bacteriologic, urologic, and epidemiologic findings. J Infect Dis 122:382–393
2. Hellerstein S (1982) Recurrent urinary tract infections in children. Pediatr Infect Dis 1:271–281
3. Spencer JR, Schaeffer AJ (1986) Pediatric urinary tract infections. Urol Clin North Am 13:661–672
4. McCracken GH, Jr (1987) Diagnosis and management of acute urinary tract infections in infants and children. Pediatr Infect Dis J 6: 107–112
5. Kunin CM (1971) Epidemiology and natural history of urinary tract infection in school age children. Pediatr Clin North Am 18:509–528
6. Bergström T, Larson H, Lincoln K, et al (1972) Studies of urinary tract infections in infancy and childhood. XII. Eighty consecutive patients with neonatal infection. J Pediatr 80:858–866
7. Ginsburg CM, McCracken GH, Jr (1982) Urinary tract infections in young infants. Pediatrics 69:409–412
8. Durbin WA, Peter G (1984) Management of urinary tract infections in infants and children. Pediatr Infect Dis J 3: 564–574

9. Busch R, Huland H (1984) Correlation of symptoms and results of direct bacterial localization in patients with urinary tract infections. J Urol 132: 282–285

10. Brundtland GH, Hovig B (1973) Screening for bacteriuria in school-girls: An evaluation of the dip-slide culture method and the urinary glucose method. Am J Epidemiol 97:246–254

11. Ellner PD, Papachristos T (1975) Detection of bacteriuria by dip-slide: Routine use in a large general hospital. Am J Clin Pathol 63:516–521

12. LaFave JB, Engel JJ, French JD, et al (1979) Office screening for asymptomatic urinary tract infections: The evaluation of a practical, economic and reliable method of screening the urines of asymptomatic girls in a busy pediatric office. Clin Pediatr 18:53–59

13. Lohr JA, Donowitz LG, Dudley SM (1986) Bacterial contamination rates for non-clean-catch and clean-catch midstream urine collections in boys. J Pediatr 109:659–660

14. Pryles CV, Eliot CR (1965) Pyuria and bacteriuria in infants and children. The value of pyuria as a diagnostic criterion for urinary tract infections. Am J Dis Child 110:628–635

15. Aronson AS, Gustafson B, Svenningsen NW (1973) Combined suprapubic aspiration and clean-voided urine examination in infants and children. Acta Paediatr Scand 62:396–400

16. Hardy JD, Furnell PM, Brumfitt W (1976) Comparison of sterile bag, clean catch and suprapubic aspiration in the diagnosis of urinary tract infection in early childhood. Br J Urol 48:279–283

17. Pryles CV (1965) Percutaneous bladder aspiration and other methods of urine collection for bacteriologic study. Pediatrics 36:128–131

18. Kass EH (1957) Bacteriuria and the diagnosis of infections of the urinary tract. Arch Intern Med 100:709–714

19. Ogra PL, Faden HS (1985) Urinary tract infections in childhood: an update. J Pediatr 106: 1023–1029

20. Slosky DA, Todd JK (1977) Diagnosis of urinary tract infection. The interpretation of colony counts. Clin Pediatr 16:698–701

21. Corman LI, Foshee WS, Kotchmar GS, et al (1982) Simplified urinary microscopy to detect significant bacteriuria. Pediatrics 70: 133–135

22. Jenkins RD, Fenn JP, Matsen JM (1986) Review of urine microscopy for bacteriuria. JAMA 255:3397–3403

23. Todd JK (1982) Diagnosis of urinary tract infections. Pediatr Infect Dis 1:126–131

24. Hellerstein S (1982) Urinary Tract Infections in Children. Yearbook Medical Publishers, Chicago

25. Stamey TA (1972) Urinary Infections. Williams & Wilkins, Baltimore

26. Fairley KF, Bond AG, Brown RB, et al (1967) Simple test to determine the site of urinary tract infection. Lancet 2:427–428

27. Hellerstein S, Duggan E, Welchert E, et al. (1981) Localization of the site of urinary tract infections with the bladder washout test. J Pediatr 98:201–206

28. Jodal U, Lindberg U, Lincon K (1975) Level of diagnosis of symptomatic urinary tract infections in childhood. Acta Paediatr Scand 64:201–208

29. Wientzen RL, McCracken GH, Petruska ML, et al (1979) Localization and therapy of urinary tract infections of childhood. Pediatrics 63:467–474

30. Hellerstein S, Duggan E, Welchert E, et al (1982) Serum C-reactive protein and the site of urinary tract infections. J Pediatr 100:21–25
31. Jones ST, Smith JW, Sanford JP (1974) Localization of urinary tract infections by detection of antibody coated bacteria in urine sediments. N Engl J Med 290:591–593
32. Thomas V, Shelokov A, Forland M (1974) Antibody-coated bacteria in the urine and the site of urinary-tract infection. N Engl J Med 290:588–590
33. Hellerstein S, Kennedy E, Nussbaum L, et al (1978) Localization of the site of urinary tract infections by means of antibody-coated bacteria in urinary sediments. J Pediatr 92:188–193
34. Schiefele DW, Smith AL (1978) Home-testing for recurrent bacteriuria, using nitrite strips. Am J Dis Child 132:46–48
35. Kunin CM, DeGroot JE (1977) Sensitivity of a nitrite indicator strip method in detecting bacteriuria in preschool girls. Pediatrics 60:244–245

10
Glomerular Disease

ROBERT C. MACDONELL, JR. and AMIN Y. BARAKAT

I. Introduction

Renal diseases can often be divided into glomerular and nonglomerular disorders on the basis of etiology, histology or major alterations in physiology. From the clinical standpoint, however, such a distinction is more subtle and may be difficult to make. Although somewhat artificial, this distinction serves a useful purpose in the approach to patient care, treatment and prognosis. Hypertension and edema occur more frequently and there is greater likelihood and severity of reduced renal function in glomerular disease. Although the clinical picture may be helpful in differentiating various glomerular diseases from each other and from nonglomerular disorders, often a renal biopsy is required to arrive at the exact diagnosis (1,2). In this chapter, we will outline the workup of the child with glomerular disease. Nephritis associated with Henoch-Schönlein purpura, hemolytic uremic syndrome and systemic and collagen diseases, as well as rapidly progressive glomerulonephritis, are discussed in Chapter 19.

II. Clinical Signs of Glomerular Disease

The major signs of glomerular disease—proteinuria, hematuria, edema, hypertension and reduced renal function—are discussed elsewhere in this text. These may occur singly or in any combination. Each of these signs may also be present in individuals with nonglomerular disorders. Nephrotic syndrome, characterized by heavy proteinuria and hypoalbuminemia with or without edema, is often present. Classification of glomerular diseases by clinical presentation is shown in Table 10-1.

III. History in Children with Glomerular Disease

The majority of children with glomerular disease have proteinuria or hematuria discovered on routine urine testing, or hypertension found on physical examination. A smaller number present with edema as the initial finding. The physician confronted with this situation should ask the following questions: 1) Are these findings significant? 2) Are they persistent? 3) Is there need for further evaluation and if so, what is the urgency? 4) How extensive an evaluation is required?

History of the patient and his or her family regarding prior or similar findings is obviously important. The specific workup for hematuria should determine the presence of deafness, trauma, dysuria and other urinary symptoms (rare in glomerular disease); family history of hematuria, renal insufficiency and nerve deafness (hereditary nephritis) family history of hematuria without complications (familial hematuria); and other conditions. Specific historical answers to be sought in the child with proteinuria include presence of periorbital, pretibial, scrotal or generalized edema (nephrotic syndrome—initially, facial edema is often prominent on awakening and becomes less evident later in the day while later in this condition generalized edema is constant); recurrent treatment for allergies (periorbital edema is often misdiagnosed as an allergic reaction); signs of recent rapid weight gain due to expansion of extracellular fluid ("clothes too tight" or abdominal enlargement); decrease in urine volume; anorexia and fatigue or listlessness. Symptoms of mild hypertension are rare. In more severe cases, anorexia, headache, vomiting or seizures may be present. Clues to the presence of renal insufficiency include anorexia,

TABLE 10-1. Classification of Glomerular
Diseases by Clinical Presentation

Isolated proteinuria
  Mild proteinuria
  Orthostatic proteinuria
Proteinuria with edema
  Idiopathic nephrotic syndrome
    Minimal change
    Focal glomerular sclerosis
    Membranous
    Membranoproliferative
  Congenital and infantile nephrotic syndrome
  Secondary nephrotic syndrome
  Chronic glomerulonephritis
Isolated hematuria
  Benign recurrent hematuria
  Familial hematuria
  Hereditary nephritis (Alport's syndrome)
  Henoch-Schönlein purpura
  IgA nephropathy
Hematuria with proteinuria
  Acute glomerulonephritis
  Chronic glomerulonephritis
Acute renal failure
  Acute glomerulonephritis
  Hemolytic uremic syndrome
  Rapidly progressive glomerulonephritis

apathy, easy fatigability, a recent decrease in growth and anemia (see Chapter 15).

IV. Physical Examination in Children with Glomerular Disease

Specific documentation of weight, height, blood pressure and presence of edema or ascites is essential. Signs of systemic disease associated with renal involvement, such as arthritis, skin rash, cardiovascular, pulmonary and central nervous system changes, should be looked for.

V. Laboratory Evaluation in Children with Glomerular Disease

If isolated proteinuria, microscopic hematuria or mild hypertension are found in a child with normal history and physical examination, documentation of the persistence of these abnormalities is indicated prior to further evaluation. Guidelines for significant levels of proteinuria, microscopic hematuria and hypertension are presented in Chapters 8 and 16. Microscopic hematuria or mild proteinuria may be transient in a significant number of children (20–40%), and in these cases they are almost always insignificant. Gross hematuria always requires further evaluation, since it may indicate more serious pathology, and is a dramatic event that usually necessitates patient and parental reassurance. Painless gross hematuria may be glomerular in origin. The combination of hematuria with or without red blood cell (RBC) casts, significant proteinuria, hypertension, edema and renal insufficiency is an indication for prompt evaluation.

Once the persistence of significant abnormalities has been documented, further workup should be performed (Table 10-2). Complete urinalysis allows a qualitative evaluation of proteinuria, detection of RBC casts and an estimation of the degree of hematuria and leukocyturia, as well as an inspection of urinary RBC morphology. A more specific assessment of eumorphic (nonglomerular origin) versus dysmorphic (glomerular origin) RBCs can be undertaken with phase-contrast microscopy (Chapter 8). Estimation of the magnitude of proteinuria can easily be accomplished using the protein/creatinine ratio on a random urine specimen. In infants, this avoids the frustration inherent in obtaining timed urine collections. Catheterization for quantitation of proteinuria is not encouraged. A 12- to 24-hour urine collection to quantify protein and creatinine excretion may be done in older chidren. The glomerular filtration rate (GFR) should be determined by measuring the creatinine clearance (Chapter 5) or cal-

TABLE 10-2. Evaluation of Children with Glomerular Disease

All patients
  Persistence of findings
  Urinalysis
  Quantitative proteinuria
  Glomerular filtration rate
  Hematocrit
  Streptozyme
  C_3 complement
  Serum albumin
Selected patients
  Urinalysis in family members
  Urine culture
  Urine calcium/creatinine ratio
  Protein selectivity index
  Renal ultrasound (kidney size and shape)
  Antinuclear antibodies
  Renal biopsy

culating it from serum creatinine using one of the formulas presented in Appendix II.

Anemia is often present in the child with acute or chronic renal insufficiency. Hematocrit should be determined in all children. Streptozyme is elevated and C_3 complement is decreased initially in 90% of chidren with acute glomerulonephritis; the C_3 usually normalizes in four to eight weeks and the streptozyme in four to six months. Serum complement may also be depressed in systemic lupus erythematosus (SLE), membranoproliferative glomerulonephritis, shunt nephritis, and glomerulonephritis associated with bacterial endocarditis. It can be used in conjunction with other serological measures of disease activity in assessing response to therapy in lupus glomerulonephritis. Antinuclear antibody levels are greatly elevated in virtually all patients with lupus glomerulonephritis and will improve with effective therapy in most patients. Determining whether hypoalbuminemia is present is important in the evaluation of any child with proteinuria.

Urinalysis and audiogram should be performed on family members to rule out familial hematuria or hereditary nephritis. Urine calcium/creatinine ratios over 0.21 (over 0.11 in postpubertal child) suggests hypercalciuria as the cause of isolated hematuria. Urine protein selectivity predicts a favorable response to steriod treatment in nephrotic syndrome; however, 10 to 20% of patients do not respond as predicted.

A renal biopsy is often necessary to make the exact diagnosis of glomerular disease. Indications for performing a renal biopsy have been presented in Table 6-2. Renal size and structure should be assessed prior to the biopsy to demonstrate the presence of two kidneys and to exclude the presence of tumor and significant structural abnormalities.

VI. Characteristic Features of Individual Glomerular Diseases

A classification of glomerular diseases is presented in Table 10-1.

A. Mild Proteinuria

Mild proteinuria in the absence of any other signs or symptoms of glomerular disease and with normal laboratory studies is common. Affected patients may be followed up in six months and then annually with respect to increases in the amount of proteinuria, edema, hypertension, hypoalbuminemia or change in renal function. Renal biopsy is not required (see Chapter 8).

B. Orthostatic Proteinuria

This is characterized by proteinuria in the upright position, and normal urinary protein excretion at rest. Orthostatic proteinuria, which rarely exceeds 1.5 to 2.0 g/day, may account for over 50% of all childhood proteinuria and even greater percentage of adolescent proteinuria. Renal function, blood pressure and serum albumin are persistently normal, and the prognosis is excellent (3). Kidney biopsy is not indicated in these cases, and when performed it may be normal or may show only minor glomerular changes. Over a 20- to 30-year follow-up, one-quarter to one-third of cases are in remission, a similar number develop fixed proteinuria with no deterioration in renal function and one-third to one-half continue to have orthostatic proteinuria. Yearly follow-up is recommended.

C. Primary (Idiopathic) Nephrotic Syndrome

The clinical findings in primary nephrotic syndrome in children are presented in Table 10-3.

1. Minimal Change Nephrotic Syndrome (see Chapter 8)

Minimal change nephrotic syndrome (MCNS), primarily a disease of childhood, represents about 80% of prepubertal nephrotic children and usually occurs between the ages of one and ten years (2,4–6). Patients, of male preponderence, usually present with dependent edema and infrequently present with asymptomatic proteinuria. They usually respond favorably to corticosteroids. Ascites, pleural effusion, generalized anasarca and various infections such as pneumonia, urinary tract infection and peritonitis may follow. Characteristic laboratory findings are proteinuria of more than 40 mg/m² an hour or 50 mg/kg a day and serum albumin <2.5 g/dL. Hematuria, hypertension, decreased renal function and a low serum C_3 complement level are unusual findings and, along with the presence of poorly selective proteinuria, suggest the possibility of glomerular structural lesion. End-stage renal disease is unusual.

Biopsy is required in patients who fail to respond to initial steroid treatment, and in whom additional immunosuppressive therapy is contemplated.

Glomerular changes on light microscopy are minimal and immunofluorescent studies are usually negative or inconclusive. Ultrastructurally, there is fusion of the pedicles of the podocytes.

2. Focal Glomerulosclerosis

Focal glomerulosclerosis (FGS) occurs in children of the same age as MCNS (2,6,7). It accounts for 10 to 15% of prepubertal nephrotic children. Although the initial features presented by the individual child often

TABLE 10-3. Clinical Findings in Primary Nephrotic Syndrome in Children

Type	Incidence (%)	Age of onset (years)	HT (%)	Hematuria (%)	GFR	C3 complement	PSI	Response to steroids	ESRD
Minimal change	75	<10	10	15	N	N	s	95%	Rare
Focal glomerulosclerosis	10	1–10	25–50	20–50	↓25%	N	ps	20% (FGO 75%)	50% (FGO 15%) by 10–15 yr
Mesangial proliferative	2.5	wr	10	80	N	N	v	40–80%	10%
MPGN Type I (43%), Type II (dense deposit, 32%), Type III (25%)	7.5	10–20	30–50	Majority	↓25–50%	↓60%	ps	25–50%	50–75% by 10 yr
Membranous	1.5	10–20	<10	80	N	N	ps	Poor; 50% spontaneous remission	20%
Infantile	Rare	<1	Rare	Rare	N	N	v	Very poor	All by 2–5 yr
Miscellaneous	3								

GFR: glomerular filtration rate; HT: hypertension; PSI: protein selectivity index; ESRD: end-stage renal disease; wr: wide range; v: variable; s: selective; ps: poorly selective; N: normal; ↓: decreased; FGO: focal global obsolescence; MPGN: membranoproliferative glomerulonephritis.

do not allow differential diagnosis from MCNS, hematuria and hypertension occur at the onset of the disease in 25 to 50% of patients with FGS. One quarter of all patients respond to a two-month course of steroids; a few respond to long-term, alternate-day steroid therapy after one to several years. Approximately 25 to 30% of those who do not respond to steroids will respond to chlorambucil or cyclophosphamide. If response to therapy results in a steroid-sensitive or steroid-dependent course, the prognosis is good. If not, the majority will develop end-stage renal disease within 10 years. Clinical findings suggesting poor prognosis include hypertension, persistent nephrosis and hematuria.

Focal global obsolescence (FGO) refers to the presence of totally fibrosed glomeruli coexisting with normal glomeruli. Of patients with FGO, 75% (vs 20% in FGS) respond to corticosteroids. Patients with FGO also have a better prognosis than those with FGS.

3. Mesangial Proliferative Glomerulonephritis

This occurs in about 2.5% of patients with idiopathic nephrotic syndrome. It is characterized by slight but diffuse increase in mesangial cells and a moderate increase in mesangial fibrils. Hematuria is common, hypertension occurs in about 10% of cases and the GFR and C_3 complement are normal. Response to steroids is variable.

4. Membranous Glomerulonephritis

Membranous glomerulonephritis (MGN) is a rare cause of idiopathic nephrotic syndrome in children accounting for 1.5 to 5.5% of cases (2,8,9). More predominant in males, the disease can occur at any age, including infancy, but it is rare below the age of two years. The clinical course is variable but rarely severe. It usually presents with proteinuria or microscopic hematuria on routine urinalysis, and edema that usually subsides in a few months. Less often, patients may have macroscopic hematuria and rarely hypertension and renal failure. Proteinuria is usually constant, although isolated hematuria can occur. Nephrotic syndrome may appear during the course of the disease and disappears within 12 to 18 months. A low serum C_4 with normal C_3 complement is suggestive of MGN. Clinically one cannot distinguish the individual child with MGN from either MCNS or FGS and only renal biopsy can give the exact diagnosis.

The majority of patients respond to steroids slowly, usually within 18 to 24 months; a few to 50% will have spontaneous remission. Hence, the benefit of steroid treatment in these patients is controversial. However, 15 to 20% of patients develop renal failure 10 to 20 years after onset, and about 25% of them continue to have significant proteinuria.

Extrarenal conditions associated with MGN include SLE, hepatitis B, streptococcal infection, sickle cell disease, syphilis, renal transplantation, renal vein thrombosis, therapy with D-penicillamine and other drugs and toxic agents.

5. Membranoproliferative Glomerulonephritis

Membranoproliferative glomerulonephritis (MPGN) is a chronic progressive glomerular disease accounting for approximately 7.5% of patients with idiopathic nephrotic syndrome (2,5,10). It is rarely encountered in Blacks and Orientals. There is no sex predominance. Most cases present before age 20 years. The disease is uncommon before age six years, and extremely rare before age 2 years. Edema and gross hematuria are the predominant presenting findings. Micro- or macrohematuria are present in almost all patients, however, the latter is rarely seen after the first year of the disease. The disease is discovered by the presence of asymptomatic hematuria or proteinuria in about one-third of patients. Hypertension is common; C_3 complement is decreased in about 60% of cases and C_5 and properdin may also be low. Long-term prognosis is considered much poorer than for either MCNS or FGS. Edema and serum creatinine readings above 2 mg% are usually associated with poor prognosis. Renal failure probably never develops in the absence of edema. In the study of Habib et al (10), about 25% of patients died from renal disease or were on chronic dialysis, 11% had chronic renal failure, 29% were nephrotic, 38% had proteinuria and only 5% had spontaneous remission.

Three types of the disease are recognized on the basis of glomerular morphology, however, the clinical presentation is similar in all three types. Type I has mesangial subendothelial, and Type III mesangial subepithelial and subendothelial deposits. Type II (dense deposit disease), which is primarily a disease of children and young adults, is characterized by the presence of dense deposits in the lamina densa and may be associated with a poorer prognosis. Over one-half of the patients with Type II disease develop renal failure. Poor prognostic signs in Type II disease include nephrotic syndrome, macroscopic hematuria, an initial decrease in renal function and no clinical remission.

The disease may be associated with various systemic disorders such as shunt nephritis with *Staphylococcus albus,* persistent viral hepatitis, visceral abscess with or without bacteremia and, in as many as 80% of patients with partial lipodystrophy.

D. Infantile and Congenital Nephrotic Syndrome

Nephrotic syndrome in the first year of life may be divided into congenital (CNS) and infantile (INS) types, the arbitrary age limit being three months (11–13). There is no single clinical or histological feature pathognomonic of CNS. In the evaluation of these patients several conditions should be considered (Table 10-4). The prototype of the idiopathic CNS is the Fin-

TABLE 10-4. Classification of Congenital and Infantile Nephrotic Syndrome

Idiopathic
  Congenital nephrotic syndrome of the Finnish type
  Diffuse mesangial sclerosis
  Other glomerular diseases
    Mesangial proliferative glomerulonephritis
    Focal glomerulosclerosis
    Minimal change
Secondary
  Perinatal infections—syphilis, toxoplasmosis, others
  Intoxication—mercury
Syndromes
  Denys-Drash (abnormal gonadal differentiation, nephropathy, Wilms' tumor)
  Nail-patella
  XY gonadal dysgenesis
  Nephropathy associated with brain malformations

nish type CNS. This disease, which is autosomal recessive, presents with birth asphyxia, prematurity, placentomegaly, growth failure and edema. Edema is seen at birth or within the first month of life. Proteinuria is initially selective; however, selectivity decreases with decrease in renal function. Most patients develop serious bacterial infections and all of them go into end-stage renal disease before age two years. The typical renal histological finding is microcystic dilation of the proximal tubules. Prenatal diagnosis is possible by demonstrating elevated alphafetoprotein in the amniotic fluid. Patients with INS differ from those with CNS by a later onset (usually after age three months), a milder course, and a more favorable prognosis.

E. Secondary Nephrotic Syndrome

Nephrotic syndrome secondary to other primary illness occurs in SLE (50–75%), Henoch-Schönlein purpura (HSP) (10–20%), subacute bacterial endocarditis (10%) and acute glomerulonephritis (10%); in a number of rare infectious diseases, other collagen diseases and drug reactions; and in congenital disorders including Alport's syndrome, diabetes mellitus and sickle cell disease. Nephrotic syndrome in AIDS nephropathy has a poor prognosis with deteriorating renal function. In each of the secondary forms of nephrotic syndrome, remission of the nephrosis follows the response to treatment of the primary condition (2).

F. Benign Hematuria

This type of hematuria is usually microscopic but may be occasionally macroscopic. It is associated with normal physical examination and laboratory studies, it follows a mild course, it may be familial and the outcome is usually good. Idiopathic hypercalciuria should be ruled out, and IgA nephropathy should be kept in mind. Renal biopsy is usually not indicated in these children (14,15) (see Chapter 8).

G. Alport's Syndrome

This is an inherited disorder characterized by familial progressive nephritis with persistent or recurrent hematuria and neural hearing loss (2,16,17). It is apparent now that there is clinical, pathological and genetic heterogeneity in this syndrome (18). X-linked, dominant and other modes of inheritance have been proposed. It accounts for approximately 3% of chronic renal failure in childhood. Microscopic hematuria occurs in almost every patient; single or recurrent episodes of macroscopic hematuria, often following an upper respiratory tract infection, occur in about 50% of patients. In most males, the disease progresses to renal failure associated with hypertension before the third decade, whereas most females have a mild disease. Neural hearing loss occurs in over three-quarters of males and about one-fifth of females. Various types of ocular defects involving the lens and retina may be seen also. Prognosis is usually poor especially in males, in patients who demonstrate regular increase in proteinuria, and in the presence of hearing loss and ocular abnormalities.

The diagnosis of this disease is suggested by the presence of hematuria with or without proteinuria, hypertension and renal failure, as well as a family history of renal disease or neural hearing loss. A urinalysis and audiogram should be performed on the proband and members of the family. The final diagnosis is histological. Light microscopic changes are not specific. The characteristic ultrastructural changes consist of glomerular basement membrane thickening with irregular outer and inner contours and splitting and splintering of the lamina densa. In some patients, especially children, extreme thinning of the lamina densa is seen. A subset of patients with this disease is characterized by typical ultrastructural glomerular basement membrane (GBM) lesions and absence or abnormality of the GBM antigen recognized by the monoclonal antibody MCA-P1 (18).

H. IgA Nephropathy

This is a clinicopathological entity characterized by the presence of hematuria and dominant or codominant mesangial IgA deposits in the glomeruli, in the absence of clinical and laboratory evidence of SLE, HSP and chronic liver disease (2,19,20). There is 2:1 male preponderance. Peak incidence is in late childhood through adult life and it rarely occurs under age five years. The disease is very closely related to HSP and has been considered by some as HSP without a rash (21). It usually presents with intermittent gross or microscopic hematuria with or without proteinuria and is associated with loin pain in 35 to 50% of cases. Although in children it is not as benign as originally thought, the disease generally has a good outcome. The disease presents with macroscopic hematuria (34%), proteinuria with or without microscopic hematuria (30%), acute nephritis (10%), malignant hypertension (8%), nephrotic syndrome (6%), chronic renal failure (6%) and acute renal failure (6%) (19). Increased serum IgA levels occur in three-quarters of adults but are unusual in children. Unfavorable prognostic signs include significant proteinuria, hypertension and severe histological changes, particularly the presence of glomerular crescents.

VII. Tubulointerstitial Nephritis

This is a focal or diffuse inflammatory reaction of the renal interstitium with secondary involvement of the tubules and, rarely, the glomeruli (2,22). The exact incidence of this disease in children is unknown, but it is thought to be present in 5 to 10% of children with end-stage renal disease. The clinical signs and symptoms are nonspecific and may include abdominal pain, anorexia, pallor, headache and edema. Hypertension is generally absent. The presence of progressive renal insufficiency associated with good urine output and urinary abnormalities such as hyposthenuria and proteinuria should suggest the diagnosis of acute tubulointerstitial nephritis (TIN). Acute TIN is usually secondary to infections or drugs (Table 10-5). Drug-induced acute TIN can occur at any age and does not seem to be related to the dose, route of administration or duration of treatment. The most common cause of chronic TIN is urinary tract obstruction with or without infection. Other causes are shown in Table 10-5.

Investigation for TIN is similar to that for glomerular diseases. Leukocytes are frequently present in the urine, and Wright's stain of the urine sediment may reveal eosinophils, particularly in drug-induced TIN. Isosthenuria is often present. Renal ultrasound serves to determine the kidney size and show the presence of obstruction or structural abnormalities. Proximal tubular dysfunction as evidenced by glucosuria, aminoaciduria and phosphaturia, and distal tubular dysfunction manifesting as inability to concentrate urine may be present also. Eosinophilia is commonly seen on the peripheral blood smear. Finally, a renal biopsy will establish the diagnosis and help assess the prognosis.

TABLE 10-5. Some Causes of Tubulointerstitial Nephritis

Acute
Infections
　　Group A, β-hemolytic streptococcal infections
　　Toxoplasmosis
　　Streptococcal pneumonia
　　Brucellosis
　　Typhoid fever
　　Infectious mononucleosis
　　Viral infections
Drugs
　　Antibiotics—penicillins (methicillin, ampicillin, oxacillin, etc.) sulfonamides,
　　　cephalosporins, nitrofurantoin, co-trimazole, etc.
　　Nonsteroidal antiinflammatory agents
　　Others—phenytoin, furosemide, phenobarbital
Allograft rejection
Idiopathic reactions

Chronic
Infections—chronic pyelonephritis, tuberculosis

Urological disorders—urinary tract obstruction, vesicoureteral reflux

Drugs—aspirin, lithium

Metabolic/hereditary
　　Oxalosis
　　Cystinosis
　　Balkan nephropathy
　　Wilson's disease
　　Nephrocalcinosis
　　Sickle cell disease

Other
　　Idiopathic
　　Allograft rejection
　　Irradiation

References

1. Silva FG (1988) Overview of pediatric nephropathy. Kidney Int 33:1016–1032
2. Holliday MA, Barratt TM, Vernier RL (eds) (1987) Pediatric Nephrology, 2nd edition. Williams and Wilkins, Baltimore, pp 407–491
3. Robinson RR (1980) Isolated proteinuria in asymptomatic patients. Kidney Int 18:395–406
4. Vehaskari VM, Robson AM (1981) The nephrotic syndrome in children. Pediatr Ann 10:42–64
5. International Study of Kidney Disease in Children (1978) The nephrotic syndrome in children. Prediction of histopathology from clinical and laboratory characteristics at the time of diagnosis. Kidney Int 13:159–165

6. Habib R, Kleinknecht C (1971) The primary nephrotic syndrome of childhood. Classification and clinicopathologic study of 406 cases. In: Sommers
SC (ed) Pathology Annual. Appleton-Century-Crofts, New York, pp 417–474
7. Southwest Pediatric Nephrology Study Group (1985) Focal segmental glomerulosclerosis in children with idiopathic nephrotic syndrome. Kidney Int
27:442–449
8. Habib R, Kleinknecht C, Gubler M-C (1973) Extramembranous glomerulonephritis in children: report of 50 cases. J Pediatr 82:754–766
9. Wiggelinkhuizen J, Sinclair-Smith C (1987) Membranous glomerulonephro-
pathy in childhood. S Afr Med J 72:184–187
10. Habib R, Kleinknecht C, Gubler M-C, et al (1973) Idiopathic membranoproliferative glomerulonephritis in children. Report of 105 cases. Clin Nephrol
1:194–203
11. Rapola J (1987) Congenital nephrotic syndrome. Pediatr Nephrol 1:441–446
12. Sibley RK, Mahan J, Mauer SM, Vernier RL (1985) A clinicopathologic study
of fourty-eight infants with nephrotic syndrome. Kidney Int 27:544–552
13. Hallman N, Norio R, Kouvalainen K (1967) Main features of the congenital
nephrotic syndrome. Acta Paediatr Scand (Suppl) 172:75–78
14. Pardo V, Berian MG, Levi DF, et al (1979) Benign primary hematuria: Clinicopathologic study of 65 patients. Am J med 67:817–822
15. Blumenthal SS, Fritsche C, Lemann J, Jr (1988) Establishing the diagnosis of
benign familial hematuria. The importance of examining the urine sediment
of family members. JAMA 259:2263–2266
16. Gubler M-C, Levy M, Broyer M, et al (1981) Alport's syndrome. A report of
58 cases and review of the literature. Am J Med 70:493–505
17. Iversen UM (1974) Hereditary nephropathy with hearing loss "Alport's syndrome." Acta Paediatr Scand (suppl) 245:1–23
18. Grünfeld JP, Grateau G, Noel L-H, et al (1987) Variants of Alport's syndrome.
Pediatr Nephrol 1:419–421
19. Clarkson AR, Seymour AE, Thompson AJ, et al (1977) IgA nephropathy: a
syndrome of uniform morphology, diverse clinical features and uncertain
prognosis. Clin Nephrol 8:459–471
20. Southwest Pediatric Nephrology Study Group (1982) A multicenter study of
IgA nephropathy in children. Kidney Int 22:643–652
21. Meadow SR, Scott DG (1985) Berger disease: Henoch-Schönlein syndrome
without rash. J Pediatr 106:27–32
22. Ellis D, Fried WA, Yunis EJ, et al (1981) Acute interstitial nephritis in children:
a report of 13 cases and review of the literature. Pediatrics 67:862–870

11
Clinical Study of Renal Tubular Disease

RUSSELL W. CHESNEY

I. Introduction

Renal tubular diseases are a group of relatively uncommon disorders that can affect children of all ages and that have in common the development of disease because of renal hyperexcretion of ions or organic molecules that are normally reabsorbed by the kidney. Several characteristics of these disorders are largely universal and worth comment (1):

1. These disorders are usually inherited; more than one child in a family may be affected.
2. The children frequently present with growth failure.
3. They can be diagnosed by a simultaneous assessment of the serum and urine concentration of the substance that is being lost.
4. The principle of treatment usually involves the replacement of the substance lost in the urine. However, some disorders relate to the hyperexcretion of a toxic substance, such as cystine, which leads to damage, because it is insoluble or a metabolic poison.
5. Some of these disorders are benign and require no therapy. Thus, it is important to make the proper diagnosis so that unnecessary therapy can be avoided.

The features of some of these disorders are shown in Table 11-1, and their evaluation is outlined in Table 11-2.

II. Glucosuria

Isolated glucosuria is defined by the presence of glucose in the urine with a normal plasma concentration of glucose (less than 120 mg/dL). Normal urine contains less than 15 mg/dL of glucose (170 mg/m^2 in a 24-hour period) as determined by enzymatic methods (glucose oxidase or hexokinase). This disorder represents the loss of a renal glucose transport system (2). Glucose threshold (tubular glucose reabsorption/glomerular filtration rate) is significantly reduced, while maximal rate of tubular maximum for glucose is variable. Glucosuria is usually not suspected and is demonstrated by a positive test result on a reagent test strip when urine glucose concentration is more than 40 mg/dL. Benedict's reagent test material (Clinitest® tablets) detects all reducing agents in the urine.

Glucosuria due to an overflow phenomenon develops because of hyperglycemia and occurs in diabetes mellitus, following intravenous dextrose-containing solutions, epinephrine injection or glucocorticoid therapy. The differential diagnosis of normoglycemic glucosuria includes certain phosphate-wasting syndromes, the renal Fanconi syndrome, nephrotic syndrome and certain tubulointerstitial nephropathies. Glucosuria may also occur during the course of renal tubular disorders induced by antibiotics, e.g. aminoglycosides, cephalosporins, or semisynthetic penicillins. Because isolated glucosuria is often familial, urine samples of siblings and parents should be evaluated with reagent test strips. No therapy is indicated for isolated or familial glucosuria. Galactose, fruc-

TABLE 11-1. Renal Tubular Disorders

Disorder	Inheritance[a]	Prevalence	Tubular abnormality	Clinical consequences
Renal glucosuria	AR	1 in 20,000	Transport system for glucose affected; altered transport concentration; benign	Glucosuria at normal blood glucose concentration
Cystinuria (3 allelic forms)	AR	1 in 7,000 to 12,000	Shared transport system for cystine and dibasic amino acids (lysine, arginine, ornithine) altered in kidney and intestine	Cystinuria results in stones and obstruction; gut defect is benign
Iminoglycinuria	AR	1 in 15,000	Shared transport system for imino acids (proline and hydroxyproline) and glycine is defective	Iminoaciduria and glycinuria; benign
Hartnup disease	AR	1 in 16,000 to 130,000	Shared transport system for neutral amino acids is defective in kidney and intestine	Neutral aminoaciduria; loss of tryptophan causes nicotinamide deficiency and symptoms of pellagra
Dicarboxylic aminoaciduria	AR?	1 in 50,000 births	Shared transport system for dicarboxylic amino acids	Aspartic and glutamic aminoaciduria; no clinical findings
Renal tubular acidosis (Type I) (several different disorders)	AD	Uncommon, but not rare	Defective acidification mechanism in distal tubule	Metabolic acidosis with or without hypercalciuria leading to nephrocalcinosis
Fanconi syndrome	AR, AD, acquired	Variable; cystinosis 1 in 40,000	Unknown	Generalized proximal tubular defect
Nephrogenic diabetes insipidus	XLR	Uncommon	Unknown	Renal tubular cells insensitive to vasopressin, leading to polyuria and polydipsia
Bartter's syndrome	AR?	Rare	Impaired chloride reabsorption, potassium wasting	Hypokalemic alkalosis, normal blood pressure, impaired pressor response to angiotensin II

[a]AR: autosomal recessive; AD: autosomal dominant; XLR: X-linked recessive.
Friedman AL, Chesney RW (1987) Isolated renal tubular defects. In: Schrier RM, Gottschalk CW (eds) Diseases of the Kidney, 4th edn. Little Brown, Boston, p 664.

TABLE 11-2. Evaluation of Renal Tubular Disorders

Test	Abnormality	Suspected diagnosis
Urinalysis	Concentration defect	Bartter, Fanconi syndromes
	Glucosuria	Glucosuria, Fanconi syndrome
	Ketonuria	Fanconi syndrome
	Proteinuria	Fanconi syndrome
	Cystine crystals	Cystinuria
	Alkaline pH	Renal tubular acidosis (RTA), Fanconi syndrome
Serum electrolytes	Hypokalemia	Fanconi, Bartter syndromes
	Reduced bicarbonate	RTA, Fanconi syndrome
	Elevated bicarbonate	Bartter syndrome
Serum chemistries	Reduced phosphate	Phosphaturias
	Reduced calcium	Vitamin D abnormality
	Elevated alkaline phosphatase	Phosphaturias, vitamin D abnormality
	Elevated phosphate	Renal failure, hypo- or pseudohypoparathyroidism
	Hypercalcemia	Primary hyperparathyroidism
	Hypomagnesemia	Renal leak, drug-induced Mg deficiency
Urine metabolic screen	Amino acids	Aminoaciduria, vitamin D deficiency, Fanconi syndrome
	Cyanide nitoprusside	Cystinuria
	Organic acids	Fanconi syndrome
	Excessive phosphaturia (TRP <85%)	Phosphaturia, Fanconi syndrome, hyperparathyroidism
	Excessive phosphate retention (TRP >85%, with hyperphosphatemia)	Hypo- or pseudohypoparathyroidism

tose, lactose, and other sugars may also be found in normal urine samples along with glucose.

III. Aminoacidurias

Amino acids are reabsorbed in the proximal tubule to such an extent that only 1 to 2% of filtered amino acids are excreted in the urine (3). Aminoaciduria is generally encountered during the evaluation of a child who has growth failure, mental retardation, convulsions and other clinical evidence of a metabolic disorder. A 24-hour urine sample should be analyzed to determine the amount of amino acids present. Amino acids can be determined by one- or two-dimensional paper chromatography or quantitated by an amino acid analyzer. Whenever urine amino acid values are determined, serum fasting amino acid levels, as well as the concentration of creatinine in the serum and urine, should also be measured. Thus, amino acid levels can be determined in relationship to creatinine [μmoles of amino acid (AA)/milligrams creatinine (Cr)] and clearance of the amino acid (C_{AA}):

$$C_{AA} = \frac{(\mu\text{mole AA/mL urine} \times \text{urine volume (mL/min)}}{\mu\text{mole AA/mL plasma}}$$

or, in terms of fractional excretion (FE_{AA}):

$$\frac{\text{Urine/plasma AA}}{\text{Urine/plasma Cr}} \text{ or } \frac{\text{Urine AA}}{\text{Plasma AA}} \times \frac{\text{Plasma Cr}}{\text{Urine Cr}}$$

The types of aminoaciduria are shown in Table 11-3. The hyperexcretion of an amino acid may occur singly (as in cystinuria), in a group, in which all amino acids of a given class are spilled (as in Hartnup disease) or generalized (as in Fanconi syndrome). The differential diagnosis of aminoaciduria includes certain inborn errors of amino acid metabolism, in which the amino acid lost is hyperexcreted, because its plasma concentration is excessive. The following disorders result in aminoaciduria from this mechanism: phenylketonuria, tyrosinemia, maple syrup urine disease (leucine, valine, isoleucine), histidinemia, hypermethioninemia, hyperprolinemia Types I and II, ketotic and nonketotic hyperglycinemia,

TABLE 11-3. Hereditary Aminoacidurias

Transport system where mutant phenotype is expressed	Amino acids affected
Dicarboxylic[a]	Aspartate, glutamate
Dibasic [a]	Lysine, arginine, ornithine
Isolated cystinuria	Cystine, cysteine
Cystinuria[a]	Cystine (primary transport defect), lysine, arginine, ornithine (hyperexcreted, since they share this transport system)
Iminoglycinuria[a]	Proline, hydroxyproline, sarcosine, glycine, N-methyl-L-alanine
Isolated glycinuria	Glycine, sometimes glucose
Hartnup disease[a]	Neutral amino acids: alanine, serum threonine, valine, leucine, isoleucine, phenylalanine, glutamine, histidine, asparagine, tyrosine, tryptophan and citruline
Taurinuria (mice)	Taurine, β-alanine, β-isobutyrate
Histidinuria[a]	Histidine
Lysinuria[a]	Lysine
Generalized (Fanconi syndrome)	All amino acids
Generalized (neonatal hyperaminoaciduria)	All amino acids

[a]Disorders in which other tissues (usually the intestine) are affected.
Adapted from Friedman AL, Chesney RW (1987) Isolated renal tubular defects. In: Schrier RM, Gottschalk CW (eds) Diseases of the Kidney, 4th edn. Little Brown, Boston, p 666

sarcosinemia and homocystinuria. These disorders are readily distinguished by measuring plasma amino acid concentrations.

Amino acids with high renal clearance and those due to errors of amino acid transport are best detected by measuring the urine amino acids in the urine. Certain diagnostic considerations are pertinent to the major aminoaciduric syndromes, which occur with normal plasma values, as follows.

A. Iminoglycinuria

Iminoglycinuria occurs because the common transport system for glycine, proline and hydroxyproline is defective. It is a benign, autosomal recessive trait in which glycine, proline and hydroxyproline are hyperexcreted (2). Its importance is that isolated glycinuria may occur in adults with hypophosphatemic bone disease, in association with glucosuria, and in inborn errors of glycine metabolism, including propionyl coenzyme A carboxylase and glycine decarboxylase deficiency. It requires no therapy.

B. Dicarboxylic Aminoaciduria

Representing the excessive urinary loss of glutamic and aspartic acids, this condition is usually clinically inapparent, but it may cause hypoglycemia due to the loss of these key gluconeogenic amino acids. A rare patient with this autosomal recessive disorder may require additional dietary aspartic and glutamic acid.

C. Histidinuria

This is a benign, autosomal recessive trait, requiring no therapy, in which histidine only is lost in the urine.

D. Cystinurias

This is a group of autosomal recessive traits in which the relatively insoluble, sulfur-containing amino acid cystine is hyperexcreted along with lysine, arginine and ornithine (the dibasic amino acids). This disorder occurs in 1 in 7,000 to 1 in 12,000 individuals, and, thus, it is not an infrequent cause of renal stones during childhood. Some patients may have isolated cystinuria or isolated dibasic aminoaciduria. The latter leads to diarrhea, malnutrition, hyperammonemia, growth retardation and mental deficiency. Failure of the dibasic amino acids to be transported into the liver could account for the hypoproteinemia and hyperammonemia (4). A diagnosis of cystinuria should be considered in any child with renal stones or frequent infections and evidence of renal colic. The diagnosis can be established by excessive urinary cystine excretion, usually more than 300 mg/day. However, a family history of stones or surgery for stones, a radiopaque stone, the finding of hexagonal crystals (determined by microscopy of a spun urine sample) and a positive urinary cyanide nitroprusside test are strong indicators of cystinuria (5).

Cystine crystals form in the urine due to the relative insolubility of this disulfide amino acid; indeed, cystine is the most insoluble amino acid. Therapy is thus directed at improving its solubility by hydration and alkalinization to raise the urine pH above 7.5, which dissolves more cystine, and the use of D-penicillamine or a methylpropionylglycine, both of which form more solubly mixed disulfides with cystine (5). Therapy must be lifelong to avoid staghorn calculi. Some success in disrupting these calculi by the use of extracorporeal shock wave lithotripsy has been reported (2).

E. Hartnup Disease

In this rare autosomal syndrome all of the neutral amino acids—alanine, threonine, valine, leucine, isoleucine, phenylalanine, glutamine, histidine, asparagine, tyrosine, tryptophan and citrulline—are lost in the urine (6). This disorder also involves intestinal malabsorption of these amino acids, as is the case in the aminoacidurias described above. The disease, named after the propositus family the Hartnups, is clinically featured by cerebellar ataxia, an intermittent red, scaly rash that is especially prominent in sun-exposed areas and a variety of psychiatric disorders, in effect, the features of nicotinamide deficiency or pellagra. The bacterial decomposition of amino acids in the bowel results in the excretion of indoles and indican in the urine. Finally, with the intestinal malabsorption of L-tryptophan, its metabolic conversion to nicotinamide via the cynurenine pathway is diminished.

Children who ingest 20 to 30 mg of nicotinamide in their diet will seldom show the clinical features of Hartnup disease; although their urine samples may contain the neutral monoamino, monocarboxylic amino acids listed previously, as well as the indoles and indicans.

F. Generalized Aminoaciduria

Massive generalized aminoaciduria usually indicates a complex proximal tubulopathy such as Fanconi syndrome (see section VII). A generalized aminoaciduria occurs whenever there is spilling of amino acids of all classes—neutral, dibasic, dicarboxylic, imino and β-amino acids (such as taurine, β-amino isobutyrate, and β-alanine)—and their presence should lead the physician to think of immaturity, heavy metal intoxication, vitamin D deficiency, high amino acid intakes in total parenteral nutrition solutions, and tubulointerstitial nephritis due to drug sensitivity (2,3).

Generalized aminoaciduria found in a developmentally delayed child should alert one to the possibility of heavy metal exposure—lead, cadmium, bismuth, organomercurials, uranium and copper—and a 24-hour urine collection should be analyzed for these substances. It is also far more likely that aminoaciduria will be evident in preterm than in term infants.

IV. Disorders of Vitamin D Metabolism

Since the renal proximal tubule is the site of the final 1 α hydroxylation of 25 hydroxyvitamin D [25(OH)D], renal disease can affect vitamin D metabolism, reducing the availability of 1,25 dihydroxyvitamin D, the most active metabolite of vitamin D in terms of its biological activity (7). Vitamin D is either ingested or arises from 7-dehydrocholesterol in the skin and is converted to 25(OH)D by a hydroxylation step in the liver.

The conditions that occur as the result of a deficiency of vitamin D— rickets and hypocalcemic tetany—can occur because of lack of exposure to sunshine, dietary inadequacy, hepatocellular disease or renal insufficiency. Rickets occurs because of a lack of sufficient minerals (calcium and/or phosphate) to adequately mineralize the organic matrix of bone, which is termed *osteoid*. Bowing and widening of the epiphyses occur due to weight bearing and in relation to hypocalcemia and/or hypophosphatemia. However, rickets and tetany are physical signs that indicate the need for further exploration to understand the real cause so that appropriate therapy can be instituted (Table 11-4; Figure 11-1).

A. Nutritional Rickets

It is rare in healthy children who receive vitamin D-supplemented milk and who are exposed to sunshine (7). Nutritional vitamin D deficiency should be suspected in children who remain indoors, e.g. those who are retarded or institutionalized, those whose skin conditions do not permit the usual sun exposure, or those who are the offspring of parents who embrace religious tenets that lead them to wear long robes and whose dietary customs include human milk (which contains insufficient amounts of vitamin D), and a vegan, nondairy product diet (8).

The diagnosis is made on the basis of history, a reduction in serum calcium and phosphate values, elevated alkaline phosphatase activity and an elevated parathyroid hormone (PTH) level. Alkaline phosphatase activity is elevated due to increased bone turnover. Hypocalcemia increases PTH levels. The concentration in serum of 25(OH)D is usually under 7 ng/mL (normal, 10–60 ng/mL; mean, 30 ng/mL); 25(OH)D is the main circulating metabolite of vitamin D and is reduced in vitamin D deficiency of all causes. In nutritional rickets, the value for 1,25(OH)$_2$D may

TABLE 11-4. Features and Laboratory Findings in Hypocalcemic Forms of Rickets

Finding	25(OH)D-deficient	Vitamin D-dependent	Vitamin D-dependent, Type II (not responsive to calcitriol)
Age of onset (months)	9–12	3–6	3–6
Inheritance	None	Autosomal recessive	Autosomal recessive; often consanguinity
Rickets	Yes	Yes	Yes
Hypocalcemia	Yes	Yes	Yes
Hypophosphatemia	Yes	Yes	Yes
Aminoaciduria	Yes	Yes	Yes
iPTH level	Elevated	Elevated	Elevated
Intestinal calcium malabsorption	Yes	Yes	Yes
Muscle weakness	Yes	Yes	Yes
Alopecia	No	No	Common
Serum 25(OH)D (normal 30 ± 5 ng/mL)	Very low	Normal	Normal (except in one case)
Serum 1,25(OH)$_2$D (normal 20–80 pg/mL)	30–50 pg/mL (normal)	3–9 pg/mL (very low)	150–300 pg/mL (very high)
Proposed defect	Deficient intake of vitamin D or sunshine	Abnormal conversion of 25(OH)D to 1,25(OH)$_2$D, ? impaired 1 α-hydroxylase activity	Refractoriness of target organs to calcitriol
Response to treatment (daily dose)			
10 μg vitamin D$_2$ or D$_3$	Curative	No response	No response
2,500 μg (100,000 units) vitamin D$_2$ or D$_3$	Hypercalcemia	May be curative	May be curative
1–2 μg calcitriol	Curative	Curative	No response
6 μg calcitriol	Hypercalcemia	Hypercalcemia	Curative in some cases

be in the "normal" range of 20–60 pg/mL but is actually low for the degree of hypocalcemia, hypophosphatemia and secondary hyperparathyroidism, all factors known to stimulate 1,25(OH)$_2$D synthesis (7). Finally, despite the normal values of 1,25(OH)$_2$D synthesis, dietary cal-

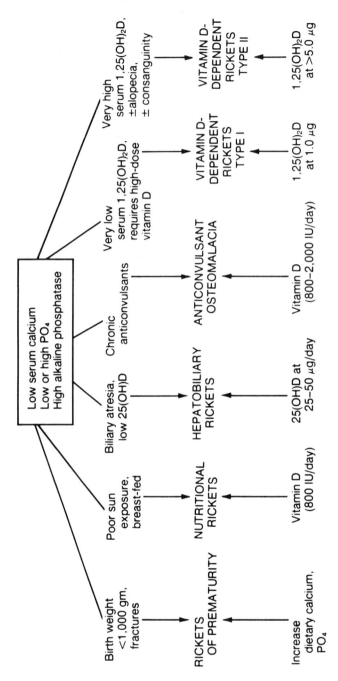

FIGURE 11-1. Diagnosis and treatment of various forms of rickets.

cium intake may be too low to attain normocalcemia and bone mineralization. Therapy is presented in Figure 11-1.

B. Neonatal Rickets

This complex disorder is mainly due to mineral deficiency. Prematurity is associated with a loss of active placental calcium and phosphate transport system needed to adequately mineralize the skeleton of the fetus (9). Most calcium and phosphate enter the skeleton during the third trimester and thus the 26- to 30-week gestational infant is at great risk for mineral deficiency. The diagnosis is made on the basis of mild hypocalcemia, hypophosphatemia (normal PO_4 in an infant, 6.0–7.5 mg/dL) and elevated alkaline phosphatase levels. Vitamin D and 25(OH)D values are normal, although 1,25(OH)$_2$D values are elevated compared to those in older children at 80 to 100 pg/mL versus a normal range of 20 to 60 pg/mL (9). Therapy includes the addition of calcium and phosphate to human milk or the use of high mineral, prepared formulas created for neonates. In infants receiving total parenteral nutrition, calcium and phosphate should be added to the intravenous solutions.

C. Anticonvulsant Osteomalacia

This disorder occurs in children who receive chronic anticonvulsant therapy and who are usually institutionalized. These children have reduced 25(OH)D levels, as well as hypocalcemia hypophosphatemia, and elevated alkaline phosphatase levels. The use of phenylhydantoins or phenobarbital stimulates the metabolism of 25(OH)D to an inactive metabolite and thus the substrate for 1,25(OH)$_2$D synthesis is diminished. These children require 800 to 1000 units of vitamin D daily.

D. Calcium-Deficient Osteomalacia

For an individual to be on a calcium-deficient diet, he would have to eat a bizarre, unbalanced or monotonous diet (7). This cause of rickets and/or osteomalacia is fortunately rare and probably represents child abuse or neglect. Patients have been fed such items as hot dogs and carbonated cola drinks or potato chips and beer exclusively. These children usually have osteomalacia or bone hypomineralization, without real evidence of rickets. Because children need sufficient protein and calories in their diet to promote growth before rickets can develop, these children have hypocalcemia, hypophosphatemia and secondary hyperparathyroidism, but their 25(OH)D levels are normal and 1,25(OH)$_2$D levels are elevated, as stimulated by hypocalcemia and increased PTH secretion. The addition of adequate calcium (800 to 1000 mg daily) will rapidly heal this bone disease.

E. Vitamin D-Dependent Rickets, Type I

This type of rickets develops as an autosomal recessive trait in children under eight months of age and is caused by a defect in the conversion of 25(OH)D to 1,25(OH)$_2$D (10). These children demonstrate all the features of classical rickets—hypocalcemia, hypophosphatemia, elevated alkaline phosphatase levels, high PTH levels, generalized aminoaciduria and severe rickets—and do not respond to conventional (400–1000 IU) or even massive doses of vitamin D. The serum 25(OH)D in these patients is normal or high if they are treated with high doses of vitamin D, and the 1,25(OH)$_2$D level is usually under 15 pg/mL. Therapy with 0.5 to 1.5 ng of 1,25(OH)$_2$D is curative.

F. Vitamin D-Dependent Rickets, Type II

This represents an end-organ nonresponsiveness to 1,25(OH)$_2$D and is characterized by a defective nuclear receptor for 1,25(OH)$_2$D as well as high circulating levels of 1,25(OH)$_2$D (1,7). Affected patients are often the offspring of first cousin matings and frequently have alopecia totalis as well as all the signs and symptoms of hypocalcemic rickets listed above. These patients sometimes, but not always, respond to extremely high, supraphysiological doses of 1,25(OH)$_2$D in the range of 6 to 25 ng daily.

G. Renal Osteodystrophy

This extremely complex metabolic bone disease is caused by a combination of reduced urinary phosphate excretion and reduced 1,25(OH)$_2$D synthesis, due to the decline in nephron mass in chronic renal insufficiency. The synthesis of 1,25(OH)$_2$D begins to fall as the glomerular filtration rate is reduced to 50% of normal and is markedly reduced to 5 to 15 pg/mL at a clearance of 15 mL/1.73 m^2 a minute (11). These children have hypocalcemia, hyperphosphatemia, elevated alkaline phosphatase levels, extremely high PTH levels and azotemia. The bone lesion consists of parathyroid bone disease (osteitis fibrosa), osteomalacia due to reduced bone mineral deposition, osteosclerosis due to high PTH levels and severe bowing of the legs with slipped epiphyses. This disorder can respond to oral 1,25(OH)$_2$D at 10 to 15 ng/kg a day and to phosphate restriction. The use of aluminum hydroxide binding gels to block intestinal phosphate absorption can lead to aluminum-induced osteopenia, which consists of extensive osteopenia with failure of mineralization (7). Because of the severity of this bone lesion, which is detected by an elevated serum aluminum content after four days of deferoxamine (40 mg/kg) (12), or by specific iron staining of a bone biopsy sample, it is best to avoid aluminum hydroxide-containing antacids. Calcium carbonate (500 to 1000 mg with each meal) can be used as a substitute phosphate binding agent, but it can produce hypercalcemia.

H. Hypoparathyroidism and Pseudohypoparathyroidism

These disorders present with tetany, hypocalcemia and hypophosphatemia. The causes of hypoparathyroidism include postsurgical, congenital, idiopathic, familial and autoimmune hypoparathyroidism, and DiGeorge syndrome (7). The diagnosis is established by measuring the immunoreactive PTH level, which is usually nondetectable or reduced, despite the hypocalcemia. Urinary cyclic adenine monophosphate levels are also reduced. Since PTH stimulates the conversion of 25(OH)D to 1,25(OH)$_2$D, the levels for this metabolite are reduced. Treatment includes a low phosphate diet, aluminum hydroxide binding gels and the administration of 1,25(OH)$_2$D (1–2 ng/day).

Pseudohypoparathyroidism is diagnosed in a patient who has the signs and symptoms of hypoparathyroidism and an elevated PTH level. Many of these patients have a round face, short stature, developmental delay, shortened fourth or fifth metacarpals or metatarsals or both and subcutaneous calcification. Some patients may appear to have rickets with bowing. These patients lack renal responsiveness to PTH and thus lack the phosphaturic response to high PTH levels; however, their bones respond to PTH. These patients develop hyperparathyroid bone disease (13). Therapy is similar to that for hypoparathyroidism.

I. Primary Hyperparathyroidism

Patients with this disorder, which is rare in childhood, present with hypercalcemia, hypophosphatemia and elevated urinary calcium values (more than 4 mg calcium/kg body weight daily), and some of the vague symptoms of hypercalcemia including fatigue, lassitude, nausea, emesis and polyuria. The bone lesion described in bone-responsive pseudohypoparathyroidism can occur in hyperparathyroidism because of extensive osteitis fibrosa. Two diagnostic features in addition to hypercalcemic hypercalciuria are elevated PTH and 1,25(OH)$_2$D levels, the latter being stimulated by PTH.

Therapy includes oral phosphate to reduce intestinal calcium absorption and surgical removal of the hyperplastic or adenomatous gland. Although no controlled study of childhood hyperparathyroidism has shown the requirement for parathyroidectomy, the fact that this problem will not disappear over the patient's long life and the potential for continuing bone resorption makes surgery a reasonable therapeutic approach.

V. Phosphaturias

Rickets in childhood is not only caused by hypocalcemia but may be the result of hypophosphatemia as well. Fraser and Scriver call this "phosphopenic rickets" (10). Rickets develops because the phosphate content of extracellular fluid is reduced. Several childhood phosphaturic syndromes have the same underlying mechanisms of osteomalacia and rickets but differ in their vitamin D metabolic profiles (14,15) (Table 11-5).

A. X-Linked Hypophosphatemic (Vitamin D-Resistant) Rickets

This is the most common form of rickets that occurs during childhood and is typified by normocalcemia, hypophosphatemia (serum phosphate 1.5 to 2.9 mg/dL; normal 3.5 to 5.5 mg/dL), elevated alkaline phosphatase levels and bowing of the lower limbs (2,7,10). This is an X-linked dominant disorder, because female hemizygotes are variably affected by the disease. The levels of $1,25(OH)_2D$ are low or low normal, and there is evidence that vitamin D metabolism is defective in this disorder. Laboratory investigation reveals normal PTH levels, a $1,25(OH)_2D$ level of 20 to 30 pg/mL (normal 20–80 pg/mL), massive urinary phosphate excretion and no aminoaciduria. The percentage of tubular reabsorption of phosphate is usually under 85% despite hypophosphatemia. The percentage tubular reabsorption of phosphate (% T.R.P.) is as follows:

$$1 - C_{Cr} \times \frac{C_{PO_4}}{100}$$

or

$$\frac{U_{PO_4}}{S_{PO_4}} \times \frac{S_{Cr}}{U_{Cr}} \times 100$$

Additional clues to the diagnosis of this disease are short stature, frontal bossing of the skull and the absence of Harrison's groove (the incurving and bowing of the rib cage found in calcium-deficient forms of rickets).

Therapy consists of oral phosphate administered over a 24-hour period, since the renal phosphate loss is continuous; hypophosphatemia can occur unless oral phosphate use is frequent (14). Because oral phosphate blocks intestinal calcium absorption and because a defect in $1,25(OH)_2D$ synthesis exists, it is also necessary to use $1,25(OH)_2D$.

This condition may sometimes be found in conjunction with polyostotic fibrous dysplasia neurofibromatosis or the epidermal nevus syndrome, which are familial. The diagnosis is made on the basis of rickets, normocalcemia, hypophosphatemia, hyperphosphaturia and a markedly low (under 10 pg/mL) serum $1,25(OH)_2D$ level (1,7). Removal of the

TABLE 11-5. Types of Primary Hypophosphatemic Rickets

Condition	Inheritance[a]	Associated findings	Salient clinical features	Age detected	Therapy
X-linked hypophosphatemic (vitamin D-resistant) rickets	XLD, rarely AD or AR	Occasional patient with parathyroid adenoma or hyperplasia	Bowing of lower segment, short stature, no myopathy, more severe in males	9–13 months	Oral phosphate 1–4 g/d in four to five doses, $1,25(OH)_2D$ at 65–75 ng/kg daily
Hypophosphatemic, nonrachitic bone disease	AD or sporadic		No radiological evidence of rickets, disease is milder, short stature may appear in late adolescence	3 years to adult	Oral phosphate and vitamin D; may be cured by $1,25(OH)_2D$
Hereditary hypophosphatemic rickets with hypercalciuria	AR; consanguinity	High calcitriol levels; increased intestinal calcium absorption; hypercalciuria, low urinary cAMP	Rickets, short stature, osteomalacia, sexes equally affected	Early childhood	Oral phosphate reverses biochemical features
Oncogenous rickets	Sporadic AD, AR	Sometimes neurofibromatosis, polyostotic fibrous dysplasia, epidermal nevus syndrome	Rickets cured by removal of tumor when serum $1,25(OH)_2D$ levels are low	Birth onwards	Oral phosphate and $1,25(OH)_2D$ reverse hypophosphatemia; surgery may be curative if tumor is totally removed
Adult sporadic hypophosphatemic osteomalacia	Sporadic	Glycinuria	Severe bone pain, vertebral flattening, severe myopathy and weakness	Adult	Oral phosphate plus vitamin D in any form

[a]AR: autosomal recessive; AD: autosomal dominant; XLD: X-linked dominant.
Adapted from Friedman AL, Chesney RW (1987) Isolated renal tubular defects. In: Schrier RM, Gottschalk CW (eds): Diseases of the Kidney, 4th edn. Little Brown, Boston, p 671.

tumor, whenever feasible, reverses all signs and symptoms of disease. If the tumor is widespread and cannot be removed completely, or if it is metastatic, then therapy with oral phosphate and $1,25(OH)_2D$ in a regimen similar to that used in X-linked hypophosphatemic rickets is appropriate.

VI. Magnesium Deficiency

Disorders of magnesium (Mg) metabolism affect calcium homeostasis. Hypomagnesemia, as a clue to Mg deficiency, can impede PTH release or alter end-organ responsiveness to PTH, thus rendering the patient hypocalcemic (16). Although many patients with chronic hereditary hypomagnesemia have an autosomal recessive disorder of intestinal Mg absorption, Mg deficiency may occur as the result of renal Mg wasting.

A. Renal Magnesium Wasting

This is an uncommon cause of hypomagnesemia, which is diagnosed by the presence of hypomagnesemia and high urinary Mg levels (normal 180 $\pm$ 10 mg/1.73 m² a day). Most patients also have renal potassium wasting and hypokalemia. The fractional excretion of Mg may exceed 20% at a time when serum Mg levels are under 1 mg/dL (17). Other manifestations of congenital Mg wasting include glucosuria, aminoaciduria, nephrocalcinosis and chondrocalcinosis and distal renal tubular acidosis. Sensorineural deafness has also been reported in familial renal Mg wasting. Some patients may also have rickets. Serum PTH and $1,25(OH)_2D$ levels are usually low.

Treatment with oral magnesium oxide at 500 to 1000 mg three times daily will generally reverse hypokalemia, hypomagnesemia and hyperkaluria. With normalization of serum Mg values, serum calcium, PTH and $1,25(OH)_2D$ concentrations usually return to normal. Since renal Mg wasting is a life-long event, patients should continue to take Mg to maintain normomagnesemia.

B. Drug-Induced Magnesuria

Renal Mg wasting may be evident in diabetic ketoacidosis, primary or secondary hypercalciuria, hyperaldosteronism, Bartter's syndrome and Fanconi syndrome, and following the use of certain drugs (16). The administration of *cis*platin, loop diuretics and aminoglycoside antibiotics, alone or in combination, can result in hypomagnesemia with renal Mg excretion patterns exceeding 20% of the filtered load. Although hypomagnesemia is infrequent after furosemide or aminoglycoside antibiotic administration, it is nearly universal following *cis*platin administration for solid tumors. The signs and symptoms of drug-induced renal Mg wasting are the same as in genetic or idiopathic renal magnesium wasting. However, the cure for this form of Mg is to stop the causative drug.

VII. Fanconi Syndrome

The urinary hyperexcretion of amino acids of all classes, glucose, bicarbonate, calcium, potassium, phosphate and other ions and low molecular weight proteins, along with vasopressin nonresponsive polyuria and renal tubular acidosis, define the proximal tubulopathy commonly called the Fanconi syndrome (1-3).

A. Causes

The diagnosis of the Fanconi syndrome is established by the urinary findings listed above, hypokalemia, metabolic acidosis with a low PCO_2 level, a reduced serum HCO_3 concentration, marked hypophosphatemia and rickets. Other features include hypokalemic myopathy, polyuria and short stature. The inherited and sporadic causes of Fanconi syndrome are listed in Table 11-6.

TABLE 11-6. Etiology of the Fanconi Syndrome

Inherited[a]
Idiopathic (AR, AD, XL)
Cystinosis (AR)
Wilson's disease (AR)
Lowe's (oculocerebrorenal) syndrome (XLR)
Galactosemia (AR)
Tyrosinemia (AR)
Hereditary fructose intolerance (AR)
Nephronophthisis-medullary cystic disease (AR, AD)
Acquired
Heavy metal poisoning (lead, cadmium, mercury, uranium)
Drugs: antibiotics (outdated tetracycline, gentamicin, cephalosporin), streptozocin, cisplatin
Chemicals (maleic acid, nitrobenzines, lysol)
Malignancies (multiple myeloma, monoclonal gammopathies)
Hyperparathyroidism, vitamin D deficiency
Renal disease
Nephrotic syndrome (e.g. focal sclerosing glomerulonephritis)
Renal transplantation
Balkan nephropathy

[a]AR: autosomal recessive; AD: autosomal dominant; XL: sex-linked; XLR: sex-linked recessive.
Adapted from Friedman AL, Chesney RW (1987) Isolated renal tubular defects. In: Schrier RM, Gottschalk CW (eds) Diseases of the Kidney, 4th edn. Little Brown, Boston, p 674

The most common cause of Fanconi syndrome in childhood is *infantile nephropathic cystinosis,* which may present with hypokalemic myopathy, features of Bartter's syndrome (see section VIII) and polyuria and polydipsia suggestive of nephrogenic diabetes insipidus. The basic defect is an abnormal efflux of cystine out of the lysosome of nearly all the cells in the body. The peculiar features of this disorder include blond hair, photophobia from crystalline cystine in the cornea, a depigmenting lesion of the retina, marked short stature, the ultimate development, by 10 years, of renal insufficiency and, at times, severe rickets (18). Patients with cystinosis may be helped by cysteamine, a cystine-depleting agent, which appears to slow the progression toward uremia.

Lowe's (oculocerebrorenal) syndrome is a rare, X-linked disorder presenting with a peculiar sloping forehead, glaucoma, hypotonia, areflexia and severe mental retardation. These patients also may develop renal insufficiency (19).

A group of autosomal recessive renal-hepatic syndromes present with features of the Fanconi syndrome and hepatocellular damage. In *galactosemia,* caused by galactose-1-phosphate uridyl transferase deficiency, hepatomegaly and icterus are evident at birth. This condition is tested for by most state genetic screening programs. If untreated, cataracts, inanition, vomiting and cirrhosis develop. Fanconi syndrome features disappear following dietary galactose restriction. Re-feeding lactose or galactose leads to hepatic dysfunction within minutes, but exposure for several days is required for the Fanconi syndrome to appear.

Hereditary fructose intolerance is caused by a fructose aldolase B deficiency. Fanconi syndrome features can develop in minutes after exposure to this sugar. Children with this disorder quickly learn to avoid fruit sugars to prevent the profound metabolic acidosis and hypophosphatemia that can develop.

Tyrosinemia or tyrosinosis presents in infancy with growth failure, hepatic damage, cataracts and hypoglycemia related to islet cell hypertrophy, which ultimately leads to cirrhosis. A defect in fumaryl acetoacetate fumaryl hydroxylase (FAH) is the cause of this disease. Affected patients with cirrhosis may develop hepatoblastoma after several years of disease (19).

In *Wilson's disease,* a copper storage disorder, cirrhosis and neurological symptoms, such as a flapping tremor, predominate, but some patients show the Fanconi syndrome features along with bicarbonate wasting, hypercalciuria and nephrocalcinosis. Patients have both distal and proximal renal tubular acidosis. Some patients with an untyped glycogen storage disease *(Fanconi Bickel syndrome)* have complex abnormalities of carbohydrate metabolism including hyperinsulinism, ketosis, glucose intolerance and hyperlipidemia. Other common features are hepatomegaly, a doll-like face, short stature and massive glucosuria (20). A renal biopsy specimen shows renal tubular glycogen storage.

Other causes of the Fanconi syndrome are sporadic, and include Bence-Jones proteinuria in multiple myeloma, after renal transplantation, an antibody-induced interstitial nephritis and renal vein thrombosis during infancy. A variety of toxins can produce the Fanconi syndrome (Table 11-6).

The full expression of the syndrome can be detected in some patients with vitamin D deficiency who have secondary hyperparathyroidism and hypocalcemia. Appropriate doses of vitamin D will reverse these features.

B. Diagnosis and Special Tests

The diagnosis of Fanconi syndrome is not difficult if the pediatrician or child care physician is aware of this disease. The features include poor growth, rickets and bowing, myopathy and other features of hypokalemia, polyuria and polydipsia, and in some forms, massive hepatomegaly (1,2). Some children have ocular findings suggestive of the etiology of the disease. Cystinotic children show severe photophobia and corneal crystal deposits, noted by slit-lamp examination: glaucoma and enlarged globes are noted in Lowe's syndrome; cataracts are found in galactosemia and the Kayser Fleischer ring is found at the limbus of the cornea in Wilson's disease. The reagent test strip (to test urine) can demonstrate the presence of this complex proximal tubulopathy, since glucosuria, ketonuria, proteinuria and, at times, an alkaline urine will be detected. The urine is also very dilute and may be clear. A serum chemistry survey by an autoanalyzer method will often show hypokalemia, reduced bicarbonate levels, hyperchloremia, hypophosphatemia, hypocalcemia, elevated alkaline phosphatase levels and two fairly uncommon findings, that is, hyperlipidemia and a reduced serum uric acid. This latter finding reflects the fact that uric acid reabsorption is reduced and serum uric acid levels of under 2 mg/dL are commonly found. In the child with features suggestive of *cystinosis*, the definitive diagnosis is made by determining leukocyte cystine concentrations, although slit-lamp examination for corneal crystals, the pressure of hexagonal cystine crystals in a bone marrow aspirate and another affected sibling may strongly suggest this diagnosis.

Lowe's syndrome is suggested by its physical features associated with the Fanconi syndrome and by its almost exclusive predominance in males.

Galactosemia often presents with many of the features of hepatic disease, including hyperbilirubinemia, icterus, elevated hepatocellular enzyme levels in serum and hepatomegaly with ascites.

Hereditary fructose intolerance is suggested by the development of acidosis, hypoglycemia and profound hypophosphatemia after an oral fructose load. Oral ingestion of 500 mg/kg of fructose will lead to acidosis, vomiting and hepatomegaly, since available phosphate is bound in fructose 1-phosphate, which cannot be further metabolized due to the defective aldolase B activity. The definitive diagnosis of both galactosemia and fructose intolerance is made from direct enzyme analysis of a hepatic biopsy sample (19).

Tyrosinemia is suggested by elevated levels of tyrosine and methionine in the plasma and urine of children with Fanconi syndrome and cirrhosis. This disorder appears at age eight months or earlier and is also associated with the excretion of Δ-amino-levulinic acid, *p*-hydroxyphenylpyruvate, and other *p*-hydroxyphenyl compounds, succinylacetate and succinyla-cetoacetate because of the FAH deficiency. As in galactosemia and hereditary fructose intolerance, patients are very ill and may die of cirrhosis, infection or inanition. Some patients have a chronic form of tyrosinosis with nodular cirrhosis, which may ultimately lead to hepatocellular carcinoma or hepatoblastoma.

Wilson's disease is specifically diagnosed by an elevated serum non-ceruloplasmin bound copper and urinary copper excretion, Kayser-Fleischer rings and a reduced serum ceruloplasmin concentration of under 20 mg/dL (19).

Untyped *glycogen storage disease* is diagnosed by the finding of massive amounts of glycogen in a liver biopsy specimen and by the ketosis and glucose intolerance of patients (20).

The Fanconi syndrome associated with heavy metal toxicity is diagnosed by a history of exposure and by plasma or urinary levels of the identified heavy metal (19). *Lead poisoning* can also be diagnosed by determining the erythrocyte-free protoporphyrin level and by the presence of anemia and basophilic stippling of erythrocytes examined by oil microscopy (1000 ×) on a Wrights' stained smear. The Fanconi syndrome associated with *vitamin D deficiency* is diagnosed by the methods described in section VI and by determining serum 25(OH)D level determinations (1–7).

VIII. Bartter's Syndrome

In 1962, Bartter and his colleageus reported a syndrome consisting of hypokalemia, chronic metabolic alkalosis, hyperreninemia, hyperaldosteronism and juxtaglomerular apparatus hyperplasia (1,7). Patients are normotensive and resist the pressor effects of norepinephrine and angiotensin II. Presenting symptoms consist of weakness, cramping of many muscle groups, abdominal pain and polyuria. Children with this condition may also have poor growth, mental retardation and nephrocalcinosis. Patients who have clinical and chemical symptoms similar to those seen in Bartter's syndrome, but without juxtaglomerular apparatus hyperplasia, have been recently described (21).

The pathophysiology of Bartter's syndrome is unclear but may involve primary renal potassium loss, a defect in chloride reabsorption with potassium loss due to enhanced sodium-potassium exchange in the distal tubule or the loss of sodium and chloride together (22,23). Finally, a group of hyperprostaglandinuric syndromes of childhood, in which urinary prostaglandin levels are extremely high, can present with all the features of Bartter's syndrome (24). All four of these mechanisms seem to be relevant in the expression of Bartter's syndrome.

The diagnosis is made on the basis of the symptoms discussed above in conjunction with the finding of a hypokalemic, hypochloremic metabolic alkalosis. If the urine chloride level is greater than 10 mEq/L, then Bartter's syndrome is likely (1), in contrast to patients with bulemia, chronic vomiting and diuretic or laxative abuse, in whom the urine chloride level is below 10 mEq/L. However, if diuretic abuse has not resulted in volume depletion, then urine chloride excretion may exceed 10 mEq/L. Since Mg deficiency may result in hypokalemic alkalosis, serum Mg levels should be measured (17). In infants, a chloride-deficient formula was associated with a Bartter-like syndrome, which reversed when adequate chloride was restored to the infant's formula (25). Urinary prostaglandin E_2 levels can be measured in a hypokalemic syndrome with low urinary chloride levels to rule out a primary hyperprostaglandinuric state (23).

References

1. Friedman AL, Chesney RW (1987) Isolated renal tubular defects. In: Schrier RM, Gottschalk CW (eds) Diseases of the Kidney, 4th edn. Little Brown, Boston, pp 663–688
2. Chesney RW, Novello AC (1987) Defects of renal tubular transport. In: Massry SG, Glassock RJ (eds) Textbook of Nephrology, 2nd edn. Williams and Wilkins, Baltimore, pp 445–460
3. Mitch WE, Chesney RW (1983) Amino acid metabolism by the kidney. Miner Electrolyte Metab 9:190–202
4. Desjeux J-F, Rajantie J, Simell O, et al (1980) Lysine fluxes across the jejunal epithelium in lysinuric protein intolerance. J Clin Invest 65:1382–1387
5. Segal S, Thier SO (1983) Cystinuria, In: Stanbury JB, Wyngaarden JB, Frederickson DS, Goldstein JL, Brown MS (eds) The Metabolic Basis of Inherited Disease, 5th edn. McGraw Hill, New York, pp 1774–1791
6. Jepson JB (1983) Hartnup disease. In: Stanbury JB, Wyngaarden JB, Frederickson DS, Goldstein JL, Brown MS (eds) The Metabolic Basis of Inherited Disease, 5th edn. McGraw Hill, New York, pp 1804–1805
7. Chesney RW (1984) Metabolic bone disease. Pediatr Rev 5:227–237
8. Chesney RW, Zimmerman J, Hamstra AJ, et al (1981) Vitamin D metabolite concentrations in vitamin D deficiency: are calcitrol levels normal? Am J Dis Child 135:1025–1028
9. Greer F, Chesney RW (1983) Disorders of calcium in the neonate. In: Moore ES, Kurtzman NA (eds) Seminars in Nephrology: Role of the Kidney in Mineral Homeostasis in Early Life. Grune and Stratton, New York, pp 110–115

10. Fraser D, Scriver CR (1976) Familial forms of vitamin D-resistant rickets: X-linked hypophosphatemia and autosomal recessive vitamin D dependency. Am J Clin Nutr 29:1315–1329

11. Chesney RW, Hamstra AJ, Phelps M, et al (1983) Vitamin D metabolites in renal insufficiency and other vitamin D disorders of children. Kidney Int 24:S63-S69

12. Salusky IB, Coburn JW, Foley J, et al (1983) Effects of oral calcium carbonate on control of serum phosphorus and changes in plasma aluminum levels after discontinuation of aluminum containing gels in children receiving dialysis. J Pediatr 108:767–770

13. Dabbagh S, Chesney RW, Langer LO, et al (1984) Renal-nonresponsive, bone responsive pseudohypoparathyroidism. A case with vitamin D metabolite levels and clinical features of rickets. Am J Dis Child 138:1030–1033

14. Olorieux FH, Scriver CR, Reade TM, et al (1972) Use of phosphate and vitamin D to prevent dwarfism and rickets in X-linked hypophosphatemia. N Engl J Med 287:481–487

15. Teider M, Modai D, Samuel R, et al (1985) Hereditary hypophosphatemic rickets with hypercalciuria. N Engl J Med 312:611–617

16. Agus ZS, Wasserstein A, Goldfarb S (1982) Disorders of calcium and magnesium homeostasis. Am J Med 72:473–488

17. Zelikovic I, Dabbagh S, Friedman AL, et al (1987) Severe renal osteodystrophy without elevated serum immunoreactive parathyroid hormone concentrations in hypomagnesemia due to renal magnesium wasting. Pediatrics 79:403–409

18. Gahl WA, Schneider JA, Thoene JG, et al (1986) Course of nephropathic cystinosis after age 10 years. J Pediatr 109:605–608

19. Brewer E (1985) Clinical aspects of the Fanconi syndrome. In: Gonick H, Buckalew VM, Jr (eds) Renal Tubular Disorders. Marcel Deckker, New York. pp 475–544

20. Chesney RW, Kaplan BS, Colle E, et al (1980) Abnormalities of carbohydrate metabolism in idiopathic Fanconi syndrome. Pediatr Res 14:209–215

21. Barakat AY, Francis YK, Mufarrij AA (1986) Hypokalemic alkalosis, hyperreninemia, aldosteronism, normal blood pressure and normal juxtaglomerular apparatus—a new syndrome of renal alkalosis. Int J Pediatr Nephrol 7:99–100

22. Roth KS, Buckalew VM, Jr, Chan JCM (1985) Renal tubular disorders. Curr Nephrol 8:87–137

23. Stein JH (1985) The pathogenetic spectrum of Bartter's syndrome. Kidney Int 28:85–93

24. Seyberth HW, Rascher W, Schweer H, et al (1985) Congenital hypokalemia with hypercalcemia in preterm infants: a hyperprostaglandinuric tubular syndrome different from Bartter syndrome. J Pediatr 107:694–701

25. Roy S III, Arant BS, Jr (1981) Hypokalemic metabolic alkalosis in normotensive infants with elevated plasma renin activity and hyperaldosteronism: Role of dietary chloride deficiency. Pediatrics 67:423–429

12
Water and Electrolyte Disturbances

VALENTINA KON and IEKUNI ICHIKAWA

I. Introduction

Disturbances in plasma sodium (Na) and potassium (K) concentrations are frequent complications of disease states that afflict the pediatric population. This chapter will first categorize and describe Na disorders and then conditions that affect the extracellular concentration of K (1-9).

II. Disturbances in Sodium Concentration

Despite great variability in daily Na intake, under normal conditions, plasma Na stays remarkably constant. There exist, however, a variety of disorders that can alter the level of measured Na to produce hypo- and hypernatremia.

A. Hyponatremia

1. Pseudohyponatremia

Hyponatremia in the face of normal osmolality (280–295 mOsm/kg) is termed pseudohyponatremia (Table 12-1). This is not associated with a change in total body Na content or redistribution of total body water. Normally, the circulating plasma is made up of 94% water and 6% solids (lipids and protein), with the Na being principally dissolved in the aqueous phase. However, when the fraction of whole plasma that is solids increases, there is an apparent decrease in plasma Na. For example, accumulation of large amounts of lipids (extreme hypertriglyceridemia in nephrotic syndrome) or protein (Waldenstrom's macroglobulinemia) displaces water so that any volume of plasma is made up of lower percentage of water and Na concentration measured in total plasma becomes lower.

Hyperproteinemia is a distinctly unusual circumstance in pediatrics. Adjustments can be made either by removing the excess plasma solids and then measuring Na concentration in plasma water or, instead of using the conventional flame photometer, measuring Na by direct potentiometry which utilizes a Na electrode to measure the actual Na content. It is also possible to estimate a correction in serum Na by the following equations:

Magnitude of reduction in Na due to lipids (mEq/L) = plasma lipids (mg/dL) × 0.002.

Magnitude of reduction in Na due to hyperproteinemia (mEq/L) = amount of protein >8 (g/dL) × 0.25

In applying these formulas it can be appreciated that the degree of hyperlipidemia/hyperproteinemia must be extreme to alter the value of plasma Na substantially.

2. Hypertonic Hyponatremia

Hyponatremia with elevated plasma osmolality is termed *hypertonic hyponatremia,* and reflects an abnormal presence of an osmotically active substance (Table 12.1). This should be suspected if hyponatremia occurs with a plasma osmolality over 295 mOsm/kg or if the osmolality is 20 mOsm/kg greater than the calculated sum of the usual osmotically active substances:

TABLE 12-1. Hyponatremia (Plasma Na <130 mEq/L)

S_{osm} 280–295 (pseudohyponatremia)	S_{osm} <280 (hypotonic hyponatremia) Establish volume status			S_{osm} >295 (hypertonic hyponatremia)
Hyperlipidemia	*Hypovolemia*	*Isovolemia*	*Hypervolemia*	Hyperglycemia
Hyperproteinemia				Mannitol
	Extrarenal (U_{Na} <20 mEq/L; FE_{Na} <1%)	Nausea, pain, stress	Extrarenal (U_{Na} <20 mEq/L; FE_{Na} <1%)	X-ray contrast media
	Vomiting/diarrhea, GI suction	Glucocorticoid insufficiency	Heart failure	Methanol
	Hemorrhage	Severe hypothyroidism	Nephrotic syndrome	Ethylene glycol (antifreeze)
	Transcutaneous losses	Excessive water intake	Liver cirrhosis	
	Burns	Drugs:	Renal (U_{Na} >20 mEq/L; FE_{Na} >3%)	
	Increased perspiration	Diuretics	Acute renal failure	
	Cystic fibrosis	Promoting ADH release (barbiturates, clofibrate, isoproterenol, nicotine, vincristine)	Chronic renal failure	
	Fluid sequestration	Prostaglandin inhibitors (aspirin, nonsteroidal anti-inflammatory drugs)		
	Peritonitis/pancreatitis	Potentiate ADH action (clorpropamide, cyclophosphamide)		
	Ileus	Others (oxytocin, vasopressin)		
	Rhabdomyolysis	SIADH		
	Renal (U_{Na} >20 mEq/L; FE_{Na} >3%)			
	Diuresis (thiazides, osmotic)			
	Adrenal insufficiency			
	Metabolic alkalosis			
	Tubulointerstitial (interstitial nephritis, obstruction, pyelonephritis)			
	Cystic diseases			

$$(2 \times Na) + (glucose/18) + (BUN/2.8)$$

Where BUN is blood urea nitrogen. An important example of this type of hyponatremia occurs with hyperglycemia. In this instance, glucose is the osmotically active substance that increases plasma osmolality. This increase in plasma osmolality then causes movement of water from the intracellular to the extracellular space. Since two-thirds of total body water is within the intracellular compartment, this transcellular movement of water can lead to substantial dilution of plasma Na. It is important to remember that in addition to water redistribution, hyperglycemia produces glycosuria, which promotes excretion of free water in the urine. Thus, the initial glucose-induced hypertonicity causes a water shift and hyponatremia, but the diuresis may normalize the Na concentration at the expense of volume. It is common for a hyperglycemic patient to present with volume depletion and normal Na concentrations. However, should the patient continue to drink or receive intravenous fluid, actual (not redistribution) hyponatremia will occur.

Adjustments in plasma Na concentration due to hyperglycemia not yet treated with insulin can be estimated:

$$\text{Expected Na (mEq/L)} = \text{measured Na (mEq/L)}$$
$$+ 0.028 \text{ (glucose} - 100)$$

Adjustments in plasma Na with insulin treatment:

$$\text{Expected Na (mEq/L)} = \text{measured Na (mEq/L)}$$
$$+ 0.16 \text{ (glucose} - 100)$$

Some of the other causes of hypertonic hyponatremia include administration of mannitol or glycerol to control intracerebral pressure and X-ray contrast material. Also, urea and ingestion of ethanol, methanol and ethylene glycol (antifreeze) may transiently raise serum osmolality and cause hyponatremia. It should be emphasized that these latter substances permeate cells so that normal serum Na concentrations in association with hyperosmolality quickly supervene after exposure.

3. Hypotonic Hyponatremia

Hyponatremia, in association with reduced plasma osmolality (<280 mOsm/kg), is termed *hypotonic hyponatremia*. This, by far, is the most common clinical condition and is characterized by an absolute or relative excess of total body water relative to total body Na. It must be emphasized that hyponatremia does not imply low total body Na, since hyponatremia can occur in the face of increased, decreased or near normal total body Na. As can be seen from Table 12-1, once hyponatremia is established to be hypotonic it is useful to further categorize it as hypovolemic, hypervolemic and isovolemic.

a. Hypotonic Hyponatremia with Hypovolemia

Since volume depletion is a frequent cause of hyponatremia, the features of volume depletion are reviewed in Table 12-2. The mechanisms of hyponatremia in volume depletion include decrease in the rate of glomerular filtration and reduced fluid delivery to distal nephron segments which normally elaborate a dilute urine. Increase in plasma osmolality and volume depletion itself also stimulate the release of antidiuretic hormone (ADH), which acts on the distal nephron segments to reduce the amount of free water formed. Because preservation of volume supercedes maintenance of normal osmolality, these mechanisms promote retention of hypotonic fluid and hyponatremia. It should be recognized that since no bodily fluid is hypertonic to plasma, hyponatremia occurs only if the patient is drinking or receiving hypotonic fluids. A rare exception has been noted with thiazide diuretics, when solute loss exceeds water loss, which effectively lowers plasma Na, independent of water intake.

Once hyponatremia is established to be associated with volume depletion, urinary Na is a useful parameter in determining if the hyponatremia is of renal or extrarenal etiology. Gastrointestinal losses (vomiting/diarrhea) are commonly associated with renal conservation of Na (urinary sodium concentration <20 mEq/L or $FE_{Na} <1\%$). Similarly, hemorrhage, transcutaneous fluid losses and fluid sequestration into third spaces (peritonitis, ileus, rhabdomyolysis) will lower the urinary Na concentration. Although volume losses through the gastrointestinal tract are typically associated with urine Na conservation, there are conditions when high urine Na excretion is observed. Vomiting sufficient to cause alkalosis, such as with pyloric stenosis, is associated with bicarbonaturia. Since bicarbonate must be excreted with a cation, there is an associated loss

TABLE 12-2. Clinical and Laboratory Features of Volume Depletion

History
  Vomiting/diarrhea
  Decreased intake

Signs/Symptoms
  Irritability, lethargy, thirst
  Decreased weight, sunken fontenelle and sunken, soft eyeballs
  Dry mucous membranes, decreased turgor and mottling of skin
  Elevated pulse, orthostatic changes in pulse and blood pressure
  Decreased central venous pressure

Laboratory
  Elevated BUN, creatinine
  Elevated hematocrit
  Elevated protein concentration, uric acid
  Decreased urine volume; urine Na <20 mEq/L; $FE_{Na} <1\%$, urine osmolality >500
    mOsm/L (these parameters are for normally functioning kidneys)

of Na and K in the urine. Thus, patients with pyloric stenosis can develop hyponatremic volume depletion due to gastrointestinal losses, decreased intake and partial replacement with hypotonic fluids but have concurrent high urinary Na.

The other category of disorders that cause hypotonic hyponatremia in the face of volume depletion are those in which losses occur primarily through the kidneys. Patients with intrinsic renal failure, in particular, disorders that affect tubules such as medullary/cystic kidney disease or interstitial nephritis, and individuals undergoing diuresis can develop hyponatremia and have high urinary Na content (urinary Na >20 mEq/L or $FE_{Na} >3\%$). Patients with proximal renal tubular acidosis lose bicarbonate in the urine, which obligates the loss of a cation, e.g. Na. High anion gap acidosis (diabetic ketoacidosis) is another example in which obligate anion loss (ketoacids) must be accompanied by a cation (Na) and contribute to a high urinary Na excretion. Finally, hypotonic hyponatremia with volume depletion and high urinary Na in the absence of renal disease, particularly in association with hyperkalemia, should suggest adrenal insufficiency.

b. Hypotonic Hyponatremia with Hypervolemia

Hypotonic hyponatremia associated with hypervolemia is seen in edema-forming states, such as congestive heart failure, liver cirrhosis, nephrotic syndrome and renal damage. Again, it is useful to divide this category into extrarenal and renal disorders.

In extrarenal disorders (congestive heart failure, nephrotic syndrome, cirrhosis), the kidney function is typically normal but there is perturbation in the regulatory mechanisms for fluid volume maintenance, which enhances retention of Na (Table 12-1). Hyponatremia occurs when there is positive balance of fluid with a relative excess of water to Na. Thus, the urinary Na excretion is low (unless the patient is taking a diuretic). Although the pathogenesis of edema formation in hyponatremia is complicated and reflects the specific underlying disorder, some of the mechanisms include decreased effective arteriolar blood volume, decreased cardiac output, hypoproteinemia, increased capillary leak, decreased glomerular filtration rate (GFR), increased proximal tubule reabsorption with decreased fluid delivery to the distal nephron segments and increased stimulation for ADH release. Individually, and in combination, these factors contribute to decreased free water clearance.

Acute and chronic renal disease that decrease the GFR are sometimes characterized by hyponatremia (urinary Na >20 mEq/L and $FE_{Na} >3\%$). The main problem is damage of the renal parenchyma, which is unable to regulate salt and water excretion and therefore volume. For example, in the case of an abrupt and severe decrease in GFR, there is little or even no production of urine so that hyponatremia becomes a direct consequence of hypotonic intake. More commonly, there develops a decrease in GFR sufficient to limit the delivery of fluid to the diluting segments of the nephron, thereby limiting excretion of free water. Since only 20% of GFR can be excreted as solute-free water, any intake above this volume is retained as positive water balance i.e. a GFR of 5 mL/minute produces about 7.2 L of filtrate each day; ingestion of more than 1.4 L (20% of 7.2 L) will be retained.

c. Hypotonic Hyponatremia with Isovolemia

The third category of hypotonic hyponatremia is associated with isovolemia (Table 12-1). In these disorders, there is normal volume and the hyponatremia reflects an increased level of ADH. The elevated level of ADH is abnormal in that it is not due to osmotic or volume stimuli that normally induce ADH release. Pain, nausea or emotional and physical stress are potent stimuli for ADH release. Under these circumstances, if water is administered or ingested, hyponatremia occurs. Endocrine disorders, such as hypopituitarism and hypothyroidism, can cause isovolemic hyponatremia. Glucocorticoid deficiency without mineralocorticoid deficiency, e.g. hypopituitarism stimulates ADH release in the absence of volume depletion. Hypothyroidism may be associated with a low GFR and, therefore, decreased fluid delivery to the diluting segments of the nephron to produce hyponatremia; however, clinically relevant hyponatremia occurs only in myxedematous hypothyroidism where ADH release is enhanced.

Various drugs are associated with isovolemic hyponatremia. Most common among these are the diuretics. Although much of the diuretic-induced hyponatremia is associated with volume contraction, some patients have low plasma Na with normal volume status. These cases may be related to severe K depletion, which increases the sensitivity of ADH secretory cells in the hypothalamus to respond to even clinically insignificant decreases in volume. Other medications which cause hyponatremia include 1) those that promote ADH release, 2) those that potentiate the renal effects of ADH by inhibiting prostaglandins which in turn decrease the antidiuretic action of ADH, 3) those that potentiate the antinatriuretic action of ADH and 4) others (Table 12-1) such as oxytocin, given to induce labor and delivery, has been reported to produce water intoxication in obstetric patients and their babies. Exogenous vasopressin given to patients with central diabetes insipidus (DI) can also cause hyponatremia.

An important and relatively frequent entity in the pediatric population is the syndrome of inappropriate ADH (SIADH) and is a prominant cause of hypotonic hypoatremia in the absence of disturbance in volume. This syndrome occurs with central nervous system disorders, such as meningitis, encephalitis, brain abscesses, brain tumors and head injuries. It can also occur with systemic diseases, such as infections. Since ADH is not routinely measured, the diagnosis of SIADH is largely made by the process of exclusion. Table 12-3 outlines the pertinent features of SIADH.

TABLE 12-3. Diagnosis of Syndrome of Inappropriate Antidiuretic Hormone (SIADH)

Hyponatremia associated with hypo-osmolality
$U_{osm} > P_{osm}$
High U_{Na} (relative criteria)
Absence of volume depletion or edema
Normal adrenal and thyroid functions (relative criteria: normal
    cardiac, renal, hepatic and pituitary function)
Correction with fluid restriction

The urine osmolality, which is inappropriately elevated relative to plasma, suggests an inappropriate release of ADH. Thus, even 200 mOsm/kg in the urine does not rule out the diagnosis of SIADH, since a 4 to 5 mEq/L fall in plasma Na concentration should completely inhibit ADH release and cause urine osmolality to fall to less than 100 mOsm/kg. The urine Na concentration is high in SIADH despite normal volume because elevated ADH levels cause decreased water excretion, water retention, expansion of total body water and dilution of serum Na. Total body water expansion stimulates volume receptors which increase urinary Na excretion. This is a relative criteria since the SIADH that occurs in a previously Na restricted/volume-depleted patient may occur in association with a very low urinary Na concentration. The hyponatremia of SIADH is corrected by strict fluid restriction.

4. Clinical Manifestations of Hyponatremia

Signs and symptoms observed in hyponatremia relate primarily to central nervous system function and are reviewed in Table 12-4. The severity of these symptoms reflect the degree and rapidity of development of hyponatremia. Thus, although symptoms can present even with modest decrease in Na, the majority of the major central nervous system symptoms occur when the serum Na concentration reaches <120 mEq/L. The symptoms are particularly profound if this hyponatremia develops within a 24-hour period. It should be emphasized that the underlying disorders contribute to and may even overshadow these clinical manifestations of the hyponatremia per se.

TABLE 12-4. Clinical Manifestations of Hyponatremia

Lethargy, fatigue, irritability, disorientation
Nausea, vomiting, muscle cramps
Abnormal sensorium, depressed deep tendon reflexes
Seizures, coma
Hypothermia
Cheyne-Stokes respiration

B. Hypernatremia

As with hyponatremia, hypernatremia indicates a relative imbalance of Na and water and occurs when the amount of Na in the extracellular fluid space is increased relative to water. Although not all hyponatremic states are hyposmolar (Table 12-1), all hypernatremic states are hyperosmolar. Normally, the body has a very effective mechanism against hyperosmolality and hypernatremia. When plasma osmolality rises above 295 mOsm/kg, thirst is stimulated and fluid intake increases, correcting the hyperosmolar hypernatremic state. In an extreme example, patients with central DI who lack ADH and are unable to conserve water are sufficiently stimulated by thirst alone to consume more than 10 L of fluid per day to prevent hyperosmolality. This example underscores the fact that except in the circumstance of an acute Na load, development of hypernatremia suggests an inability to obtain adequate volumes of fluid in the face of ongoing losses or an impairment in the thirst mechanism.

Hypernatremia may occur in the face of hypovolemia, isovolemia or hypervolemia (Table 12-5).

TABLE 12-5. Approach to Hypernatremia (Plasma Na >150 mEq/L)

Establishing the volume status is an important step in the workup of the etiology of hypernatremia

Hypovolemia
  Extrarenal
    Vomiting/diarrhea
    Excessive sweating
  Renal
    Diuretics/decreased intake
    Osmotic diuresis (glucose, urea)
    Nonoliguric acute renal failure

Isovolemia
  Extrarenal
    Hyperventilation
    Fever
    Sweating
    Phototherapy/radiant warmers
  Renal
    Diabetes insipidus (central, nephrogenic)

Hypervolemia
  Sodium gain
    NaHCO$_3$ therapy during cardiac resuscitation or acidosis
    Hypertonic saline in the treatment of extreme hyponatremia
    Ingestion of improperly diluted baby formula
    Seawater near-drowning

1. Hypernatremia with Hypovolemia

Hypernatremia associated with hypovolemia develops when water losses exceed solute losses. Total body Na here is low. This can occur from excessive losses of any of the body fluids that are hypotonic to plasma and occur through extrarenal or renal routes. Extrarenal losses include gastrointestinal tract (vomiting/diarrhea) and transcutaneous losses (excessive sweating, phototherapy and radiant heat warmers). Primary renal disorders include excessive urinary fluid losses such as during treatment with diuretics or mannitol or in disorders which include urinary losses of glucose or urea. As noted, the thirst mechanisms are very effective in dictating the ingestion of water and the maintenance of water balance; therefore, hypernatremia associated with volume depletion suggests that, in addition to hypotonic fluid losses, there is also impaired water intake. This impairment can occur in comatose patients, those without access to water or persons otherwise unable to effectively communicate thirst, such as infants. Additional factors that make infants particularly vulnerable to hypernatremic volume depletion is the high ratio of surface area to weight, which amplifies insensible skin loss of fluid. Furthermore, the relative renal immaturity in infants, with respect to the ability to excrete a solute load, contributes to their susceptibility to hypernatremic volume depletion.

2. Hypernatremia with Isovolemia

Hypernatremia, in association with isovolemia, results when relatively more water than Na is lost from the body but is not sufficient as to cause appreciable decrease in volume. Total body Na here is normal. Extrarenal routes include insensible water loss through the respiratory system, e.g. hyperventilation, improperly humidified ventilators, fever, phototherapy and radiant warmers. The urinary osmolality is expected to be high under these conditions.

The primary cause of isovolemic hypernatremia, in which hypotonic losses occur through the kidneys, includes disorders in the production or release of ADH, i.e. central DI or in an abnormal renal response to ADH, i.e. nephrogenic DI. Patients with DI may present with polyuria, polydipsia and hypernatremia. Other salient features of DI are listed in Table 12-6. Central DI may be congenital or acquired. Head trauma, brain tumors and complications from neurosurgical procedures constitute the majority of cases. Nephrogenic DI may also be congenital or acquired. The congenital form is complete only in males, but girls manifest full-blown symptoms when there is water deprivation. Acquired nephrogenic DI may be due to intrinsic renal disease, particularly diseases that affect the papillary and medullary regions of the kidney, such as polycystic

TABLE 12-6. Causes of Diabetes Insipidus

Central	Nephrogenic
Hereditary: autosomal dominant, sex-linked recessive	Decreased water permeability of renal tubules to ADH
Infectious: meningitis/encephalitis	Hereditary (sex-linked)
Neoplasm: craniopharyngeoma, pinealoma, optic glioma, melanoma, metastases	Hypokalemia
	Hypercalcemia
	Drugs (lithium, demeclocycline)
Head trauma, basilar skull fracture	Decreased medullary tonicity
Neurosurgical complication	Renal failure, particularly tubulointerstitial disease
Hypoxic encephalopathy	"Medullary washout" (forced diuresis, postobstructive diuresis)
Idiopathic	Diuretics
	Other
	Sickle cell disease
	Methoxyfluorene

kidney disease, nephronophthesis, sickle cell disease, obstructive nephropathy and chronic pyelonephritis. Certain electrolyte disorders, such as hypokalemia and hypercalcemia, have also been reported to cause nephrogenic DI.

A history of enuresis and nocturia can often be elicited, particularly in patients with central DI. Affected children tend to avoid foods with a high protein content (e.g. prefer water over milk) and favor foods with a high carbohydrate content to decrease their daily osmolar load contributed by the proteins. Constipation, due to the avid colonic water reabsorption, and growth retardation, secondary to repeated bouts of dehydration, chronic hypernatremia and spontaneous avoidance of proteins in the diet are also seen. Marked bladder distenstion and hydronephrosis may be observed due to the high urine flow rate.

Quantitation of the daily urine output, determination of specific gravity (sp gr) and osmolality on the first-morning urine are quick screening tests that help in the diagnosis of DI. Elevated serum Na and osmolality are strongly suggestive of this condition, although normal values are not unusual, especially in the older child with free access to water. The classic test used in diagnosing DI is the *water deprivation test*. This test should be performed in a hospital setting so that the patient's vital signs can be closely monitored; it should be performed with caution in small infants, since water deprivation in these individuals may lead to circulatory collapse. The procedure may be performed as follows:

1. In the morning, empty bladder and weigh patient. Patient should have had nothing orally.

2. Obtain hourly weights; urine volume, sp gr and osmolality; plasma Na and osmolality.
3. Stop this part of the test if:
   body weight decreases by $>3\%$
   plasma Na >150 mEq/L
   plasma osmolality >300 mOsm/kg water

Upon the completion of the above steps:

1. Collect blood for ADH level.
2. Give aqueous vasopressin (1–10 μ) intramuscularly or DDAVP (1–10 μg) intranasally depending on the age of the child.
3. Obtain two consecutive 30-minute specimens for urine sp gr and osmolality as well as plasma osmolality

In normal individuals, water deprivation leads to a progressive decrease in urine flow and increased urine osmolality to 500 to 1400 mOsm/kg water; plasma osmolality remains normal. In the newborn, the concentration mechanism is not fully developed, and urine osmolality cannot increase over 700 to 800 mOsm/kg water in response to dehydration. Following a dose of 10 μg of DDAVP, infants have been found to increase their urine osmolality to 385 ± 25 mOsm/kg water (359 in prematures) by age one to three weeks, and to 566 ± 50 mOsm/kg water (524 in prematures) by age four to six weeks (10).

Following dehydration, U_{osm} remains $< P_{osm}$ in complete central and nephrogenic DI ($U_{osm} <200$ mOsm/kg water), and U_{osm} increases in partial central DI ($U_{osm} > P_{osm}$). Patients with psychogenic polydipsia will always have $U_{osm} >> P_{osm}$.

Antidiuretic hormone administration in normal individuals produces no further increase in urine sp gr and osmolality ($\leq 5\%$ change) or decrease in urine volume. In the child with complete central DI, urine osmolality increases less than 50% and serum osmolality gradually increases. Patients with nephrogenic DI do not respond to ADH and there is no change in urine osmolality, volume or plasma osmolality. In patients with nephrogenic DI, a 10-fold dose of ADH should be tried to differentiate between the partial and complete form.

When the water deprivation test is inconclusive, a *hypertonic saline infusion test* may distinguish between central DI, nephrogenic DI and primary polydipsia; here 5% saline is given intravenously for two hours at the rate of 0.04 to 0.05 mL/kg/minute. Plasma samples for osmolality and ADH assays are collected at 30-minute intervals and results are plotted on a nomogram (11).

In patients with central DI, plasma ADH is subnormal relative to plasma osmolality and volume, but it is normal in patients with primary polydipsia and nephrogenic DI.

3. Hypernatremia with Hypervolemia

A Na gain is an uncommon cause of hypernatremia, since an increase in extracellular fluid volume activates mechanisms that increase renal Na excretion. However, acute infusion of hypertonic saline or ingestion of salt may precipitate hypernatremia. For example, administration of hypertonic solutions of sodium bicarbonate ($NaHCO_3$) during cardiac resuscitation or treatment of lactic acidosis delivers 50 mEq of Na in each 100 mL of 3% $NaHCO_3$. Other examples of hypernatremia associated with increased volume include administration of hypertonic sodium chloride in the treatment of extreme hyponatremia, ingestion of improperly diluted baby formula, and near-drowning in seawater. Total body Na here is increased.

4. Clinical Manifestations of Hypernatremia

Hypernatremia due to loss of hypotonic fluid often presents with symptoms of volume depletion (Table 12-2). It should be noted that hypernatremic volume depletion causes movement of water out of cells into the extracellular compartment (including the plasma space); therefore, it is associated with relative preservation of the circulation for any given amount of volume lost when compared to isotonic dehydration. This is very important, since all the clinical symptoms related to the circulation e.g. blood pressure and orthostatic changes, are attenuated in hypernatremic volume depletion and may be overlooked. Hypernatremia associated with increased volume will have symptoms such as edema, hepatomegaly and venous congestion.

In addition, signs and symptoms referable to the hypernatremia itself relate mostly to disturbances in the central nervous system. Lethargy, weakness, irritability, hypertonicity, nuchal rigidity, muscle twitching, focal and generalized convulsions and even paresis have been described. The neurological symptoms are related to water movement out of the brain cells. Thus, when an osmotic gradient is created, water instantly moves out of the brain cells and other cells to adjust to the solute concentration. The consequence is that the brain shrinks. Since the brain is encased in a rigid skull and the veins are under continuous pressure from the cardiac pump, they may rupture. It has been estimated that a 30 to 35 mOsm/kg is required to cause neurological symptoms. Thus, plasma Na >155 to 160 mEq/L (15–20 mEq of Na + the accompanying anion) puts the patient at risk for clinically apparent neurological symptoms.

III. Disturbances in Potassium Concentration

Total body K concentration (TBK) varies with sex, age and muscle mass. In general, TBK is estimated at about 50 mEq/kg body weight. Of this total, 98 to 99% is intracellular (primarily within muscle), having an average concentration of about 125 mEq/L. Extracellular K normally remains in the 3.5 to 4.5 mEq/L range. The transcellular K distribution can be modified by several factors including the acid-base status, insulin, catecholamine levels and plasma osmolality. In addition to redistribution of transcellular K, plasma K concentration is also regulated by the kidneys. Thus, although some of the ingested K is eliminated in sweat and stool, over 90% is excreted by the kidney. The renal excretion of K also varies with the plasma K concentration, the level of glomerular filtration, the acid-base status and various hormone levels.

A. Hypokalemia

Hypokalemia is defined as a plasma K concentration of less than 3.0 mEq/L. It has been estimated in adults that a decrease in plasma K concentration from 4.0 to 3.0 mEq/L reflects an approximately 10% reduction in TBK, and a decrease from 4.0 to 2.0 mEq/L suggests a 15 to 20% reduction in TBK. Table 12-7 summarizes the causes of hypokalemia.

1. Artifactual Hypokalemia

Hypokalemia without K depletion may be fictitious. For example, leukemic patients with a white blood cell count over 100,000 may have artifactual hypokalemia because white blood cells can extract K from plasma.

2. Redistribution Hypokalemia

Redistribution of K from the extracellular into the intracellular spaces produces hypokalemia. Alkalemia or an increase in HCO_3 can redistribute K and lead to an apparent hypokalemia. It should be noted that severe K depletion (serum K <2.0 mEq/L) itself causes metabolic alkalosis; therefore, the finding of alkalosis may be either the cause of redistribution hypokalemia or the result of true K depletion. Administration of glucose, glucose and insulin or insulin alone can cause hypokalemia because insulin drives K intracellularly. It should be noted that diabetic hyperglycemia also causes true hypokalemia due to osmotic diuresis, vomiting and decreased K intake. Beta-adrenergic agents such as metaproterenol used in the treatment of asthma can cause redistribution hypokalemia. Redistribution hypokalemia can occur in a rare autosomal dominant disorder of periodic paralysis. It presents in the first or second decade and is believed to be an abnormality in the excitation-contraction coupling mechanism in the muscle. The paralysis occurs at variable intervals in association with hypokalemia and lasts between 6 to 24 hours, at which time K returns to normal levels. The attacks can be precipitated by high carbohydrate diet, exercise, infections and alcohol ingestion and is relieved by carbonic anhydrase inhibitors, such as acetozalamide. Other causes of redistribution of K are presented in Table 12.7.

3. True Hypokalemia

True K depletion constitutes the largest and most important category of hypokalemia. The causes can be divided into primarily extrarenal and renal.

a. Hypokalemia of Extrarenal Etiology

Within the extrarenal category, inadequate intake is an unusual cause of hypokalemia but may occur in the setting of malnutrition, particularly kwashiorkor, anorexia nervosa or homemade infant formulas having a low K or chloride content. Unlike Na deprivation which leads to the virtual absence of urinary Na, renal K conservation takes time and is never complete. Thus, urinary K losses usually do not fall below 5 mEq/day and stool losses often continue between 5 to 10 mEq/day. In this setting, inadequate K intake may lead to K depletion over a period of time. Relatively inadequate intake of K can occur soon after initiation of treatment of severe anemias in which the increased demand for K from accelerated production of red blood cells precipitates hypokalemia. Transfusion of frozen washed cells may cause hypokalemia, since these cells are low in K and may leach plasma K.

Gastric losses (vomitus/gastric drainage) contain only about 10 mEq/L of K; however, loss of the acid gastric fluids can lead to alkalosis, volume depletion and elevated levels of aldosterone. The alkalosis decreases proximal HCO_3 reabsorption and increases HCO_3 delivery to the distal nephrons where, in the presence of increased aldosterone levels there is enhanced K secretion. Here, although the primary loss occurs through the gastrointestinal tract, there is also substantial renal K wasting and the urine K will be >20 mEq/L. In contrast to gastric losses, diarrhea losses are relatively high in K and, therefore, represent a direct route for K loss. However, unlike Na losses that parallel the volume of diarrhea, stool K tends to decrease as the stool volume increases. Volume depletion that often accompanies these situations stimulates aldosterone, which acts to conserve Na, and promotes K excretion in renal and intestinal epithelia. In addition to K, diarrhea losses include HCO_3 and the organic anions that are metabolized HCO_3. The resultant hyperchloremic metabolic acidosis also contributes to K wasting; however, since acidosis redistributes K extracellularly, the severity of hypokalemia may not be appreciated. Uncommon causes of hypokalemia in children include gastrointestinal fistulae, geophagia and laxative and enema abuse.

b. Hypokalemia of Renal Etiology

Renal K wasting should be suspected in the face of hypokalemia and urinary K over 20 mEq/L. It is useful to consider hypokalemia depending on the presence of accompanying acid-base disturbance (Table 12-7).

TABLE 12-7. Hypokalemia

Artifactual
  Extreme leukocytosis
Redistribution
  Alkalemia, increased bicarbonate
  Insulin
  Beta-adrenergic agonists
  Toxins: Toluene (paint and glue sniffing), barium salts (contaminated food), lithium salts
    (antidepressants)
  Extreme thyrotoxicosis
  Hypokalemic periodic paralysis
True Hypokalemia
  Extrarenal
    Inadequate intake
      Malnutrition (kwashiorkor)
      Anorexia nervosa
      Homemade formula with low K or Cl concentration
      Treatment of severe anemia
      Transfusion of frozen washed red blood cells
    Gastrointestinal
      Vomiting/gastric drainage
      Diarrhea
      Fistulae
      Laxative abuse
  Renal
    Associated with metabolic acidosis
      Proximal and distal renal tubular acidoses
      Ketoacidosis
      Ureterosigmoidostomy
    Associated with metabolic alkalosis
      Mineralocorticoid excess
        Primary hyperaldosteronism (bilateral adrenal hyperplasia, adenoma)
        Secondary hyperaldosteronism (renovascular disease, renin-secreting tumor such
          as hemangiopericytoma, Wilms' tumor)
      Glucocorticoid non-aldosterone mineralocorticoid excess
        Endogenous/exogenous excess of glucocorticoids
        Adrenogenital syndrome (17 alpha-hydroxylase/1 beta-hydroxylase deficiency)
    Variable acid-base status
      Licorice/chewing tobacco
      Liddle's syndrome
      Bartter's syndrome
      Diuretic phase of ATN/postobstructive diuresis
      Hypomagnesemia
      Drugs: Diuretics, penicillins, aminoglycosides, netilmicin, vitamin D, Amphotericin
        B, probenecid, *cis*platinum

Hypokalemia with acidosis occurs in renal tubular acidoses (RTA).
Proximal (Type II) RTA describes an abnormal reabsorptive capacity of
the proximal tubule for HCO_3. It is frequently accompanied by defective
reabsorption of other substances such as glucose, amino acids, phosphate

and uric acid. Initially, these patients are usually not hypokalemic, but the HCO_3 treatment for acidemia increases $NaHCO_3$ delivery to the distal nephron, which stimulates Na-K exchange and enhances kaluresis predisposing to hypokalemia. Secondary hyperaldosteronism due to concomitant volume depletion can amplify this exchange and exacerbate kaluresis. Distal (Type I) RTA describes an abnormality in the hydrogen secretion in the distal tubule and collecting duct where K wasting results from impairment of Na^+-H^+ exchange. This impairment also augments the Na^+-K^+ exchange. Acidosis of any cause depresses proximal tubule reabsorption, thereby increasing distal solute delivery, which augments the exchange of Na for K.

Ketoacidosis on presentation often has a normal serum K that reflects movement for K out of cells in response to the acidosis, insulinopenia and hyposmolality. However, true K deficiency is usually already established because of osmotic diuresis (glycosuria/nonreabsorbable ketoacids) and vomiting. This hypokalemia usually becomes evident when treatment with insulin and fluids is initiated.

Urinary tract diversion, using the sigmoid colon, can lead to hypokalemia, since Na and chloride are reabsorbed and exchanged for K and HCO_3 by the colonic segment. Thus, an increase in quantity of watery stools leads to hyperchloremic metabolic acidosis and hypokalemia. As noted above, hypokalemia due to gastrointestinal disorders can cause renal K losses, through volume depletion, acidosis and hyperaldosteronism.

Hypokalemia with alkalosis may be due to an excess amount of mineralocorticoids. This is characterized by metabolic alkalosis, salt retention, expansion of the extracellular space and frequently, hypertension without edema. Volume expansion leads to increased Na delivery to the distal nephron, which, in the presence of high mineralocorticoid activity, results in increased K losses. Some of the conditions leading to mineralocorticoid excess are noted in Table 11-7. Primary aldosteronism involves excess aldosterone secretion by a benign tumor, hyperplasia or, occasionally, carcinoma within the adrenal glands. Renin levels are low, aldosterone levels are high, and hypertension is a characteristic feature, with hypokalemic alkalosis being a prominent finding. In addition to primary aldosteronism, overproduction hyperaldosteronism can be caused by stimulation of the renin-angiotensin system. This stimulation is not related to the volume status and occurs with renin-secreting tumors and with vascular disease (e.g. hemangiomata, Wilms' tumor and renovascular disease (e.g. diabetic or hypertensive nephropathy). Unlike primary aldosteronism, the renin level here is high. The mechanism of hypokalemia in these conditions is also due to increased delivery of Na and/or elevated aldosterone levels, that promote urinary K wasting.

In addition to excess mineralocorticoids, excess glucocorticoids can cause hypokalemia with alkalemia, e.g. adrenocorticotropic hormones

(ACTH)-producing malignancies in the pituitary or with adrenal glucocorticoid overproduction. In these instances, aldosterone levels are normal and renal K wasting and hypokalemia are due to increased Na
delivery because of the higher rate of glomerular filtration, rather than
to increased Na^+-K^+ exchange in the distal tubule.

Adrenogenital syndrome, or congenital adrenal hyperplasia, is a genetic
defect in adrenal biosynthesis of cortisol and sex hormones. In 17-alpha-
hydroxylase deficiency, cortisol deficiency increases ACTH, corticosterone and deoxycorticosterone secretion. Excess mineralocorticoids in this
condition suppress both renin and aldosterone. This condition presents
as a pseudohermaphrodism in males; and females who appear normal at
birth, subsequently fail to develop secondary sexual characteristics. In
11-beta-hydroxylase deficiency, there is abnormal production of cortisone
and excessive production of adrenal androgens; renin and aldosterone
are not increased. Girls present with hermaphrodism, and boys who appear normal at birth develop early virilization.

Miscelleneous disorders that cause hypokalemia but are not associated
with acid-base disturbances are noted in Table 12.7. Licorice and chewing
tobacco have been associated with a mineralocorticoid-excess picture,
complete with hypokalemia but without an actual excess in corticosteroids. Liddle's syndrome is a familial disorder characterized by failure
to thrive, hypokalemia, Na retention, hypertension, alkalosis, low renin
and low aldosterone, without an increase in other mineralocorticoids.
The defect in this syndrome is believed to be a generalized increase in
the permeability of cell membranes, including renal tubules, to Na.

Bartter's syndrome is a rare disease characterized by hyperaldosteronism, metabolic alkalosis, severe hypokalemia and normotension with
a resistance to the pressor actions of angiotensin II and norepinephrine
(see Chapter 11).

The diuretic phase of acute tubular necrosis (ATN) can cause hypokalemia that may relate to increased Na and water delivery to the distal
nephron segments and increase the Na-K exchange. There may also be
a defect in the K reabsorption by a previously damaged proximal segment
of the nephron. Similarly, postobstructive diuresis may precipitate excessive electrolyte losses, including K.

Diuretics cause hypokalemia by increasing delivery of solutes and water
to distal nephron segments, which enhances K secretion. Many of the
circumstances that warrant the use of diuretics, e.g. congestive heart failure or nephrotic syndrome or the volume contraction induced by the
diuretics themselves, cause secondary hyperaldosteronism, which, in the
face of diuretic-induced increased distal tubal delivery, will amplify K
wasting. Concomitant alkalosis, which can accompany diuretic therapy,
causes transcellular movement of K and urinary K wasting. Penicillins
can cause hypokalemia by acting as nonreabsorbable anions causing urinary K losses. Aminoglycosides cause K wasting. Aminoglycosides also

cause magnesium (Mg) wasting, which in itself causes hypokalemia. Unexplained hypokalemia warrants investigation of the Mg level. Diuretics, gentamicin and *cis*platinum can cause both hypokalemia and hypomagnesemia.

4. Clinical Manifestations of Hypokalemia

The clinical manifestations of hypokalemia are summarized in Table 12-8, and the associated electrocardiographic features are shown in Figure 12-1.

TABLE 12-8. Clinical Manifestations of Hypokalemia

Cardiac
    Electrocardiographic abnormalities (flattening of T wave, ST depression, prolonged PR
       interval)
    Ventricular ectopy
    Predisposition to digitalis intoxication

Neuromuscular
    Skeletal: weakness, cramps, rhabdomyolysis, paralysis (including respiratory)
    Smooth muscles: gastric distention, ileus, constipation, urinary retention

Renal/metabolic
    Polyuria/polydipsia
    Azotemia—decreased in renal blood flow and GFR, interstitial nephritis
    Metabolic alkalosis
    Decreased blood pressure, decreased peripheral vascular resistance
    Decreased level of aldosterone
    Increased level of renin
    Glucose intolerance due to decreased insulin secretion

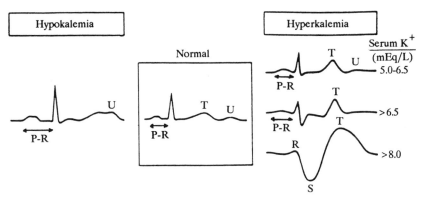

FIGURE 12-1. Electrocardiographic manifestations of hypo- and hyperkalemia. Hypokalemia: Flattening of T wave, prolonged PR interval, and appearance of U wave. Hyperkalemia: Tall narrow T wave, widened and flattened P wave, widening of PR interval and QRS complex. From Tannen RL (1987) The patient with hypokalemia and hyperkalemia. In: Schrier RW (ed) Manual of Nephrology. 2nd Ed. Little, Brown and Co., Boston, p 35, with permission.

B. Hyperkalemia

Hyperkalemia is defined as plasma concentration of K greater than 5.5–6.5 mEq/L, depending on age. In newborns up to three weeks of age, serum K up to 7 mEq/L is accepted as normal. Hyperkalemia may be classified into artifactual, redistribution and true K excess (Table 12-9).

1. Artifactual Hyperkalemia

Since hyperkalemia is a potentially lethal condition, there must be strong evidence that the elevated K value is artifactual. If there is any doubt, an electrocardiogram should be obtained for evidence of hyperkalemia, while a repeat sample is drawn. A common cause of artifactual hyperkalemia in the pediatric population is ischemic blood drawing. Prolonged and severe tourniquet application can release K from muscles of the extremity. The serum does not appear pink. Hemolysis, particularly from heel sticks, is another cause of hyperkalemia, since K is released from the lysed red blood cells. This can be seen by examining the serum, which will be pink. In vitro release of K from leukocytes, platelets and red blood cells during clot retraction process can also cause hyperkalemia, i.e. leukocytosis ($>100,000$) and thrombocytosis (platelets $>1,000,000$) can artifactually increase K. Potassium assayed in a heparanized sample will be normal. Abnormal red cell membrane or fragility can also cause an apparent increase in K. Infectious mononucleosis can increase membrane permeability of the cellular components of blood and cause movement of K out of cells thereby causing artifactual hyperkalemia.

2. Redistribution Hyperkalemia

As noted in the beginning of this section, changes in pH affect plasma K. It is commonly estimated that 0.1 unit decrease in pH will increase K concentration by 0.6 mEq/L. However, the relationship depends upon several factors including the type of acidosis (metabolic acidosis changes K concentration more than respiratory acidosis); the nature of the anion accompanying the accumulating hydrogen ion (mineral acids, such as HCl or NH_4Cl, change K concentration more than organic acids, such as lactate or ketoacids); duration of acidosis (acute acidemia directly inhibits distal tubule K secretion but a longer duration decreases proximal tubule reabsorption and causes a greater distal delivery which stimulates K secretion) and extent of intracellular buffering (unless there is profound hypokalemia, acidemia will cause K to move out of cells and hydrogen ions to move in).

Hyperglycemia, in diabetes mellitus, promotes movement of intracellular K into the extracellular space, and in the absence of insulin, which normally stimulates cellular uptake of K, hyperkalemia develops. Although ketoacidosis is not as powerful a stimulus as mineral acid acidosis

TABLE 12-9. Hyperkalemia

Artifactual
  Ischemic blood drawing
  Hemolysis
  Leukocytosis/thombocytosis
  Abnormal red blood cell membrane
  Infectious mononucleosis

Redistribution
  Acidosis
  Hyperglycemia:
    Insulin insufficiency
  Poisoning: drugs/toxins
    Digitalis
    Beta-adrenergic blockers (Inderal, Corgard)
    Succhinylcholine (muscle relaxant used in anesthesia)
    Arginine and lysine HCl (with insulin used in provocative testing for growth hormone release)
    Chemotherapeutic agents
    Fluoride (component of rat poisoning)

True K Excess

Increased K load	Decreased K excretion	
Exogenous load	Reduced GFR	Relatively preserved GFR
Potassium supplements	Acute renal failure	Low aldosterone
Salt substitutes	Chronic renal failure	Addison's disease
Penicillin K		Adrenal biosynthetic defect
Stored blood		Hyporeninemic hypoaldosteronism
Riverbed clay		Drugs: indomethacin, heparin, ACE inhibitors (captopril, enalapril), cyclosporine
Endogenous load		
Tissue necrosis		Normal/high aldosterone
Internal hemorrhage		Pseudohypoaldosteronism
Intravascular coagulopathy		Obstructive nephropathy
Tumor lysis syndrome		Sickle cell nephropathy
		SLE
		Drugs (spironolactone triamterene, amiloride)

in causing cellular translocation, it may contribute to hyperkalemia in diabetic ketoacidosis. Drugs that cause transcellular movement of K from intracellular stores include cardiac glycosides, most prominently digitalis; beta adrenergic blockers (propranolol); the depolarizing muscle relaxant succinylcholine; arginine or lysine hydrochloride (together with insulin, these agents are used in provocative tests for growth hormone secretion); cancer therapeutic agents and sodium fluoride (which is a component of rat poison). All of these agents may be potentially more dangerous in patients predisposed to increased TBK stores including those with renal failure or diabetes mellitus.

3. True Hyperkalemia

True hyperkalemia may be due to increased K intake or more commonly decreased ability to excrete K. Increased K load, in the face of normal renal function, is a distinctly unusual cause of hyperkalemia. A common source of exogenous K is oral and parenteral K supplements. Oral K preparations usually contain 5 to 25 mEq/tablet or packet. Other substances that present a K load include salt substitutes (contain ~ 12 mEq/g of K), penicillin K (1.7 mEq of $K/10^6$ units), stored blood, which after three weeks can have a K concentration of 30 mEq/L and riverbed clay (ingested). Endogenous routes for K load include tissue necrosis (rhabdomyolysis, trauma, burns), massive intravascular coagulopathy, extreme catabolic states, gastrointestinal bleeding and reabsorption of hematoma (cephalohematoma in the newborn). Finally, initiation of therapy in certain cancers having large tumor burdens (Burkitt's lymphoma, Hodgkin's disease and certain leukemias) can lead to hyperkalemia from the rapid destruction of large numbers of cells.

Decreased K excretion occurs when kidney function is profoundly impaired, but can also occur in the face of relative preservation of kidney function (Table 12-9). In acute renal failure, hyperkalemia occurs because the reduced GFR limits the elimination of K. In addition, since distal tubules secrete K, decreased distal delivery of solutes and water limits K-Na exchange and decreases K excretion. Acute renal failure is also frequently associated with tissue breakdown and acidosis, which present an extra K load. Chronic renal failure also causes hyperkalemia. Progressive renal impairment that occurs over a period of time induces the remaining functioning nephrons to excrete more K per nephron, hence, hyperkalemia is unusual in chronic renal failure until the GFR falls to 5 to 10% of normal. Chronic renal failure also induces several other adaptive mechanisms to dispose of a K load: there is increased K loss in the stool and more rapid redistribution of a given K load into cells.

Potassium regulation is under profound mineralocorticoid influence. Therefore, even in the face of relatively preserved renal function, a reduced level of mineral-corticoid or responsiveness to mineralocorticoids can precipitate hyperkalemia. Decreased mineralocorticoid activity, regardless of etiology, causes hyperkalemia (Table 12-9). Addison's disease describes the combined mineralocorticoid and glucocorticoid deficiency that occur with adrenal aplasia/hypoplasia or adrenal destruction (autoimmune processes, infection, tumors). Presentation of this condition relates mainly to deficiency in mineralocorticoids including hyponatremia, hyperchloremic acidosis and hyperkalemia, which is exacerbated during episodes of stress. Adrenal biosynthetic defects can result in mineralocorticoid overproduction and K wasting (see causes of hypokalemia), or mineralocorticoid deficiency and hyperkalemia. The most common mineralocorticoid deficiency is 21-hydroxylase deficiency. Here, there is a deficiency of both mineralocorticoids and glucocorticoids, together with an overproduction of adrenal androgens. Affected patients present with salt wasting, hyperkalemia, viralization and failure to thrive. Three-β-ol-dehydrogenase deficiency is another mineralocorticoid deficiency characterized by decreased aldosterone, cortisone and testosterone production. In addition to ambiguous genitalia, these patients exhibit salt wasting and hyperkalemia. Finally, isolated aldosterone deficiency has been described and results from a defect in the enzyme required to convert corticosterone to aldosterone. It usually presents early in life with salt wasting and hyperkalemia.

Hyporeninemic hypoaldosterone states are a relatively common cause of hyperkalemia. Secondary hypoaldosteronism results from an impairment in renin production and is well recognized in chronic renal insufficiency, especially with diabetic nephropathy or tubulointerstitial disease (obstruction nephropathy, pyelonephritis). The characteristics of this syndrome are low renin, low aldosterone, an adequate level of glomerular filtration and normal cortisone levels. Diagnosing this syndrome can be difficult, since hyperkalemia itself lowers aldosterone levels. Thus, aldosterone levels may be normal while the patient is hyperkalemic and the diagnosis can only be confirmed when the serum K is normalized and a low aldosterone level is observed.

Drugs can decrease renin/aldosterone and lead to hyperkalemia. The prostaglandin synthetase inhibitor indomethacin can decrease renin secretion and cause the syndrome of hyporeninemic hypoaldosteronism. In addition, prostaglandin inhibition may lower distal tubule delivery of salt and water by decreasing the GFR, inhibiting K secretion. Converting enzyme inhibitors (enalapril, captopril) decrease angiotensin II generation and, therefore, aldosterone production, producing the picture just described. It should be noted that converting enzyme inhibition does not lower plasma renin activity. Heparin directly inhibits the enzymes in aldosterone synthesis. Cyclosporine has also been observed to produce hyperkalemia; however, the mechanism is not yet clear.

If the GFR is not profoundly reduced and the mineralocorticoid levels are not depressed, hyperkalemia suggests resistance of the renal tubule to mineralocorticoids. Pseudohypoaldosteronism describes an abnormality in the adrenal biosynthesis that causes failure to thrive, acidosis, salt wasting, hyponatremia and hyperkalemia. However, plasma renin and aldosterone level are elevated and there is no response to mineral-ocorticoid replacement. This syndrome represents a relative insensitivity of the renal tubule to aldosterone. Pseudohypoaldosteronism II presents in late childhood and adulthood with hyperkalemia, acidosis, low plasma renin activity, normal or low aldosterone with salt wasting and usually hyperkalemia. The underlying defect may be increased tubule chloride reabsorption, which results in low plasma renin activity, low aldosterone and impaired K secretion.

Hyperkalemia in sickle cell disease relates to damage of the distal and collecting tubules and/or the disruption of the normal medullary architecture. Some patients with sickle cell disease may have the syndrome of hyporeninemic hypoaldosteronism. Other disorders in which impaired tubule secretion of K has been described include systemic lupus erythematosis, obstructive nephropathy, interstitial nephritis and renal transplantation. Diuretic drugs, such as spironolactone, which is an aldosterone antagonist, impair K secretion, whereas triamterine and amiloride impede K secretion by an aldosterone-independent action.

4. Clinical Manifestations of Hyperkalemia

The electrocardiagraphic manifestations of hyperkalemia are shown in Figure 12-1. The important clinical manifestations of hyperkalemia relate to increased excitability of the cell membrane, particularly within the heart. The earliest electrocardiographic changes include increased amplitude of the T-wave and sometimes ST depression. Next may be an increased PR interval and widening of the QRS complex; the P wave may be flattened or may completely disappear. It should be noted that, although ventricular fibrillation is the typical arrhythmia, any arrhythmia may be seen. Furthermore, cardiac toxicity may occur without any preceding EKG changes. Finally, it must be noted that the hyperkalemia that occurs rapidly is associated with greater toxicity at any given level of K than the hyperkalemia that develops gradually. Furthermore, hyperkalemia is known to be potentiated by certain conditions such as hyponatremia, hypocalcemia and acidemia.

References

1. Finberg L, Krarath RE, Fleischman AR (1982) Water and Electrolytes in Pediatrics. Pathophysiology and Treatment. WB Saunders, Philadelphia
2. Holliday MA, Barratt TM, Vernier RL (1987) Pediatric Nephrology, 2nd edition. Williams and Wilkins, Baltimore
3. Paneth N (1980) Hypernatremic dehydration of infancy. Am J Dis Child 134:785–792
4. Rodriguez-Soriano J, Vallo A, Castillo G, et al (1981) Renal handling of water and sodium in infancy and childhood: a study using clearance methods during hypotonic saline diuresis. Kidney Int 20:700–704

5. Rose BD (1984) Clinical Physiology of Acid-Base and Electrolyte Disorders. McGraw-Hill, New York
6. Santosham M, Daum RS, Dillman L, et al (1982) Oral rehydration therapy of infantile diarrhea. N Engl J Med 306:1070–1076
7. Spitzer A (1981) The role of the kidney in sodium homeostasis during maturation. Kidney Int 21:539–545
8. Winters RW (1982) Principles of Pediatric Fluid Therapy, 2nd edition, Winters RW (ed). Little, Brown & Co., Boston
9. Ichikawa I (ed) (1989) Pediatric Textbook of Fluids and Electrolytes. Williams and Wilkins, Baltimore (in press)
10. Svenningsen NW, Aronson AS (1974) Postnatal development of renal concentration capacity as estimated by DDAVP-test in normal and asphyxiated neonates. Biol Neonate 25:230–241
11. Felig P, Baxter JD, Broaders AE, et al (eds) (1987) Endocrinology and Metabolism, 2nd edition, McGraw-Hill, New York

13
Acid-Base Disturbances

JUAN RODRIGUEZ-SORIANO

I. Introduction

Acid-base abnormalities are extremely common in pediatrics. There are two fundamental types of acid-base disorders, metabolic and respiratory. Metabolic acidosis and alkalosis are abnormal conditions caused by a primary decrease or increase, respectively, of the metabolic component of the Henderson-Hasselbach equation, i.e. plasma bicarbonate (HCO_3^-) concentration. Respiratory acidosis and alkalosis are abnormal conditions caused by a primary increase or decrease, respectively, of the respiratory component of the Henderson-Hasselbach equation, i.e. partial pressure of carbon dioxide (pCO_2). The clinician is often faced with the problem of distinguishing between single and mixed acid-base disorders. An understanding of basic concepts of acid-base physiology and the limits of physiological compensation for each primary abnormality will generally permit an easy approach to diagnosis and therapy (1–5).

II. Basic Physiology

A. Hydrogen Ion Concentration and pH

Blood pH is regulated within narrow physiological limits of 7.35 to 7.45, with a mean value of 7.40. Although pH represents a measure of hydrogen ion (H^+) activity rather than concentration, it has become customary to use it for clinical purposes. Normal H^+ ranges between 45 and 35 nEq/L, with a mean of 40 nEq/L (1 nEq = 10^{-6} mEq). It is important to know that in the usual range of observed acid-base disturbances (blood pH from 7.2 to 7.5), there is an almost linear relationship between parameters: each 0.01 unit change in pH represents a change in H^+ concentration of about 1 nEq/L. Beyond those limits, the relationship is curvilinear, and conversion should be made by using a nomogram (Figure 13-1).

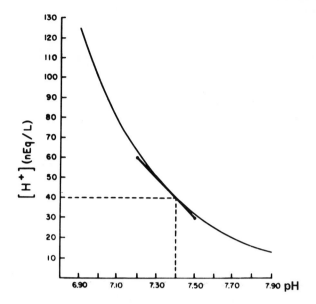

FIGURE 13-1. Relationship between pH and H⁺ concentration (nEq/L). Over the pH range of 7.20 to 7.50, each 0.01 unit change in pH represents a change in H⁺ concentration of about 1 nEq/L. A normal blood pH of 7.40 corresponds to a H⁺ concentration of 40 nEq/L. From Cohen JJ (1979) Disorders of hydrogen ion metabolism. In: Early LE, Gottschalk CW (eds) Strauss and Welt's Diseases of the Kidney. Little, Brown and Co, Boston, pp 1543–1579, with permission.

B. Buffer Systems and Regulation of Blood pH

The Brønsted-Lowry concept defines an acid as a H⁺ (or proton) donor, and a base as a H⁺ (or proton) acceptor. Acids and bases may be classified as strong or weak according to whether they dissociate completely or partially in a solution. A buffer is a substance that, by its presence in a solution, can counteract changes in pH in a solution, when acid or alkali is added, by converting strong acids or alkalis (bases) to more weaker compounds. A buffer system, or pair, is formed by a weak acid and the conjugate base of this weak acid. Buffering occurs immediately; it constitutes the first line of defense against abnormalities of acid-base equilibrium in the body.

Buffers in body fluids may be divided into bicarbonate (HCO_3^-) and non-bicarbonate systems. In man, the pair carbonic acid (H_2CO_3)/bicarbonate (HCO_3^-), represents the principal buffer system, contributing to 53% of the total buffering capacity of the blood. This is due to the capacity of the lungs and kidneys to regulate the components of the blood: the lungs can volatilize the weak acid (H_2CO_3) of the buffer pair and maintain a constant blood carbon dioxide (CO_2) concentration, and the kidneys can regenerate the conjugate base lost in the buffer reaction and maintain the plasma HCO_3^- concentration within normal limits. Total nonbicarbonate buffering of the blood amounts to 47%, of which hemoglobin and oxyhemoglobin contribute about 35%, and organic phosphates, inorganic phosphates and plasma proteins the remaining 12% (1).

Blood pH is dependent on the relationship between the metabolic component (HCO_3^-) and respiratory component (CO_2) of the buffer system. This relationship is expressed by the Henderson-Hasselbach equation:

$$pH = pK + \log \frac{[HCO_3^-]}{[H_2CO_3] \text{ (or } \alpha pCO_2)}$$

where α represents the constant of solubility of CO_2, which corresponds to 0.03 at 37 °C. The pK (a constant) is related to the strength of the weak acid. In the case of the H_2CO_3 dissolved in plasma, the value is 6.10. Thus in a normal individual, the corresponding values of the Henderson-Hasselbach equation will be as follows:

$$7.40 = 6.10 + \log \frac{24}{1.2}$$

In infants and young children, HCO_3^- concentration is slightly lower (20–22 mEq/L) because the immature kidney reclaims less HCO_3^- than the mature kidney. Blood pH, however, remains close to 7.40 because the plasma pCO_2 undergoes a compensatory decrease (6,7).

It should be remembered that most clinical laboratories do not actually measure HCO_3^- concentration but rather total CO_2 concentration. Bicarbonate concentration can be easily calculated by subtracting the amount corresponding to dissolved CO_2 ($pCO_2 \times 0.03$) or by using the Sigaard-Andersen nomogram (Figure 13-2). This nomogram also can be used to obtain one of the three variables of the Henderson-Hasselbach equation when the other two are known.

The Henderson-Hasselbach equation can be rearranged by expressing H^+ concentration (instead of pH) in terms of pCO_2 and HCO_3^- concentration:

$$[H^+] = 24 \times \frac{pCO_2}{[HCO_3^-]}$$

This equation can be used clinically to estimate the concentration of one component when any two components are known, if the Sigaard-Andersen nomogram is not available. A nomogram is also available for the graphic interpretation of these acid-base relationships (4) (Figure 13-3).

Although the measurements of pH, HCO_3^- concentration and pCO_2 permit one to determine the the acid-base equilibrium, it must be remembered that nonbicarbonate buffer systems also play an important role in homeostasis. The *total buffer base* is the sum of all the conjugate

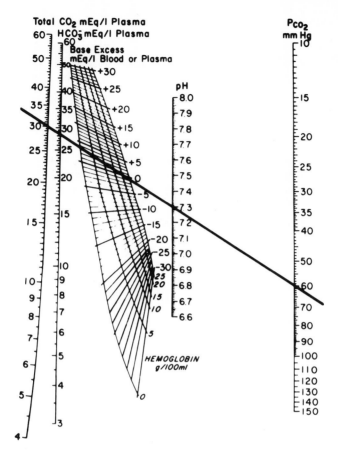

FIGURE 13-2. Siggaard-Andersen nomogram. The nomogram is copyrighted by Radiometer, Copenhagen, with permission.

bases present in 1L of whole blood, which, in normal adults, is about 48 mEq/L at a hemoglobin concentration of 15 g/100 mL. The *base excess* indicates possible changes from this normal value, and is positive or negative according to whether the measured value is greater or smaller than the normal value expected for the concentration of hemoglobin. The normal value of base excess should be around zero in adults and children, but it may be slightly negative in infants (-3 mEq/L). Base excess can also be obtained using the Sigaard-Andersen nomogram.

C. Anion Gap

The anion gap (*AG*) is the difference between the plasma concentration of sodium (Na^+) and the sum of the plasma concentrations of chloride (Cl^-) and bicarbonate (HCO_3^-):

$$AG = [Na^+] - ([Cl^-] + [HCO_3^-])$$

These "unmeasured" anions (normally 8 to 16 mEq/L) include negatively charged proteins, phosphate, sulfate and organic anions.

The value of the anion gap is used to evaluate acid-base abnormalities (8,9). In the absence of renal insufficiency, an *elevated anion gap* (>16 mEq/L) usually reflects an accumulation of organic acids (lactate, hydroxybutyrate, acetoacetate, etc.) in the body fluids, whereas a *normal anion gap*, as observed in hyperchloremic metabolic acidosis, indicates the loss of endogenous HCO_3^- via the gastrointestinal system or the kidney. This rule does not hold when hydrochloric acid or salts which are metabolically converted to hydrochloric acid (ammonium chloride, arginine hydrochloride, lysine hydrochloride, etc.), have been administered. The classic teaching is that the anion gap is normal during metabolic alkalosis. However, recent studies have shown that an elevated anion gap may be observed due to the fact that plasma proteins are generally increased

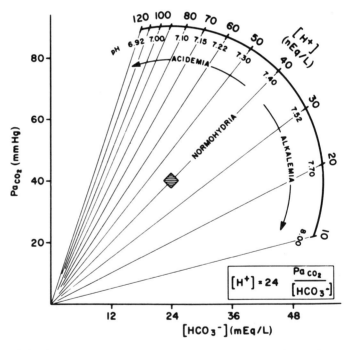

FIGURE 13-3. The Cohen nomogram shows plasma concentrations of carbon dioxide tension (Pa_{CO_2}), bicarbonate (HCO_3^-) and hydrogen ion (H^+) at chemical equilibrium. The algebraic form of these relationships is depicted at lower right. From Cohen JJ (1979) Disorders of hydrogen ion metabolism. In: Early LE, Gottschalk CW (eds) Strauss and Welt's Diseases of the Kidney. Little, Brown and Co, Boston, pp 1543–1579, with permission.

because extracellular fluid (ECF) is depleted and because of the increase in their net anionic equivalency as a result of their titration during the coexisting alkalemia (10). Thus, an elevated anion gap during metabolic alkalosis does not necessarily imply a simultaneous metabolic acidosis. A *low anion gap* (< 8 mEq/L) is very rarely observed in pediatrics; when present, it frequently represents a laboratory error in the measurement of plasma electrolytes. However, it must be recognized that a low anion gap may be seen in cases of hypoproteinemia. On the average, a decrease in plasma albumin concentration of 1 g/100 mL reduces the anion gap by about 3 mEq/L (11).

D. Regulation of Acid-Base Equilibrium

A second line of defense against an abnormal acid-base equilibrium involves the physiological responses of respiratory or renal systems. Normally, the catabolism of food and the process of growth produces approximately 1.5 to 2.0 mEq/kg of H^+ daily (12), which must be immediately buffered and eliminated through the kidneys. Also, CO_2 is produced in enormous quantities in the tissues (about 200 mmol/kg daily) by the combustion of fat and carbohydrates. Carbon dioxide behaves as a weak acid and maintains an equilibrium with its hydrated form (H_2CO_3). Thus, the regulating system must not only be able to excrete the H^+ accumulated by the kidneys but also the CO_2 accumulated by the lungs. Both regulatory systems are complex, and less efficient than the buffer mechanisms. Minutes or hours are required for respiratory adjustment, whereas hours or days are required for renal adjustment. Both systems tend to work together to maintain the normal ratio of the Henderson-Hasselbach equation: the lungs act to regulate of the respiratory component (pCO_2), while the kidneys regulate the metabolic component (HCO_3^-) concentration.

E. Respiratory Regulation

Under normal conditions, plasma pCO_2 remains constant at about 40 mm Hg because the loss of CO_2 through alveolar ventilation is exactly equivalent to its metabolic production. If CO_2 production remains constant, a change in alveolar ventilation will change the plasma pCO_2; if alveolar ventilation remains constant, changes in CO_2 production will be followed by changes in plasma pCO_2 (13).

The stimuli acting at the level of the respiratory centers are pH, pCO_2 and the partial pressure of oxygen (O_2) (pO_2). Assuming normal oxygenation, an increase in CO_2 would increase alveolar ventilation because both the low pH and the high pCO_2 would stimulate the respiratory centers. If blood pH falls without a primary change in CO_2 production, alveolar ventilation will increase and this will induce a secondary lowering of plasma pCO_2. The final result will be less than expected because the fall in pCO_2 will offset, in part, the effect of acidemia (low pH).

The mechanism is reversed when the blood pH is elevated. The inhibition of the respiratory center exerted by the alkalemia will be almost completely reversed by the secondary increase in pCO_2. This phenomenon may explain in part why respiratory compensation for a state of metabolic alkalosis is less effective than the compensation observed after a comparable degree of metabolic acidosis.

F. Renal Regulation

Regulation of systemic pH is critically dependent upon the ability of the kidneys to maintain the plasma HCO_3^- concentration within normal limits. Given a normal glomerular filtration rate (GFR) of 180 L/day and a plasma HCO_3^- concentration of 24 mEq/L, the kidneys filter approximately 4300 mEq/day of HCO_3^-, which must be reclaimed through tubular reabsorption. Also, the amount of HCO_3^- lost buffering the endogenously produced H^+, or through losses via the gastrointestinal tract, must be compensated for by the kidneys.

Roughly 90% of filtered HCO_3^- is reabsorbed in the proximal tubule by a high capacity, low gradient system, which facilitates H^+ secretion (and HCO_3^- reabsorption) but cannot lower the luminal pH below 6.7 because of the activity of the luminal carbonic anhydrase. Reclamation of the remaining 10% of filtered HCO_3^-, and the regeneration of HCO_3^- via the titration of the luminal nonbicarbonate buffers phosphate (HPO_4^{-2}) and ammonia (NH_3), take place in the distal nephron. Secretion of H^+ depends on a low capacity, high gradient system catalyzed by a powerful H^+ translocating ATPase. The excretion of titrable acid (mainly in the form of $H_2PO_4^-$ and NH_4^+ minus the excretion of HCO_3^-) expresses the *net acid excretion* , or real contribution of the kidneys to the regeneration of HCO_3^-. The amount of H^+ utilized in this process represents only about 3% of the total tubular secretion of H^+, since most of the H^+ has been utilized to reabsorb filtered HCO_3^-. For a more detailed description of the cellular mechanisms involved in renal H^+ and HCO_3^- transport, the reader is referred to a recent review (14).

III. Single Acid-Base Abnormalities

A correct approach to diagnosis and treatment of acid-base abnormalities requires a knowledge of both the type and the degree of physiological compensation that takes place in each primary abnormality. The change in blood pH resulting from primary metabolic or respiratory disorders depends on the adjusted change in the ratio HCO_3^-/pCO_2 once compensation has occurred. This compensation can be *complete* or *partial,* according to whether the pH of the blood has been completely or partially restored to the normal range, respectively. It is important to differentiate properly the *single* from the *mixed* disorders of acid-base equilibrium (Table 13-1). A single metabolic or respiratory disorder involves secondary compensation in the component that is not primarily affected (Table 13-2). In a mixed disorder, two components are primarily affected at the same time, and compensation is not possible. Careful determinations of the appropriate degree of secondary compensation for any type of primary disorder has permitted the better diagnosis of mixed disorders (Figure 13-4). Physiological compensation is quantitatively limited, and distinguishing between a compensated single disorder and a mixed disorder is only possible if we know the confidence limits of the secondary compensation for the primary disorder of a given severity.

As pointed out by Winters (1), the clinician should also differentiate between physiological language and laboratory language when discussing to acid-base abnormalities. Physiologically, the terms *acidosis* and *alkalosis* are synonymous with abnormal conditions caused by the buildup or loss of acid or base from the ECF. In laboratory language, the terms *acidosis* and *alkalosis* are synonymous with a measured change in blood pH. Although acidosis generally leads to a low pH, and alkalosis to a high pH, this does not always occur because the pH of the blood may be normal if complete compensation has occurred or if another primary disorder is also present. The use of the terms *acidemia* and *alkalemia* (instead of acidosis and alkalosis) to define changes in blood pH will obviate this nosologic confusion in part.

TABLE 13-1. Classification of Acid-Base Abnormalities

I. Single disorders
  A. Metabolic
    1. Acidosis
    2. Alkalosis
  B. Respiratory
    1. Acidosis
      a. Acute
      b. Chronic
    2. Alkalosis
      a. Acute
      b. Chronic
II. Mixed disorders
  A. Mixed metabolic and respiratory acidosis
  B. Mixed metabolic and respiratory alkalosis
  C. Mixed metabolic acidosis and respiratory alkalosis
  D. Mixed metabolic alkalosis and respiratory acidosis

TABLE 13-2. Physiological Compensation of Primary Acid-Base Abnormalities

Disorder	Primary disturbance	Secondary compensation	Adjusted HCO_3^-/pCO_2	Expected range of compensation
Metabolic acidosis	Metabolic component: HCO_3^- loss	Respiratory component: pCO_2 decreases	$\downarrow\downarrow HCO_3^-/\downarrow pCO_2$	$\Delta pCO_2 = 1.0 - 1.3 \times \Delta HCO_3^-$
Metabolic alkalosis	Metabolic component: HCO_3^- gain	Respiratory component: pCO_2 increases	$\uparrow\uparrow HCO_3^-/\uparrow pCO_2$	$\Delta pCO_2 = 0.6 \times \Delta HCO_3^-$
Respiratory acidosis	Respiratory component: CO_2 gain	Metabolic component: HCO_3^- increases	$\uparrow HCO_3^-/\uparrow\uparrow pCO_2$	Acute: $\Delta HCO_3^- = 0.1 \times \Delta pCO_2$ Chronic: $\Delta HCO_3^- = 0.35 \times \Delta pCO_2$
Respiratory alkalosis	Respiratory component: CO_2 loss	Metabolic component: HCO_3^- decreases	$\downarrow HCO_3^-/\downarrow\downarrow pCO_2$	Acute: $\Delta HCO_3^- = 0.2 \times \Delta pCO_2$ Chronic: $\Delta HCO_3^- = 0.5 \times \Delta pCO_2$

$\downarrow$ = decrease; $\uparrow$ = increase; Δ = change in concentration or partial pressure.

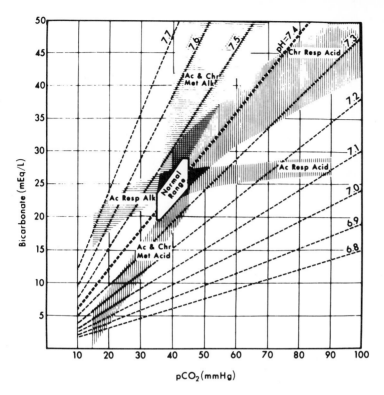

FIGURE 13-4. The Arbus nomogram shows bands of physiological compensation for single metabolic or respiratory acid-base disorders. From Arbus GS (1973) An in vivo acid-base nomogram for clinical use. Can Med Assoc J 109: 291–293, with permission.

IV. Metabolic Acidosis

Metabolic acidosis refers to an abnormal physiological process when either a gain of acid or loss of base from the ECF exceeds the renal capacity to regenerate HCO_3^-. The primary decrease in plasma HCO_3^- concentration causes a fall in blood pH, which can be partly compensated for by a secondary increase in alveolar ventilation (Table 13-2). The chemoreceptors in the respiratory centers of the medulla respond to changes in blood pH, but this response achieves its maximal level in 12 to 24 hours, possibly because H^+ passes slowly across the blood-brain barrier. Most patients with metabolic acidosis would already have achieved a steady state with respect to their maximal respiratory compensation by then. Thus, the degree of the ventilatory response can be assessed in terms of its adequacy to the degree of metabolic acidosis present.

The fall of plasma HCO_3^- concentration is linearly related to the secondary fall of plasma pCO_2 (Figure 13-4), as shown by the following equation:

$$\text{Expected } pCO_2 = 1.5 \text{ (measured } HCO_3^-) + 8 \pm 2$$

In general, for each 1 mEq/L decrease in plasma HCO_3^- concentration, there is a decrease of 1 to 1.3 mm Hg in plasma pCO_2 (2). When pCO_2 values fall outside the confidence limits, the presence of a superimposed respiratory acidosis (above) or alkalosis (below), should be suspected. In most cases, such a fall in pCO_2 permits only a partial correction of blood pH, since fully compensated metabolic acidosis only occurs with mild degrees of acidosis. A normal blood pH during physiological metabolic acidosis should suggest the presence of an associated primary respiratory alkalosis.

A delay H^+ equilibration between the blood and the cerebrospinal fluid (CSF) may explain the presence of a transient respiratory alkalosis when patients with sustained metabolic acidosis are acutely treated with exogenous alkali. This respiratory "overshoot" lasts about 12 hours and reflects the lag in the respiratory center adjustment.

A. Clinical and Laboratory Characteristics of Metabolic Acidosis

The clinical manifestations of metabolic acidosis generally reflect the primary causes of the disorder. However, a state of severe metabolic acidosis may directly suppress cardiac contractility, potentiate ventricular arrythmias or cause peripheral vascular resistance to fall.

Kussmaul respiration is specially evident when plasma HCO_3^- concentration is under 15 mEq/L. A very profound acidemia may result in lethargy or coma. In children, chronic metabolic acidosis may also be responsible for anorexia and failure to grow. Buffering of excess H^+ by bone salts and a concomitant inhibition of 1,25-dihydroxy vitamin D_3 may cause osteomalacia or osteoporosis.

The laboratory workup should always include the study of plasma electrolytes and calculation of the anion gap. Knowing the potassium ion plasma (K^+) levels is of great value in the differential diagnosis of renal tubular acidosis. It is important to know that, even in the face of some body K^+ deficiency, plasma K^+ concentration may be normal or slightly increased due to intracellular K^+ outflow. Urinary studies must always include determination of pH and excretion of the ammonium ion. The finding of a highly acid urine with an elevated NH_4^+ in a patient with an increased anion gap practically rules out the diagnosis of renal tubular acidosis.

B. Differential Diagnosis of Metabolic Acidosis

The etiological mechanisms involved in the development of metabolic acidosis are summarized in Table 13-3. In general, when faced with a patient with this disorder, it is very useful to differentiate patients with

TABLE 13-3. Causes of Metabolic Acidosis

I. With normal anion gap
  A. Renal loss of bicarbonate
    1. Administration of carbonic anhydrase inhibitors
    2. Renal tubular acidosis
    3. Posthypocapnic acidosis
  B. Gastrointestinal loss of bicarbonate
    1. Diarrhea
    2. Ileostomy drainage, digestive fistulae
    3. Ureterosigmoidostomy or ileal bladder or conduits
    4. Administration of cation exchange resins
  C. Miscellaneous
    1. Administration of HCl, NH_4Cl, arginine-HCl, lysine-HCl
    2. Parenteral nutrition
    3. "Dilution" acidosis
II. With elevated anion gap
  A. Increased production of acid
    1. Ketoacidosis (e.g. starvation, diabetes mellitus, ketogenic hypoglycemia, ethanol ingestion
    2. Lactic acidosis and other organic acidemias
    3. Toxins (e.g. salicylate, methanol, ethylglycol, paraldehyde)
  B. Decreased excretion of acid
    1. Acute renal failure
    2. Chronic renal failure

a normal anion gap from patients with an elevated anion gap. A *normal anion gap* is associated with hyperchloremia and reflects a loss of HCO_3^- from the ECF via the gastrointestinal tract or the kidney.

An *elevated anion gap* is mainly observed when ketoacids, lactic acid or other organic acids accumulate through a variety of metabolic mechanisms and when inorganic acids (phosphoric acid and sulfuric acid), which are normally excreted by the kidney, are retained because of acute or chronic renal insufficiency. The finding of hypochloremia in patients with elevated anion gap acidosis does not necessarily imply the presence of metabolic alkalosis, since it may be due to an expansion of the ECF compartment secondary to the extrusion of cellular cation during buffering (17).

C. Renal Tubular Acidosis

The term *renal tubular acidosis* (RTA) is applied to a group of tubular transport defects in the reabsorption of filtered HCO_3^-, the excretion of H^+ or both, which can result from a large number of etiologies. Renal tubular acidosis is characteristically associated with hyperchloremia and a normal anion gap; it occurs in patients with relatively normal glomerular function. On clinical and pathophysiological grounds, RTA can be classified as follows:

1. Proximal Renal Tubular Acidosis (Type 2)

Under ordinary circumstances, virtually all filtered HCO_3^- is reabsorbed by the renal tubules. If the plasma HCO_3^- concentration exceeds the level of the renal threshold (because of exogenous administration of alkali, for example), HCO_3^- reabsorption is incomplete so that the plasma concentration is gradually lowered to a level below the threshold; then HCO_3^- reabsorption ceases and a new steady state is reached. The level of the HCO_3^- threshold varies with age (25–26 mEq/L in adults, 23–24 mEq/L in children, ~ 22 mEq/L in infants) (6).

Patients with proximal RTA present with a diminished renal HCO_3^- threshold, and HCO_3^- is present in the urine when the HCO_3^- plasma level is lower than for normal individuals of a similar age; accordingly, a steady state is maintained with the plasma HCO_3^- concentration in the acidemic range. A characteristic feature of this disorder is the intact ability to lower urine pH and to excrete adequate amounts of titrable acid and NH_4^+ when the plasma HCO_3^- concentration is below the particular renal threshold of the patient. Conversely, when the plasma HCO_3^- concentration is normalized by exogenous administration of alkali, the urine is highly alkaline and contains a large amount of filtered HCO_3^- (> 10–15%).

Proximal RTA can be observed under a variety of circumstances (Table 13-4). In children, it is most frequently observed in association with the Fanconi syndrome but it may also appear as an isolated entity, which can be either transient or persistent. The possible influences of extrinsic renal factors (hyperkalemia, ECF volume expansion, chronic hypocapnia, secondary hyperparathyroidism) should be excluded before making the diagnosis of an intrinsic tubular disease.

2. Distal Renal Tubular Acidosis (Type 1)

This type of RTA is characterized by an inability to lower urine pH maximally (<5.5) during systemic acidemia. Diminished excretion of titrable acid and NH_4 is secondary to such a defect. In general, HCO_3^- reabsorption is quantitatively normal, but as consequence of the elevated urine pH, a certain degree of bicarbonaturia may be obligatorily present ($<5\%$ of the filtered load). Pathogenetically, distal RTA can be classified into several subtypes (20), as follows:

a. Distal RTA with a "Secretory Defect"

This is due to the failure of the distal nephron to secrete H^+ because of the reduced number or impaired function of the H^+ secretory pumps.

b. Distal RTA with a "Voltage-Dependent Defect" (Hyperkalemic Distal RTA)

This is due to the inability of the distal nephron to generate and maintain a negative intratubular potential difference because of a defect in distal Na^+ delivery or transport. Abolishment of the transtubular electric gra-

TABLE 13-4. Causes of Renal Tubular Acidosis

I. Proximal RTA (Type 2)
   A. Primary
      1. Sporadic (transient in infancy)
      2. Familial (persistent)
   B. Secondary
      1. Associated with Fanconi syndrome
      2. Drugs and toxic substances (e.g. carbonic anhydrase inhibitors, degraded tetracyclines, heavy metals, "experimental" maleic acid administration in animals)
      3. Associated with other clinical entities (e.g. hyperparathyroidism, nephrotic syndrome, cyanotic heart disease)
II. Distal RTA (Type 1)
   A. Primary
      1. Persistent (adult type, associated with bicarbonate wasting in infants, associated with nerve deafness)
      2. Transient (in infancy?)
   B. Secondary
      1. Disorders of mineral metabolism
      2. Hyperglobulinemic states
      3. Drugs and toxins (e.g. amphotericin B, toluene, lithium, amiloride)
      4. Associated with other renal diseases (e.g. renal transplantation, medullary sponge kidney, obstructive uropathy)
      5. Associated with genetic disorders (e.g. salt-losing congenital adrenal hyperplasia, osteopetrosis, sickle-cell disease)
III. Hyperkalemic RTA (Type 4)
   A. Primary
      1. "Early-childhood" hyperkalemia (transient)
   B. Secondary
      1. States of aldosterone deficiency without renal disease
      2. Hyporeninemic hypoaldosteronism in patients with chronic renal disease
      3. "Chloride-shunt" syndrome
      4. Primary or secondary pseudohypoaldosteronism
      5. Drugs (e.g. heparin, potassium-sparing diuretics, prostaglandin-inhibitors, captopril, cyclosporine)

dient will also reduce K^+ secretion in the cortical collecting tubule; thus, patients with this type of defect present with hyperkalemia.

c. Distal RTA with a "Gradient Defect"

This is due to the inability of the kidney to create a steep H^+ gradient across the distal nephron, because of a leakage of the secreted H^+ back into the cell or the entry of cellular HCO_3^- into the lumen. This type of RTA could result from an increased permeability of the luminal membrane to H^+, H_2CO_3 or HCO_3^-.

The "secretory" defect is characteristic of primary distal RTA; "voltage-dependent" and "gradient" defects have different and varied etiologies (Table 13-4).

3. Hyperkalemic Renal Tubular Acidosis (Type 4)

This type of RTA is seen in many hyperkalemic states and probably is not a single pathophysiological entity. It is characterized by a normal ability to acidify the urine after an acid load and to increase urinary pCO_2 after a HCO_3^- load, provided that glomerular function is not greatly impaired. The defect is characterized by the inability of the tubules to excrete enough NH_4^+ as a direct consequence of the increased cellular stores of K^+. Aldosterone deficiency, ECF volume contraction and renal insufficiency may be contributing factors.

In children, hyperkalemic RTA is observed in hyporeninemic hypoaldosteronism, "chloride-shunt" syndrome, salt-losing congenital adrenal hyperplasia, and primary or secondary pseudohypoaldosteronism. It is also an idiopathic, transient condition in infants and young children (Table 13-4).

V. Functional Tests to Assess Urine Acidification Defects

A. Functional Evaluation of Bicarbonate Reabsorption

1. Bicarbonate Titration (6,7)

Tubular reabsorption of HCO_3^- is tested by measuring the rate of reabsorption and excretion of this substance at different filtered loads. This is achieved by infusing sodium bicarbonate ($NaHCO_3$) at a rate that slowly increases plasma HCO_3^- concentration. Simultaneous determinations of concentrations of HCO_3^- and creatinine (or inulin) in blood and urine permit the calculation of the rates of reabsorbed and excreted HCO_3^-, which are plotted against the corresponding plasma HCO_3^- concentration (Figure 13-5). Ideally, the study should be initiated at low plasma HCO_3^- concentrations, when reabsorption of filtered HCO_3^- is complete and no HCO_3^- is present in the urine. The ECF volume expansion should be minimized and it should not be necessary to increase the plasma HCO_3^- concentration above 25 to 26 mEq/L. Calculating the Tm reabsorption is useless since it would reflect only volume expansion. A simple calculation of the renal HCO_3^- threshold allows a diagnosis of a HCO_3^- reabsorption defect to be made.

Our protocol consists of a 2.8% $NaHCO_3$ solution (0.33 mEq/mL) infusion. The infusion rate necessary to increase plasma HCO_3^- concentration by about 3 mEq/hour can be calculated by the following formula:

$$\text{Rate (mL/hr)} = \frac{3 \times 0.4 \times \text{body weight (kg)}}{0.33}$$

Blood and urine samples should be taken every 30 to 60 minutes. Bladder cathererization can be avoided if HCO_3^- excretion rates are expressed as

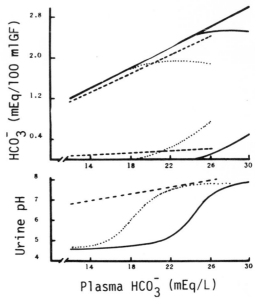

FIGURE 13-5. Functional evaluation of bicarbonate (HCO_3^-) reabsorption in the renal tubules. —— Normal subjects (> 2 years of age); ––– distal renal tubular acidosis; ⋯ proximal renal tubular acidosis.

percent of amount filtered, since an accurate estimate of urine volume is not required.

2. Plasma Bicarbonate-Urine pH Relationship

A practical approach to study tubular handling of HCO_3^- consists of simply monitoring the urine pH during the $NaHCO_3$ infusion. If the urine pH is consistently alkaline before the plasma HCO_3^- concentration returns to normal, the patient has a reduced renal HCO_3^- threshold. If the plasma HCO_3^- concentration is normalized before the urine pH becomes clearly alkaline, the patient has a normal renal HCO_3^- threshold. The diagnosis is best established by comparing the observed relationship to the normal relationship between plasma HCO_3^- concentration and urine pH (21) (Figure 13-5).

3. Bicarbonate Excretion at Normal Plasma Concentration

If large amount of alkali is required to correct the plasma HCO_3^- concentration at about 22 mEq/L, and excretion at this plasma concentration is more than 15% of the filtered load, there is probably a proximal tube defect in HCO_3^- reabsorption (22). Although most patients with severe proximal RTA will be identified by this method, milder forms of the disorder, or the presence of a concomitant distal defect, could be missed. In our opinion, the diagnosis of proximal RTA always requires the demonstration of a normal capacity to excrete acid urine when an appropriate stimulus is applied.

B. Functional Evaluation of Distal Hydrogen Ion Secretion

1. Assessment of Urine pH

The measurements of minimal urine pH and maximal rates of titrable acid and NH_4 in acidemia are basic to assessing the integrity of the mechanisms of distal urinary acidification. It should be recalled that urine pH represents the activity in the urine of free H^+, which is less than 1% of the total amount of protons excreted in the distal nephron. A normally low urine pH does not mean that the distal acidification mechanism is normal if NH_4 is low; and vice versa, a patient in whom NH_4 excretion has been stimulated may have a urine pH as low as 6.0 without having a defective acidification mechanism. Urine pH must always be evaluated in conjunction with the urinary NH_4 content to assess the distal acidification process adequately (23). Traditionally, distal H^+ secretion is assessed during spontaneous metabolic acidemia or following the acute oral administration of ammonium chloride (NH_4Cl). In general, urine pH and net acid excretion are evaluated at plasma HCO_3^- concentrations a few milliequivalents below the renal HCO_3^- threshold (about 18–20 mEq/L, depending on the age of the subject) when the low capacity, high gradient distal system is functioning maximally. In the short NH_4Cl loading test proposed by Edelmann et al (24) 100 mEq/m² of NH_4Cl is administered orally. The dose for a given subject should be calculated on the basis of the plasma HCO_3^- concentration prior to the administration of the acid load, which is given by mouth over one hour. It must be taken either as gelatin capsules or dissolved in water flavored with lemon juice or sugar so that the patient does not vomit. Urine must be collected for at least the following six hours. A practical protocol is to administer the load at home, at midnight, and to study the patient early in the morning. The response of normal infants and children is presented in Table 13-5.

In cases of hepatic or gastric intolerence to NH_4Cl, oral calcium chloride (2 mEq/kg) (25) or intravenous arginine-HCl (200–250 ml/m² of 10% solution) over two to three hours (26) may be used, respectively. Even though these short tests do not increase NH_4 excretion maximally, they are reliable clinically.

Urine pH also falls abruptly to less than 5.5 during the infusion of sodium sulfate (Na_2SO_4) or following the acute administration of furosemide (27). Both substances enhance H^+ and K^+ secretion in the cortical collecting tubule by increasing distal Na^+ delivery and by generating a high electronegative luminal charge at that nephron segment. The ability to reabsorb Na^+ in the cortical collecting tubule may be enhanced by administering 9-α-fluorocortisone (0.1 mg), 12 hours before the test is started. Sulfate is given as a 0.2 M Na_2SO_4 solution. After a control period, a priming dose is administered [5 mL × 0.3 × weight (kg)], followed by

TABLE 13-5. Urinary Hydrogen Ion Excretion after Ammonium Chloride Loading[a]

	Infants (1–12 months)	Children (4–15 years)
Urine pH	≤ 5.0	≤ 5.5
Titrable acid[b] (μEq/min/1.73 m²)	62 (43–111)	52 (33–71)
Ammonium[b] (μEq/min/1.73 m²)	57 (42–79)	73 (46–100)

[a]Edelmann CM Jr, Rodriguez-Soriano J, Boichis H, Gruskin AB, Acosta MI (1967) Renal bicarbonate reabsorption and hydrogen ion excretion in normal infants. J Clin Invest 46: 1309–1317; and Edelmann CM Jr, Boichis H, Rodriguez-Soriano J, Stark H (1967) The renal response of children to acute ammonium chloride acidosis. Pediatr Res 1: 452–460
[b]Mean ± 2 SD.

the 90-minute infusion, at a rate of 0.75 mL/1.73 m² a minute. Urine collections are continued for three hours from the start of the infusion.

Furosemide (1 mg/kg) is given as an intravenous bolus. Although maximal natriuresis and kaliuresis occur immediately, the maximal acidification effect is observed 120 minutes after administration of the drug. Urine collections should be continued for at least three hours following administration. The simultaneous determination of plasma renin activity and aldosterone concentration before, and three hours after drug administration, also permits an assessment of the renin-aldosterone axis. This test is very useful in clinical practice but it should not be used in place of the classic NH$_4$Cl loading test because failure to acidify the urine after furosemide administration does not necessarily imply an irreversible defect.

2. Urine pCO$_2$ as an Index of Distal Acidification

a. Urine pCO$_2$ During Bicarbonate Administration

When the urine is highly alkaline, such as following a massive load of NaHCO$_2$, urine pCO$_2$ increases as a direct result of cortical collecting duct H$^+$ secretion. Hydrogen ion reacts with luminal HCO$_3^-$ to form H$_2$CO$_3$. Since carbonic anhydrase is not present in the lumen, H$_2$CO$_3$ in the medullary collecting duct slowly forms CO$_2$, which is trapped in this area of the kidney. A necessary requirement of the test is that urine pH and HCO$_3^-$ concentration increase above 7.6 and 80 mEq/L, respectively. A 1 M solution of NaHCO$_3$ may be given intravenously (3 mL/1.73 m² a minute) or NaHCO$_2$ orally (4 g/1.73 m² as a single dose). Normal children increase the urine minus blood pCO$_2$ gradient to values of 46 ± 3.7 (SEM) mm Hg, at a mean urine pH of 7.74 + 0.10 (28).

b. Urine pCO₂ During Neutral Phosphate Administration

Neutral phosphate directly stimulates cortical collecting duct H^+ secretion to increase urinary pCO_2, provided that the urine pH is close to the pK of the phosphate buffer system (i.e. 6.8). At this urine pH, half of the phosphate is in the monobasic form ($H_2PO_4^{-2}$), which can titrate HCO_3^-, to increase the pCO_2 in the urine. The increase in urinary pCO_2 observed after phosphate administration is greater than that observed after HCO_3^- loading. We have found that an oral phosphate load is as effective as infused phosphate to significantly increase the in urinary pCO_2. A total dose of 54 mg/kg of elemental phosphorus (P) is divided into three aliquats, which are given at eight-hour intervals. If the urine pH is under 6.8 at the time the third dose is given, an oral $NaHCO_3$ load (2 g/1.73 m²) is also given. In a study of 18 normal children, we found that urine phosphate excretion increased to 44.8 ± 4.7 (SEM) mmol/L and that urine minus blood pCO_2 gradient increased to 68.8 ± 7.00 mm Hg, with a urine pH of 6.87 ± 0.07 (29). With a urine phosphate concentration above 20 mmol/L, all normal children achieved a urine minus blood pCO_2 above 40 mm Hg.

VI. Diagnostic Workup of the Patient with Renal Tubular Acidosis

Renal tubular acidosis should be suspected, in general, when there is a hyperchloremic, normal anion gap metabolic acidosis of obscure extrarenal etiology. As depicted in Figure 13-6, the first step in the diagnostic workup is the measurement of plasma K^+, to determine whether the RTA is normo-, hypo-, or hyperkalemic. The urinary anion gap ($Na^+ + K^+ - Cl^-$), as a rough index of urinary NH_4^+, has been suggested for an initial evaluation of hyperchloremic metabolic acidosis (30). A positive anion gap suggests a decrease in distal urinary acidification.

A. Renal Tubular Acidosis with Normokalemia or Hypokalemia

Proximal and distal RTA should be differentiated. The initial, and more important step is the measurement of urine pH. This should be performed by a pH electrode (not by simple dipstick method, which is greatly inaccurate). Urine pH may be alkaline in the presence of urinary tract infection with urea-splitting organisms. If acidemia is present, determining urine pH in the first- or second-morning urine is very useful and a preliminary acid loading is not necessary.

When the urine pH is less than 5.5, the diagnosis of distal RTA can be firmly ruled out. The suspicion of proximal RTA is frequently strength-

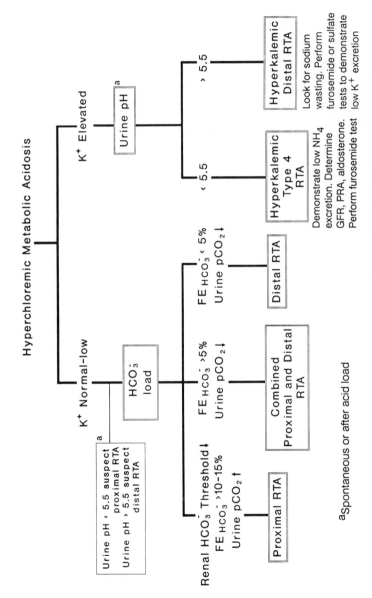

FIGURE 13-6. Diagnostic workup of the patient with hyperchloremic metabolic acidosis.

ened by other signs of proximal tubular dysfunction (glycosuria, phosphaturia, amino aciduria). Bicarbonate loading will confirm the diagnosis either by demonstrating a low renal HCO_3^- threshold (directly measured or assumed because of an abnormal plasma HCO_3^- − urine pH relationship) or by a high urine pCO_2 and an elevated fractional excretion of HCO_3^- at normal plasma HCO_3^- concentrations. When the patient is not able to decrease urine pH to less than 5.5 during mild or moderate degrees of spontaneous acidemia, the diagnosis of proximal RTA is not completely excluded and an acid loading test should be performed to bring the plasma HCO_3^- concentration below the patient's threshold.

The inability to lower urine pH to less than 5.5 suggests a diagnosis of distal RTA. Bicarbonate loading will support this diagnosis when the urine pCO_2 does not increase appropriately in highly alkaline urine. The associated presence of a defect in tubular HCO_3^- reabsorption should be suspected when fractional HCO_3^- excretion exceeds 5% of the filtered load at normal HCO_3^- concentrations. A persistent inability to lower urine pH during acid loading will definitely establish the diagnosis of distal RTA alone, or along with proximal RTA. Assessing plasma K^+, urine pH and urine pCO_2 under different functional conditions will distinguish the different pathogenetic types of distal RTA (Table 13-6).

B. Renal Tubular Acidosis with Hyperkalemia

In hyperkalemic patients, the first step is to determine the pH of the urine. A finding of an elevated urine pH during spontaneous or induced metabolic acidosis identifies a small group of patients with hyperkalemic distal RTA caused by a voltage-dependent defect. In our experience, children frequently have associated salt wasting and, accordingly, the etiologies to be suspected are salt-losing congenital adrenal hyperplasia or pseudohypoaldosteronism, primary or secondary to obstructive uropathy.

TABLE 13-6. Pathogenetic Diagnosis of Distal Renal Tubular Acidosis

	Secretory defect	Voltage-dependent defect		Gradient defect
		Mild	Severe	
Urine pH during acidosis	↑	↑	↑	↑
Urine pH during sodium sulfate infusion	↑	↓	↑	↓
Urine pH after furosemide administration	↑	↓	↑	↓
Urine/blood pCO_2 gradient in alkaline urine	↓	↓	↓	N ↓
Urine/blood pCO_2 gradient during phosphate administration	↓	↑	↓	↑
Plasma potassium ion	N ↓	N ↑	N ↑	N ↓

N = normal; ↑ = increase; ↓ = decrease.

When the ability to acidify the urine to less than 5.5 is normal, and NH_4^+ excretion is low, the diagnosis of hyperkalemic (Type 4) RTA is established, and the workup should be directed to determine its etiology. A study of glomerular filtration rate and the renin-aldosterone axis will determine the cause of the hypoaldosteronism or the pseudohypoaldosteronism.

VII. Metabolic Alkalosis

This refers to an abnormal physiological process caused by either an excess of HCO_3^- in or a loss of acid from the ECF. Elevating the plasma HCO_3^- concentration will increase blood pH, which will be partly compensated by depressed alveolar ventilation (Table 13-2). The alkalemia depresses respiratory drive by inhibiting the respiratory centers. As in metabolic acidosis, respiratory compensation is not immediate and may take 12 to 24 hours to reach its maximal efficacy.

In contrast to the highly predictable relationship present in metabolic acidosis, the 95% confidence limits for respiratory compensation in metabolic alkalosis are wide, and many patients, especially those with a profound K^+ deficiency, do not undergo an appreciable degree of respiratory compensation. The following equation has been proposed to predict changes in pCO_2 for each primary change in plasma HCO_3^- concentration (31):

$$\text{Expected } pCO_2 = 0.9 \text{ (measured } HCO_3^-) + 9$$

In practical terms, for each 1 mEq/L increase in plasma HCO_3^- concentration, plasma pCO_2 increases 0.6 mm Hg. If this is not seen, despite the passage of adequate time, another primary acid-base abnormality should be sought. The diagnosis of a mixed disorder is easy when the pCO_2 is less than normal, but not so when the pCO_2 is normal or slightly increased, given an irregular, unpredictable respiratory response.

A. Generation, Maintenance and Correction of Metabolic Alkalosis

One characteristic of metabolic alkalosis is its persistence even after the original cause has been corrected. In some circumstances, as in metabolic alkalosis caused by a mineralocorticoid excess, there is volume expansion (volume-expansion alkalosis); recovery here does not require the administration of Cl^- but rather requires the administration of K^+ ("chloride-resistant" metabolic alkalosis). In contrast, metabolic alkalosis caused by vomiting or prolonged diuretic therapy is associated with volume contraction; although K^+ is depleted, its correction requires the obligatory administration of Cl^- salts ("chloride-responsive" metabolic alkalosis).

The kidney plays a critical role in the generating and maintaining metabolic alkalosis, except for that caused by the exogenous administration of alkali (32). Volume-expansion alkalosis is generated and maintained by increased distal H^+ and K^+ secretion in exchange for Na^+. Potassium depletion increases the excretion of acid by producing an intracellular acidosis and by increasing the lumen-negative transtubular potential difference in the cortical collecting tubule. Generation of volume-contraction alkalosis also depends on increased distal H^+ secretion in exchange for Na^+, to compensate for the amount of Na^+ that has not been reabsorbed with Cl^- in the proximal tubule. Its maintenance, however, is critically dependent on volume contraction and K^+ deficiency. Volume contraction increases proximal HCO_3^- reabsorption and contributes to the decrease in distal HCO_3^- delivery by reducing the absolute amount of HCO_3^- filtered. Potassium deficiency presumably also contributes to an increase in the proximal HCO_3^- reabsorption and, as mentioned earlier, stimulates distal H^+ secretion. This classic interpretation of the pathogenesis of volume-contraction (or chloride-depletion) alkalosis has recently been disputed. Data obtained in rats with chloride-depletion alkalosis without volume depletion strongly suggest that the maintenance and correction of this type of metabolic alkalosis primarily depend upon total body Cl^- and its influence on intrarenal mechanisms, not on the demands of Na^+ or fluid homeostasis (33).

B. Clinical and Laboratory Characteristics of Metabolic Alkalosis

No specific signs or symptoms point to a diagnosis of metabolic alkalosis. The physical signs that are occasionally present are tetany or generalized convulsions, which are more related to the associated hypocalcemia or hypomagnesemia than to the alkalosis itself. Since K^+ deficiency is regularly seen in chronic metabolic alkalosis, this electrolyte abnormality may be predominant.

The laboratory workup should always include the study of plasma and urine electrolytes. Increased plasma HCO_3^- concentration is associated with hypochloremia and hypokalemia. The anion gap may increase 5 to 6 mEq/L, but, in contrast with metabolic acidosis, this increase has no diagnostic significance. Volume contraction elevate plasma concentrations of urea and creatinine and stimulate the renin-aldosterone axis. The urine pH is generally under 6.0 because of increased proximal HCO_3^- reabsorption and distal H^+ secretion. The urine pH may be over 6.0 when metabolic alkalosis is caused by the exogenous administration of alkali or when the renal mechanisms that permit the persistence of the alkalosis are not yet fully operative. Determination of urine Cl^- concentration is especially helpful in establishing the etiology of metabolic alkalosis. For reasons not clearly understood, many patients with chloride-depletion alkalosis also may present with moderate hypercalcemia and/or hypercalciuria.

C. Differential Diagnosis of Metabolic Alkalosis

There are many causes of metabolic alkalosis (Table 13-7). The urinary concentration of Cl⁻ is also very useful in determining whether volume contraction is present and whether Cl⁻ depletion has contributed to the alkalosis (34) (Table 13-8). When urine Cl⁻ concentration is less than 10 mEq/L, one must search for a dietary deficiency of Cl⁻ or for a loss of Cl⁻ through the gastrointestinal tract or the skin. The dietary chloride-deficiency syndrome has been observed in infants on low-chloride for-mulas (35). Excessive sweating in infants with cystic fibrosis may also lead to Cl⁻ depletion, if Cl⁻ intake is limited (36). Chronic diuretic ad-ministration may produce volume-contraction alkalosis with low urine Cl⁻. Posthypercapnic alkalosis is observed when a state of chronic res-piratory acidosis is abruptly corrected (by mechanical ventilation, for example) due to the continuing ability of the kidney to reabsorb HCO_3^- actively despite the normalization of plasma pCO_2. This posthypercapnic

TABLE 13-7. Causes of Metabolic Alkalosis

I. Increased intake or production of bicarbonate
   A. Administration of bicarbonate or its precursors (e.g. lactate, citrate, acetate)
   B. Combined ingestion of "nonabsorbable" antacids and cation-exchange resins in patients with end-stage renal disease
   C. Posthypercapnic alkalosis
II. Decreased intake of chloride
   A. Chronic ingestion of low chloride formulas
III. Increased excretion of hydrogen ion and/or chloride
   A. Gastrointestinal
      1. Vomiting secondary to pyloric stenosis or obstruction proximal to entrance of bile duct
      2. Gastric suction
      3. "Chloride-wasting" diarrhea
   B. Skin
      1. Cystic fibrosis (sweat losses)
   C. Renal
      1. Diuretic administration
      2. Renal tubular disorders (Bartter's syndrome, familial hypokalemia-hypomagnesemia, RTA with metabolic alkalosis)
      3. Mineralocorticoid and glucocorticoid excess (e.g. primary or secondary aldosteronism, Cushing syndrome, Liddle syndrome, licorice ingestion, creams or nasal sprays containing mineralocorticoids)
      4. Hypercalcemic states
      5. Potassium deficiency
IV. Miscellaneous
   A. "Contraction" alkalosis
   B. Hypoproteinemic alkalosis

TABLE 13-8. Urine Chloride Concentration as a Tool in the Differential Diagnosis of Metabolic Alkalosis

Urine chloride concentration <10 mEq/L	Urine chloride concentration >10 mEq/L
Ingestion of low chloride formulas	Bartter's syndrome
Loss of stomach contents	Familial hypokalemia-hypomagnesemia
"Chloride-wasting diarrhea"	Mineralocorticoid, glucocorticoid excess
Cystic fibrosis	Hypercalcemia
Chronic diuretic administration	Severe potassium deficiency
Posthypercapnic alkalosis	Hypoproteinemic alkalosis

state can be avoided if Cl$^-$ sufficient to permit the rapid excretion of the retained HCO_3^- is given. When the urine Cl$^-$ concentration is higher than 10 mEq/L, a renal tubular abnormality in Cl$^-$ reabsorption (Bartter's syndrome, familial hypokalemia-hypomagnesemia) or mineralocorticoid excess should be suspected. Clinicians should also be aware of cases caused by the use of creams or nasal sprays containing 9-α-fludrocortisone (37).

In the so-called hypoproteinemic alkalosis, plasma proteins behave as weak acids and alkalosis develops when their concentration in plasma is reduced. On average, a decrease in the plasma albumin concentration of 1 g/100 ml increases the HCO_3^- concentration by 3.7 mEq/L and reduces the anion gap by about 3 mEq/L (11).

VIII. Respiratory Acidosis

In respiratory acidosis, there is a primary elevation of plasma pCO_2. Any compromise in alveolar ventilation will cause a retention in CO_2 as a result of an imbalance between CO_2 production and excretion. The pCO_2 will stabilize at a higher level when the excretory rate of CO_2 equals its production rate. The retention of CO_2 in ECF will lead to a parallel increase in H_2CO_3. As in metabolic acidosis, the first line of defense will be the titration of nonbicarbonate buffers (Buf$^-$) by H_2CO_3.

$$CO_2 + H_2O \leftrightarrow H_2CO_3 + Buf^- \rightarrow HBuf + HCO_3^-$$

Although HCO_3^- is formed in this reaction, the total amount of buffer base remains unchanged because for each molecule of Buf$^-$ consumed, one molecule of HCO_3^- is produced. About six to twelve hours after the acute titration of tissue buffers a compensatory renal response begins, which is manifested by a further, gradual rise in plasma HCO_3^-. The kidney generates new HCO_3^- to maintain as normal a ratio of HCO_3^-/pCO_2 as possible. This process takes several days to attain its maximal efficacity. As HCO_3^- stores are being augmented, Cl^- stores are correspondingly depleted, since the excretion of NH_4^+ and Cl^- is increased. This hypochloremia counterbalances the increased plasma HCO_3^- concentration.

When the secondary physiological response is being assessed, it is important to distinguish between acute and chronic respiratory acidosis. During acute respiratory acidosis, there is virtually no significant renal compensation and the modest elevation in plasma HCO_3^- concentration is only due to titration of Buf^-. The amount of HCO_3^- produced in this manner is very small, and in general, plasma HCO_3^- concentration never exceeds 29 to 30 mEq/L. For each 10 mm Hg increase in pCO_2, plasma HCO_3^- concentration only rises about 1 mEq/L (2). If we look to values of base excess, however, we may find a paradoxical decrease of a few milliequivalents per liter. This is due to differences in the CO_2 "titration curves" of blood in vitro and in vivo. Part of the HCO_3^- formed in the in vivo buffer reaction leaks into the interstitial fluid, but when blood is titrated in vitro in the Astrup apparatus, such a loss will be recognized as a small negative base excess (1).

Chronic respiratory acidosis is associated with an important increment in plasma HCO_3^- concentration, which modifies the fall in blood pH, but is never sufficient to return it to its normal range. In general, for each 10 mm Hg increase in pCO_2, plasma HCO_3^- concentration increases by approximately 3.5 mEq/L (2). Increases in plasma HCO_3^- concentration below or above this expected range indicate a superimposed metabolic acidosis or alkalosis, respectively.

A. Clinical and Laboratory Characteristics of Respiratory Acidosis

The clinical picture of respiratory acidosis is related to the accompanying hypoxia and varies according to how fast hypercapnia develops. Acute respiratory acidosis is associated with marked anxiety, a sensation of breathlessness, reduced mental capacity and stupor.

Coma will appear when the pCO_2 rises to 70 to 100 mm Hg. Signs of hypoxia are more evident when the patient is breathing room air than when oxygen is being administered. Also, sedatives or muscle relaxants may mask the clinical picture. Paradoxically, when pCO_2 increases markedly, the patient may look more comfortable due to the depressant effect of CO_2 on the central nervous system (CNS). Carbon dioxide is a vasodilator and may produce flushing of the skin, dilation of retinal and brain vessels or even a rise in intracranial pressure with papilledema. Chronic respiratory acidosis will also increase hemoglobin concentration, and pulmonary hypertension can initiate right atrial and ventricular hypertrophy. In a patient with long-standing respiratory acidosis, hypoxia may help maintain respiration; thus, administration of high concentrations of oxygen may increase the hypercapnia, since there is no hypoxic stimulation of the respiratory centers.

Laboratory diagnosis of respiratory acidosis is based on demonstrating an increase pCO_2 associated with some degree of acidemia. The finding of hypercapnia in association with alkalemia would suggest either metabolic alkalosis or a mixed respiratory acidosis and metabolic alkalosis. A useful way to determine the presence of metabolic alkalosis in addition to a respiratory acidosis is to measure urinary Cl⁻; if it is more than 10 mEq/L, and no diuretic has been given in the hours preceding the test, an additional chloride-depletion alkalosis is unlikely.

B. Differential Diagnosis of Respiratory Acidosis

Table 13-9 shows the various etiological factors that can csuse acute or chronic respiratory acidosis. In general, any of these fall in one of the following groups: a) respiratory center depression, b) neuromuscular disorders, c) thoracic cage limitation and impaired lung motion, d) acute airway obstruction, and e) chronic obstructive lung disease. Interference

TABLE 13-9. Causes of Respiratory Acidosis

I. Depression of respiratory centers
  A. Sedatives, hypnotics
  B. Head injury
  C. Sleep apnea
II. Neuromuscular disorders
  A. Myopathies (e.g. myasthenia gravis, muscular dystrophy, botulism, potassium depletion)
  B. Neuropathies (e.g. Guillain-Barré syndrome, Werdnig-Hoffman disease, poliomyelitis, phrenic nerve palsy)
III. Thoracic cage limitation and impaired lung motion
  A. Pleural effusion
  B. Pneumothorax
  C. Severe pneumonia or pulmonary edema
  D. Chest injury
  E. Obesity (Picwick syndrome)
IV. Acute airway obstruction
  A. Aspiration
  B. Foreign body
  C. Severe laryngospasm or bronchospasm
  D. Acute laryngitis or laryngeal edema
  E. Bronchiolitis
V. Chronic obstructive lung disease
  A. Cystic fibrosis and advanced bilateral emphysema
  B. Hyaline membrane disease
  C. Bronchopulmonary dysplasia
VI. Miscellaneous
  A. Ventilator malfunction
  B. Cardiopulmonary arrest

with respiration at any of these levels reduces alveolar ventilation and elevates plasma pCO_2. In pediatrics, respiratory acidosis occurs frequently in the neonate during delivery, especially if the mother has been sedated. It is also observed in acute airway obstruction (acute laryngitis or epiglottitis, bronchiolitis, status asthmaticus), pleural effusion, pneumothorax, hyaline membrane disease, severe pneumonia, pulmonary edema or advanced cystic fibrosis.

IX. Respiratory Alkalosis

This refers to an acid-base abnormality characterized by a primary decrease in plasma pCO_2. An increase in alveolar ventilation produces a negative balance between CO_2 production and excretion. The falling pCO_2 will stabilize, albeit at a lower level, when CO_2 production equals CO_2 excretion. Hypocapnia, and the subsequent decrease in H_2CO_3 concentration, is followed by a lower plasma HCO_3^- concentration, due to the immediate response of tissue buffering:

$$HCO_3^- + HBuf \rightarrow Buf^- + H_2CO_3 \leftrightarrow CO_2 + H_2O$$

Although the decreased plasma HCO_3^- concentration counterbalances the alkalemia, the total buffer base remains unchanged because for each molecule of HCO_3^- consumed, one molecule of Buf^- is produced. This adaptive fall of plasma HCO_3^- concentration is not associated with any renal compensation, which takes several hours to occur. Changes in cellular metabolism will increase lactic acid and other organic acid concentrations.

Renal compensation will reduce the rate of HCO_3^- reabsorption and suppress NH_4^+ and Cl^- excretion. The decreased rate of NH_4^+ excretion is counterbalanced by increased excretion of Na^+ and K^+, and mild hypokalemia ensues. Plasma HCO_3^- concentration stabilizes at minimal low levels within two to four days of initiation of the hypocapnia. As in respiratory acidosis, it is important to distinguish between acute and chronic respiratory alkalosis. In acute respiratory alkalosis, the fall in plasma HCO_3^- concentration only reflects the consumption of HCO_3^- in the buffer reaction; it is not enough to prevent the increase in HCO_3^-/pCO_2 ratio and blood pH. The change in plasma HCO_3^- concentration is somewhat greater than that observed during a comparable acute respiratory acidosis: for each 10 mm Hg decrease in pCO_2, there is a decrease in plasma HCO_3^- concentration of about 2 mEq/L (2).

In chronic respiratory alkalosis, there is a highly predictable relationship between the degree of chronic hypocapnia and the fall in plasma HCO_3^-. The 95% confidence limits of the renal adaptation have been established in natives living at high altitudes, who are hypocapnic due to anoxia-induced hyperventilation. Plasma HCO_3^- concentration falls by

5 mEq/L for every 10 mm Hg fall in pCO_2 (2). This response appears to be more effective than that following chronic respiratory acidosis. Part of the HCO_3^- fall is due not to renal compensation but rather to the buffering action of lactic acid, which accumulates during hypoxia. This "lactic acid effect" is probably small and accounts for only a 0.5 to 1 mEq/L fall in plasma HCO_3^- concentration.

A. Clinical and Laboratory Characteristics of Respiratory Alkalosis

Respiratory alkalosis produces dizziness, numbness and tingling paresthesias of the lips and extremities. Occasionally, carpopedal spasm, seizures or even coma may occur. Hypocapnia produces cerebral vessel vasoconstriction and hypotension and decreases pulmonary vascular resistance. The most frequent electrocardiogram (ECG) changes are inversion of the ST segment and T waves; more rarely, alterations of the QRS complex may mimic the presence of myocardial ischemia. Hyperventilation may also induce electroencephalographic (EEG) changes, increasing the number of slow, high-voltage waves. It is noteworthy that marked hypocapnia may be present without clinical labored respiration.

The laboratory diagnosis of respiratory alkalosis is based on the demonstration of a decreased plasma pCO_2 associated with some degree of alkalemia. When hypocapnia is associated with acidemia, the diagnosis should be metabolic acidosis or mixed respiratory alkalosis and metabolic acidosis, as in cases of salicylate intoxication. Plasma electrolytes are normal, but hyperchloremia and mild hypokalemia may be present in cases of chronic hypocapnia. Blood lactic acid and pyruvic acid concentrations may be modestly increased.

B. Differential Diagnosis of Respiratory Alkalosis

Table 13-10 lists some of the more common causes of respiratory alkalosis. The factors leading to hyperventilation may operate at the level of respiratory centers of the CNS, or by stimulating peripheral chemoreceptors (hypoxia) or intrathoracic stretch receptors (localized pulmonary disease). In pediatrics, respiratory alkalosis is frequently seen as a consequence of respiratory stimulation produced by the anxiety and pain brought on by the blood sampling. Other frequent causes are fever, mild asthma, pneumonia, Gram-negative sepsis or brain trauma. Hyperventilation is also characteristically observed in salicylate intoxication (38,39), hepatic insufficiency (40) and necrotizing encephalopathy or Leigh's syndrome (41).

TABLE 13-10. Causes of Respiratory Alkalosis

I. Stimulation of respiratory centers
   A. Anxiety
   B. Drugs (e.g. salicylate, analeptic drugs, epinephrine)
   C. Fever
   D. Gram-negative sepsis
   E. Liver insufficiency
   F. Central nervous system (e.g. meningitis, encephalitis, tumors, head trauma, cerebral hemorrhage, Leigh's syndrome)
II. Stimulation of peripheral chemoreceptors
   A. Hypoxia (e.g. severe anemia. residence at high altitude, cyanotic congenital heart disease)
III. Stimulation of intrathoracic stretch receptors
   A. Localized pulmonary disease (e.g. mild bronchial asthma, pneumonia, pulmonary embolism, mild pulmonary edema)
IV. Miscellaneous
   A. Ventilator malfunction

X. Mixed Acid-Base Abnormalities

In a mixed acid-base abnormality, two single acid-base disorders occur simultaneously, one affecting the metabolic component or plasma HCO_3^- concentration, the other the respiratory component or plasma pCO_2. There are four possible mixed acid-base abnormalities. The directional change in blood pH depends upon the combination of changes of the metabolic and respiratory components and the final adjusted HCO_3^-/pCO_2 ratio (Table 13-11). Mixed metabolic and respiratory acidosis or alkalosis will induce a marked fall or increase in blood pH, respectively; mixed metabolic acidosis or alkalosis and respiratory alkalosis or acidosis will be followed by unpredictable changes in the blood pH, since the effects of each disorder are opposed. The final blood pH will reflect the relative severity of the two disturbances.

To diagnose mixed acid-base abnormalities, one must know how each disorder alters the metabolic and respiratory component and to what degree of the respiratory and the metabolic response, respectively, ought to occur for any change in the primary disorder. For example, a high plasma HCO_3^- concentration can be caused by a metabolic alkalosis or it can reflect the renal compensation during chronic respiratory acidosis. Determining the clinical condition of the patient will permit a differential diagnosis. If the patient has chronic obstructive pulmonary disease, metabolic alkalosis has probably been superimposed on a preexisting chronic respiratory acidosis. Recognizing the limits of renal adaptation for the degree of hypocapnia present will rapidly distinguish a single disorder from a mixed disorder.

TABLE 13-11. Changes in Mixed Acid-Base Abnormalities

Disorder	Primary or superimposed disturbances		Adjusted HCO_3^-/pCO_2	Directional change in blood pH
	Metabolic component	Respiratory component		
Metabolic and respiratory acidosis	HCO_3^- loss	CO_2 gain	$\downarrow HCO_3^-/\uparrow pCO_2$	$\downarrow\downarrow$
Metabolic and respiratory alkalosis	HCO_3^- gain	CO_2 loss	$\uparrow HCO_3^-/\downarrow pCO_2$	$\uparrow\uparrow$
Metabolic acidosis and respiratory alkalosis	HCO_3^- loss	CO_2 loss	$\downarrow HCO_3^-/\downarrow pCO_2$	$\downarrow N \uparrow$
Metabolic alkalosis and respiratory acidosis	HCO_3^- gain	CO_2 gain	$\uparrow HCO_3^-/\uparrow pCO_2$	$\downarrow N \uparrow$

N = Normal; $\uparrow$ = increase; $\downarrow$ = decrease.

A. Differential Diagnosis of Mixed Acid-Base Abnormalities

Some of the more frequent clinical situations causing a mixed acid-base disorder are listed in Table 13-12. *Mixed metabolic and respiratory acidosis* is generally observed in acute pulmonary diseases that lead to severe tissue hypoxia and the rapid accumulation of lactic acid: cardiopulmonary arrest or pulmonary edema, for example. Patients with stable chronic obstructive lung disease rarely present with elevated lactic acid, although an abrupt increase in lactic acid production may follow acute hypoxemia. Carbon monoxide intoxication not only causes acute pulmonary changes but also, by the formation of carboxyhemoglobin, compromised tissue oxygenation, and lactic acid production (42).

Mixed metabolic and respiratory alkalosis may occur in patients with severe liver disease. Since these patients hyperventilate and have per-

TABLE 13-12. Causes of Mixed Acid-Base Abnormalities

Clinical disorder	Primary acid-base disorder	Superimposed acid-base disorder
I. Metabolic and respiratory acidosis		
A. Cardiopulmonary arrest	Acute respiratory acidosis	Metabolic acidosis
B. Pulmonary edema	Acute respiratory acidosis	Metabolic acidosis
C. Chronic obstructive lung disease with hypoxemia	Chronic respiratory acidosis	Metabolic acidosis
D. Carbon monoxide intoxication	Acute respiratory acidosis	Metabolic acidosis
II. Metabolic and respiratory alkalosis		
A. Liver insufficiency with vomiting or diuretic therapy	Chronic respiratory alkalosis	Metabolic alkalosis
B. Chronic obstructive lung disease with acute hyperventilation	Posthypercapnic metabolic alkalosis	Acute respiratory alkalosis
III. Metabolic acidosis and respiratory alkalosis		
A. Salicylate intoxication	Acute respiratory alkalosis	Metabolic acidosis
B. Septic shock	Acute respiratory alkalosis	Metabolic acidosis
C. Subacute necrotizing encephalomyelopathy (Leigh's syndrome)	Chronic respiratory alkalosis	Metabolic acidosis
IV. Metabolic alkalosis and respiratory acidosis		
A. Chronic obstructive lung disease with salt restriction or diuretic therapy	Chronic respiratory acidosis	Metabolic alkalosis

sistent hypocapnia, vomiting or the use of diuretics can superimpose a metabolic alkalosis on the respiratory alkalosis. (40). Patients with obstructive pulmonary disease who present a compensated chronic respiratory acidosis may shift to a mixed alkalosis when rapid mechanical ventilation is administered.

Mixed metabolic acidosis and respiratory alkalosis is observed in salicylate intoxication, septic shock or Leigh's syndrome. The appearance of superimposed ketoacidosis in patients hyperventilating because of salicylate ingestion is characteristic of young children but is rarely observed in older subjects (38). A mixed disorder may be also observed in Leigh's syndrome, due to the accumulation of lactic and pyruvic acids along with the hyperventilation seen in this disease (41).

Mixed metabolic alkalosis and respiratory acidosis is observed in patients with chronic obstructive pulmonary disease who have been put on a salt-restricted diet or who have been given diuretics to treat edema. The elevation of blood pH, which results from superimposed metabolic alkalosis, may suppress ventilation and worsen the respiratory disorder (43). Aggressive therapy should be initiated to correct the alkalosis in these patients with compromised respiratory function.

References

1. Winters RW (1973) The Body Fluids in Pediatrics. Little, Brown and Co, Boston
2. Narins RG, Emmett M (1980) Simple and mixed acid-base disorders: a practical approach. Medicine 59: 161–187
3. Finberg L, Kravath RE, Fleischman AR (1982) Water and Electrolytes in Pediatrics. WB Saunders, Philadelphia
4. Cohen JJ (1979) Disorders of hydrogen ion metabolism. In: Earley LE, Gottschalk CW (eds) Strauss and Welt's Diseases of the Kidney. Little, Brown and Co, Boston, pp 1543–1579
5. Cogan MG, Rector FC Jr (1986) Acid-base disorders. In: Brenner BM, Rector FC Jr (eds) The Kidney, 3rd edn, WB Saunders, Philadelphia, pp 457–517
6. Edelmann CM Jr, Rodriguez-Soriano J, Boichis H, et al (1967) Renal bicarbonate reabsorption and hydrogen ion excretion in normal infants. J Clin Invest 46: 1309–1317
7. Broyer M, Proesmans W, Royer P (1969) Le titration des bicarbonates chez l'enfant normal et au cours des diverses néphropathies. Rev Fr Etud Clin Biol 6: 556–567
8. Emmett M, Narins RG (1977) Clinical use of the anion gap. Medicine 56: 38–54
9. Gabow PA, Kaehny WD, Fennessey PV, et al (1980) Diagnostic importance of an increased serum anion gap. N Engl J Med 303: 854–858
10. Madias NE, Ayus JC, Androgué HJ (1979) Increased anion gap in metabolic alkalosis. The role of plasma-protein equivalency. N Engl J Med 300: 1421–1423

11. McAuliffe JJ, Lind LJ, Leith DE, et al (1986) Hypoproteinemic alkalosis. Am J Med 81: 86–90
12. Chan JCM (1980) Acid-base and mineral disorders in children: a review. Int J Pediatr Nephrol 1: 54–63
13. Gray JS (1950) Pulmonary Ventilation and its Physiological Regulation. Thomas, Springfield, Illinois
14. Breyer MD, Jacobson HR (1987) Mechanisms and regulation of renal H⁺ and HCO₃⁻ transport. Am J Nephrol 7: 150–161
15. Arbus GS (1973) An in vivo acid-base nomogram for clinical use. Can Med Assoc J 109: 291–293
16. Albert MS, Dell RB, Winters RW (1967) Quantitative displacement of acid-base equilibrium in metabolic acidosis. Ann Intern Med 66: 312–322
17. Madias NE, Homer SM, Johns CA, et al (1984) Hypochloremia as a consequence of anion gap metabolic acidosis. J Lab Clin Med 104: 15–23
18. Batlle DC, Arruda JAL (1981) Renal tubular acidosis syndromes. Mineral Electrolyte Metab 5: 83–99
19. McSherry E (1981) Renal tubular acidosis in childhood. Kidney Int 20: 799–809
20. Batlle DC, Sehy JT, Roseman MK, et al (1981) Clinical and pathophysiologic spectrum of acquired distal renal tubular acidosis. Kidney Int 20: 389–396
21. Rodriguez-Soriano J (1971) The renal regulation of acid-base balance and the disturbances noted in renal tubular acidosis. Pediatr Clin North Am 18: 529–545
22. Morris RC Jr , Sebastian A, McSherry E (1972) Renal acidosis. Kidney Int 1: 322–340
23. Halperin ML, Goldstein MB, Richardson RMA, et al (1985) Distal renal tubular acidosis syndromes: a pathophysiological approach. Am J Nephrol 5: 1–8
24. Edelmann CM Jr, Boichis H, Rodriguez-Soriano J, et al (1967) The renal response of children to acute ammonium chloride acidosis. Pediatr Res 1: 452–460
25. Oster JR, Hotchkiss JL, Carbon M, et al (1975) A short duration renal acidification test using calcium chloride. Nephron 14: 281–292
26. Loney LC, Norling LL, Robson AM (1982) The use of arginine hydrochloride infusion to assess urinary acidification. J Pediatr 100: 95–98
27. Batlle DC (1986) Segmental characterization of defects in collecting tubule acidification. Kidney Int 30: 546–554
28. Rodriguez-Soriano J, Vallo A, Castillo G, et al (1985) Pathophysiology of primary distal renal tubular acidosis. Int J Pediatr Nephrol 6: 71–78
29. Vallo A, Rodriguez-Soriano J (1984) Oral phosphate-loading test to the assessment of distal urinary acidification in children. Mineral Electrolyte Metab 10: 387–390
30. Batlle DC, Hizon M, Cohen E, et al (1988) The use of the urinary anion gap in the diagnosis of hyperchloremic metabolic acidosis. New Engl J Med 318: 594–599
31. Fulop M (1976) Hypercapnia in metabolic alkalosis. NY State J Med 76: 19–22
32. Jacobson HR, Seldin DW (1983) On the generation, maintenance, and correction of metabolic alkalosis. Am J Physiol 245: F425-F432

33. Galla JH, Bonduris DN, Luke RG (1987) Effects of chloride and extracellular fluid volume on bicarbonate reabsorption along the nephron in metabolic alkalosis in the rat. J Clin Invest 80: 41–50
34. Gruskin AB, Polinsky MS, Baluarte HJ, et al (1982) Metabolic alkalosis in infancy. In: Strauss J (ed) Hypertension, Fluid Electrolytes, and Tubulopathies in Pediatric Nephrology. Developments in Nephrology, vol 5. Martinus Nijhoff, The Hague, pp 9–21
35. Rodriguez-Soriano J, Vallo A, Castillo G, et al (1983) Biochemical features of dietary chloride deficiency syndrome: A comparative study of 30 cases. J Pediatr 103: 209–214
36. Laughlin JJ, Brady MS, Eigen H (1981) Changing feeding trends as a cause of electrolyte depletion in infants with cystic fibrosis. Pediatrics 68: 203–207
37. DeStefano P, Bongo IG, Borgna-Pignatti C, et al (1983) Factitious hypertension with mineralocorticoid excess in an infant. Helv Paediatr Acta 38: 185–189
38. Winters RW, White JS, Hughes MC, et al (1959) Disturbances of acid-base equilibrium in salicylate intoxication. Pediatrics 23: 260–285
39. Hill JB (1973) Salicylate intoxication. N Engl J Med 288: 1110–1113
40. Karetzky MS, Mithoefer JC (1967) The cause of hyperventilation and arterial hypoxia in patients with cirrhosis of the liver. Am J Med Sci 254: 797–804
41. Hirschman GH, Chan JCM (1978) Complex acid-base disorders in subacute necrotizing encephalomyelopathy (Leigh's syndrome). Pediatrics 61: 278–281
42. Buehler JH, Berns AS, Webster JR Jr, et al (1975) Lactic acidosis from carboxyhemoglobinemia after smoke inhalation. Ann Intern Med 82: 803–805
43. Hodgkin JE, Balchum OJ, Kass I, et al (1975) Chronic obstructive airway disease: current concepts in diagnosis and comprehensive care. JAMA 232: 1243–1260

14
Acute Renal Failure

LEONARD G. FELD and JAMES E. SPRINGATE

I. Introduction

Acute renal failure (ARF) is defined as an abrupt, severe reduction in glomerular filtration rate (GFR). Although its course can be protracted, this potentially fatal disorder is usually temporary. With careful management, most patients can be successfully supported until renal function improves. Accurate evaluation forms the foundation for successful treatment of ARF. This evaluation has four major objectives: 1) establish the diagnosis, 2) determine the cause, 3) recognize immediately reversible cases, and 4) identify complications. These topics are emphasized in this chapter. Detailed discussions of pathophysiology and management are available elsewhere (1–4).

II. Overview

Acute renal failure occurs in 2 to 5% of hospitalized adults and is associated with a mortality rate of approximately 50%. There is a general impression that the incidence of and mortality from this disorder are lower in childhood except during the neonatal period (2,5). We reviewed 13 studies of pediatric ARF published from 1977 to 1987. Of 701 children with renal failure, 34% died. In those studies, the mortality rate in newborn infants was 62% as compared to 28% in older children. These figures probably overestimate mortality from childhood ARF because several studies included only patients requiring dialysis. Most children who survive ARF regain adequate renal function and do not require chronic dialysis or kidney transplantation. However, residual chronic renal insufficiency, hypertension or persistent renal tubular dysfunction can occur. Newborn infants appear particularly susceptible to these problems (5).

The prognosis for children with ARF has improved over the past decade. Our analysis of studies published before 1980 showed a mortality rate of 46%; the mortality rate after 1980 was 27%. A similar optimistic trend has been documented for ARF secondary to hemolytic uremic syndrome. It is hoped that advances in supportive and dialytic treatment of pediatric renal failure will continue to influence the course of this disorder favorably, especially in infants. However, it is also possible that modern renal failure management will not be able to improve prognosis significantly in the future. Acute renal failure often develops during the course of complex medical illnesses or surgical procedures. Although loss of renal function certainly complicates management of these critically ill patients, chances for recovery ultimately rest on the prognosis of their underlying diseases (6). Efforts to reduce the morbidity and mortality associated with ARF should emphasize prevention as well as early diagnosis and treatment.

III. Diagnosis

A. Azotemia

Documentation of an abrupt, severe reduction in GFR is required for the diagnosis of ARF. Loss of glomerular filtration is characterized by progressive azotemia or accumulation of nitrogenous waste products. Elevated serum concentrations of blood urea nitrogen (BUN) and/or creatinine (Cr) define the presence of azotemia. Measurement of these two substances is therefore the initial step in evaluation, but it should be remembered that normal values vary with age and sex (see Appendix I).

Azotemia is necessary, but insufficient evidence to make the diagnosis of ARF (Figure 14-1). Increased BUN or Cr levels can occur independently of changes in GFR. Conditions that increase hepatic urea production (high protein diet, hypercatabolism, steroid administration) or renal tubular urea reabsorption (intravascular volume depletion, renal hypoperfusion) will elevate BUN levels out of proportion to any change

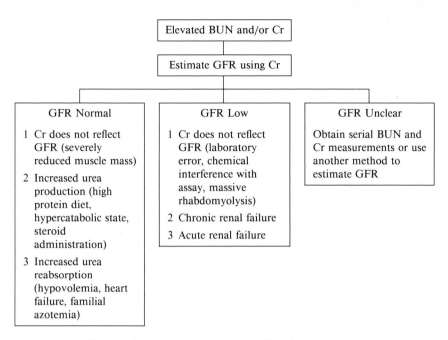

FIGURE 14-1. Approach to the child with azotemia.

in GFR. These conditions should be suspected as the only cause of azotemia in an appropriate clinical setting when BUN is high and Creatinine is normal. They should also be considered as factors contributing to azotemia when both BUN and Cr levels are elevated and the BUN/Cr ratio exceeds 20. Suspicions are confirmed by documenting a fall in BUN when the underlying condition is eliminated. Serum Cr concentration provides a much more accurate estimation of GFR than BUN. Abnormally high levels of Cr almost always indicate a significant reduction in GFR. Rarely, Cr loads (meat-based formulas, massive rhabdomyolysis) or laboratory error (assay interference from ketones or cephalosporins) may be responsible for an elevated Cr (see Chapter 5).

Azotemia can reflect either an acute or chronic loss of renal function. Distinguishing between these two forms of renal failure is important and occasionally difficult. Growth retardation, a history of underlying renal disease and radiological evidence of renal osteodystrophy or small "end-stage" kidneys suggest chronic renal failure. The distinction is most reliably made by establishing the temporal evolution of impaired renal function either retrospectively (from earlier BUN and Cr levels) or prospectively (from time of admission serial BUN and Cr levels). In general, a daily rise in Cr and BUN of at least 0.5 mg/dL and 10 mg/dL, respectively, indicates ARF.

B. Urine Volume and Composition

Oliguria (hourly urine flow rate < 0.5 mL/kg) has traditionally been considered a major feature of ARF. It is now clear that urine flow rate does not reliably reflect GFR. Up to 80% of adults and 50% of infants with ARF are not oliguric and any of the major types of ARF (prerenal, renal and postrenal) can present in an oliguric or a nonoliguric form (3). Nevertheless, documentation of urine volume remains an important part of the evaluation of suspected ARF.

Oliguria is never a normal finding and its differential diagnosis includes ARF. Careful analysis of the clinical setting and readily available laboratory tests will usually lead to an accurate working diagnosis (Figure 14-2) (1,3,7,8). Oliguria is usually the result of intravascular volume depletion, heart failure or other causes of diminished renal perfusion. Although oliguric children may be azotemic, their kidney function is otherwise normal and reflects an appropriate physiological response to hypoperfusion and avid renal salt and water retention. Their urine is therefore

Urine flow rate < 0.5ml/kg/hr

Consider urinary tract obstruction or renovascular occlusion. Obtain radiologic consultation if necessary.

Analyze clinical setting, BUN, Cr, osmolalities, and FE_{Na}

Typical clinical setting	CNS or lung disease, postoperative or traumatic stress	Dehydration, heart failure, respiratory distress syndrome	Severe renal insult
BUN	Normal	High	High and increasing
Cr	Normal	Normal or slowly increasing	High and increasing
Uosm (mOsm/L)	$> 500^c$	$> 500 (>350\text{--}400)^b$	< 350
Uosm/Posm	$> 2^c$	$> 1.5 (> 1.2)^b$	< 1.2
FE_{Na} (%)[a]	usually > 1	$< 1 (< 2.5)^b$	$> 2 (> 3)^b$
Diagnosis	SIADH	Volume depletion/ renal hypoperfusion	ATN

[a]FE_{Na} (Fractional excretion of sodium) $= (U_{Na}/P_{Na})/(U_{Cr}/P_{Cr}) \times 100\%$
[b]For neonates > 32 weeks conceptional age
[c]Uosm is inappropriately high in a state of positive water balance

FIGURE 14-2. Approach to the child with oliguria (1,3,6,7).

concentrated and relatively sodium free. This response is best assessed by calculating the fractional excretion of sodium (Na) (FE_{Na}). Urine osmolality more reliably measures urine concentrating ability than specific gravity because it is less affected by extraneous solutes (glucose, radiographic dyes) (see Chapter 3). The urine/plasma osmolar ratio helps exclude the possibility that an abnormal plasma osmolality is passively altering urine osmolality so that it does not reflect true urine concentrating ability. The FE_{Na} describes reabsorption of water and Na from glomerular filtrate by renal tubule cells. Defined as the quotient of the urine/plasma Na ratio divided by the urine/plasma Creatinine ratio multiplied by 100% ($U_{Na}/P_{Na} \div U_{Cr}/P_{Cr} \times 100\%$) obtained from simultaneous urine and blood samples, FE_{Na} represents the proportion of filtered sodium not reabsorbed and therefore excreted in the urine. A spot urine chloride (Cl) concentration of less than 20 mEq/L appears to be diagnostically equivalent to FE_{Na} of less than 1% and more accurately measures tubule cell function during metabolic alkalosis (9).

In general, oliguric children with concentrated urine and a FE_{Na} less than 1% are suffering from intravascular volume depletion (or another condition producing renal hypoperfusion) rather than ARF. Their oliguria will promptly resolve after volume repletion or after therapy designed to restore normal renal blood flow. Exceptions do occur (Table 14-1) (10,11). Diagnostic and therapeutic decisions should always be based on an overall clinical impression, not on isolated laboratory results. Once the diagnosis of ARF is established, serial measurements of urine volume will help guide appropriate fluid management. Urine volume is also an important prognostic factor in ARF. In most cases, renal failure is more severe and of longer duration if oliguria or anuria is present.

IV. Causes

Prompt identification and elimination of the cause(s) of renal failure will limit renal injury and promote recovery. A working knowledge of the various etiologies of ARF is essential to appropriate evaluation. The large number of causes of ARF can be conveniently grouped into three major categories: prerenal failure, renal parenchymal disease and urinary tract obstruction (Table 14-2).

Renal ischemia or prerenal failure occurs when extrarenal processes severely compromise blood flow to the kidney. The intricate pathophysiology of this form of ARF has recently been reviewed (12). Its causes include intravascular volume depletion, heart failure, bilateral renal artery/vein occlusion or various conditions producing abnormally high levels of renal vasoconstriction relative to systemic vascular resistance (septic shock, vasopressor agents, prostaglandin synthesis inhibitors). Ischemia from various perinatal insults accounts for most neonatal ARF.

TABLE 14-1. Fractional Excretion of Sodium in Various Oliguric Conditions (10,11)

$FE_{Na} < 1\%$[a]	$FE_{Na} > 2\%$[b]
Intravascular volume depletion	Acute renal failure (ARF)
Heart failure	Diuretic use
Acute glomerulonephritis	Chronic renal disease
Hemolytic uremic syndrome	Obstructive uropathy
Hepatorenal syndrome	Mineralocorticoid deficiency
Acute urinary tract obstruction	Intravascular volume depletion/renal
Myoglobin/hemoglobin-induced ARF	hypoperfusion in newborn or premature
Radiocontrast-induced ARF	infant
Sepsis-induced ARF	

[a]In newborns >32 weeks gestation $<2.5\%$;
[b]In newborns $>3.0\%$.

Gastroenteritis-induced intravascular volume depletion remains an important cause of childhood ischemic ARF in underdeveloped areas.

Renal parenchymal disorders associated with ARF include chemical injury, glomerulur disease and small renal vessels and interstitial nephritis. Hemolytic uremic syndrome and acute glomerulonephritis are the leading causes of ARF in children. These entities were responsible for 55% of childhood ARF cases in the studies we reviewed. Although congenital anomalies of the kidney can present as ARF in the neonatal period, they are usually irreversible and progress to chronic renal failure.

Finally, obstruction of both ureters, the bladder or urethra can result in ARF. These lesions appear to account for about 10% of childhood ARF cases. Male infants with posterior urethral valves predominate.

Although the cause of ARF is usually obvious, confusion and uncertainty do occur in complex situations in which multiple etiological factors can be present. For this reason, the evaluation of every child with ARF should include consideration of each major category of causes (prerenal, renal parenchymal disorders and urinary tract obstruction). Because the number of causes of and diagnostic tests for ARF is virtually limitless, a disciplined systematic approach is required. Without exception, this approach is based on a thoughtful analysis of information obtained from an accurate medical history, physical examination and urinalysis.

A knowledge of events preceding the development of ARF can be extremely helpful, with a careful history and medical record review emphasizing recent illnesses or insults (including medications) and laboratory data. Physical examination must be thorough and always include assessment of intravascular fluid volume, cardiac function and peripheral perfusion, as well as detection of flank masses or bladder distension. Identification of skin lesions or other organ system abnormalities can provide valuable etiological clues.

TABLE 14-2. Causes of Acute Renal Failure

Ischemia (prerenal)
  Intravascular volume depletion
    Dehydration
    Third-space losses
    Hemorrhage
  Heart failure
  Bilateral renal artery or vein occlusion
  Renal vasoconstriction/systemic vasodilation
    Septic shock
    Prostaglandin synthesis inhibitors
    Anaphylaxis
    Angiotensin-converting enzyme inhibitors
    Hepatorenal syndrome
    Acute increased intraabdominal pressure
    Antihypertensive medications
    Vasopressor agents
Renal parenchymal disease (renal)
  Chemical injury
    Endogenous
      Myoglobin
      Acute tumor lysis syndrome
      Hemoglobin
      Oxalate
      Uric acid
    Exogenous
      Antibiotics
      Acetaminophen
      Radiographic contrast material
      Dextran
      Fluorinated anesthetics
      Heavy metals
      Ethylene glycol
      Chemotherapeutic drugs
  Glomerular/vascular disease
    Hemolytic uremic syndrome
    Rapidly progressive glomerulonephritis
    Acute postinfectious glomerulonephritis
    Henoch-Schönlein purpura
    Systemic lupus erythematosus
    Malignant hypertension
  Interstitial nephritis
    Medication induced
      Antibiotics
      Nonsteroidal antiinflammatory agents
    Parainfectious
      Streptococcus and other microorganisms
    Infiltrating diseases
      Malignancy
      Pyelonephritis
    Idiopathic (with or without uveitis)
  Congenital nephropathy

TABLE 14-2. *Continued*

Urinary tract obstruction (postrenal)
  Posterior urethral valves
  Stones
  Intraabdominal lesions occluding ureters
  Blood clots
  Ureteroceles
  Bilateral ureteropelvic obstruction

It is essential to obtain a fresh urine sample as soon as renal disease is suspected. Bladder catheterization may occasionally be needed for this purpose. In addition to determining the urine concentration and FE_{Na}, dipstick testing for albumin and heme pigments and microscopy should be performed. In the absence of gross hematuria, 3^+ to 4^+ albuminuria suggests glomerular disease. Red blood cell (RBC) casts or RBCs that appear dysmorphic by phase-contrast microscopy indicate glomerulo-nephritis, hemolytic uremic syndrome or vasculitis. Reddish urine or a strongly positive dipstick reaction for heme pigments without a significant number of RBCs suggests rhabdomyolysis or hemolysis. The distinctions between these two conditions has been recently reviewed (13), and is discussed in Chapter 8. Sterile pyuria and leukocyte casts are commonly found in interstitial nephritis; detection of eosinophilia using Hansel's stain can help confirm this diagnosis (14). The urine sediment in ARF secondary to ischemia or obstruction may be relatively bland or loaded with coarse granular and tubule epithelial cell casts. Numerous football-shaped uric acid crystals are commonly found in ARF from tumor lysis syndrome, whereas envelope-shaped calcium oxalate crystals suggest eth-ylene glycol toxicity. An aliquot of the initial urine sample should always be saved in case additional tests are needed.

This basic evaluation will establish the cause of ARF or at least narrow the possibilities. Subsequent diagnostic tests are then selected to confirm or more clearly define the initial clinical impression. For example, ab-dominal masses require expeditious sonographic evaluation whereas the presence of RBC casts and proteinuria may indicate a need for serum complement levels and various serological studies. Occasionally, the cause of ARF remains unclear even after a meticulous medical history, physical examination and urinalysis. Radiological consultation may be helpful in this situation (see Chapter 6).

The widespread availability of sonography and radionuclide scanning has eliminated the use of intravenous pyelography in ARF, avoiding the risks of anaphylaxis and nephrotoxicity of the dye used in this study. Ultrasonography allows documentation of the presence of one or two kidneys, measurement of renal size and assessment of the urinary col-lecting system, renal parenchyma and vessels. Sonographic renal size varies with age and body size (see Appendix III). Azotemia associated with small kidneys suggests underlying chronic renal disease. Enlarged kidneys are characteristic of hydronephrosis, renal vein thrombosis, nephrotic syndrome, cystic disease, acute glomerulonephritis and various infiltrative diseases. Sonography is particulary useful in detecting urinary tract obstruction. If hydronephrosis is found, further ultrasonographic evaluation of the ureters and bladder will often establish the level and cause of obstruction. Unfortunately, a normal sonogram does not always exclude the diagnosis of urinary tract obstruction because significant collecting system dilation may not be present in early acute obstruction or if anuria has occurred because of superimposed renal parenchymal disease (15,16). Serial sonographic examinations or retrograde pyelography should be considered if this diagnosis is still suspected. An attempt should also be made during sonography to identify and establish the patency of renal arteries and veins and the inferior vena cava and aorta to exclude the possibility of vascular occlusion. Simultaneous Doppler flow studies enhance the accuracy of this assessment.

Radionuclide scanning provides an excellent means of assessing renal perfusion and function and complements anatomical information obtained from sonography. Radionuclide studies can help define urinary tract obstruction, renal vein thrombosis or various inflammatory conditions of the kidney. They are also useful when renal artery disease is suspected. Given the proper clinical setting, renal failure secondary to renal artery embolism or thrombosis (mainly following umbilical artery catheterization) can be confirmed by the absence of blood flow or the presence of multiple perfusion defects that represent parenchymal infarcts.

In selected cases, evaluation of ARF may require a renal biopsy (17). This procedure should be considered when the cause of ARF remains unclear, when interstitial nephritis is suspected or when a specific etiology for acute glomerulonephritis or vasculitis-induced ARF cannot be determined (Table 6-4). Renal biopsy should be performed only when there is reasonable expectation that its result will alter therapy.

V. Reversibility

A major reason for determining the cause of ARF is the possibility that a specific therapeutic intervention can be used to arrest or reverse renal injury. All forms of ARF, regardless of cause, tend to evolve through four basic phases (6). The first phase *anticipation* is defined as that interval of time preceding nephrotoxic insult when a clinical setting associated with the risk of ARF is identified; examples include dehydration, open heart surgery or use of potentially nephrotoxic medications. The *initiation* phase begins at the time of nephrotoxic insult and generally lasts from

minutes to hours. During this phase, impaired renal function is immediately reversible if the underlying cause is rapidly eliminated. If intervention during the anticipation or initiation phases is neglected or
unsuccessful, the *maintenance* phase is entered. In this phase, relatively
permanent renal damage has occurred. Even if the underlying causes are
corrected, renal function will not return to normal until the kidneys heal.
The final phase, *recovery*, begins when GFR improves and typically ends
with renal functional recovery, usually several weeks to months after the
initial insult.

The temporal evolution of ARF through these various phases depends
on the severity, duration and number of insults sustained by the kidney.
Clearly, measures to avoid or attenuate the anticipation phase will prevent renal failure. These measures include proper hydration, alternative
medications or radiographic procedures in high-risk patients and various
diuretic regimens during antineoplastic therapy. Intervention in the initiation phase is also highly desirable. At this time, elimination of the
cause of ARF can rapidly restore normal renal function, avoiding the
serious complications that ensue during the maintenance phase. Although
treatment of the underlying cause in the maintenance phase will not
immediately normalize renal function, continued (or additional) insult
will impair renal healing and jeopardize recovery. Therefore, prompt
identification and elimination of causes are appropriate in any phase of
ARF. Intervention is particularly crucial during the anticipation or initiation phases if established ARF is to be prevented.

Distinguishing between initiation and maintenance phases of ARF can
be difficult. Attempts to develop laboratory tests to help with this distinction have emphasized renal tubular cell function. The basic premise
of these tests is that renal tubular function is normal in the anticipation
and initiation phases and abnormal in the maintenance phase of ARF,
reflecting the extent of renal parenchymal damage. Therefore, documentation of normal renal tubular function would indicate a potentially rapidly reversible renal failure.

Clinically, studies of tubule function are most useful for evaluating
oliguric ARF caused by renal ischemia. In this setting, a concentrated,
Na-free urine (urine osmolality >500 mOsm/L and FE_{Na} $<1\%$ in children; urine osmolality >350 mOsm/L and FE_{Na} $<2.5\%$ in newborn infants of less than 32 weeks conceptional age) indicates a normal tubule
response to hypoperfusion and suggests that the GFR can be rapidly
normalized if the underlying insult is promptly eliminated (1,3,8). In
contrast, isosthenuria and an elevated FE_{Na} ($>2\%$ in children or $>3\%$ in
newborns) imply that significant renal damage has already occurred. Recently developed tests for urinary levels of renal tubule epithelial antigens
may also be used to distinguish between the initiation and maintenance
phases of ARF (18). These tests are not infallible (Table 14-1) (11,19).

They are meant to guide not dictate clinical decisions and must always be interpreted in the context of the clinical setting.

Various medications including dopamine (1–5 mcg/kg a minute), mannitol (0.5 g/kg, maximum 25 g) and furosemide (2–4 mg/kg) have also been used to distiguish rapidly reversible ARF from established ARF in oliguric, nonobstructed patients (2,4,20). Conversion to a nonoliguric state is felt to reflect either an actual therapeutic benefit or intrinsically less severe renal damage. In general, clinical studies have not convincingly demonstrated an important role for these agents in the diagnosis or treatment of renal failure (4,20). A trial of these medications should be considered only after hypotension and fluid deficits have been corrected. These medications require careful monitoring for adverse effects.

In our opinion, the issue of reversibility in ARF is best addressed by 1) determining its cause and instituting specific treatment if available, 2) maintaining normal intravascular volume and cardiac function and 3) eliminating exposure to additional nephrotoxic insults. The possibility that new medications such as adenosine nucleotides, thyroxine or calcium channel blockers can attenuate or actually hasten recovery in ARF is clearly exciting but requires further clinical investigation (21).

VI. Complications

Innumerable problems can arise during the course of ARF both from kidney failure itself and from associated underlying diseases (Table 14-3) (22). An abrupt severe loss of renal function invariably impairs the body's abilities to maintain water and solute homeostasis. Most complications result from this impairment. Evaluation of all children with ARF must include initial and ongoing assessment for the following problems.

A. Hypervolemia or Hypovolemia

Maintenance of euvolemia is an important part of ARF care. Once normal intravascular fluid volume has been achieved, careful attention to fluid balance (intake, evaporative loss, urine volume and tube drainage), body weight and serum Na concentration will ensure continued euvolemia. In general, body weight will decrease approximately 1% per day and the serum Na concentration will remain normal if fluid intake is appropriate. Hyponatremia commonly occurs in ARF and is usually caused by excessive free water administration. Appropriate treatment involves fluid restriction rather than Na administration.

B. Hyperkalemia and Other Electrolyte Disturbances

Life threatening hyperkalemia is common in oliguric or severely catabolic ARF patients. Appropriate evaluation for this complication includes serial measurements of serum potassium (K) concentration and elimination

TABLE 14-3. Complications of Acute Renal Failure

Cardiovascular
  Arrhythmias
  Hypervolemia/hypovolemia
  Heart failure
  Uremic pericarditis
  Hypertension
Respiratory
  Pneumonia
  Uremic pleuritis
  Pulmonary edema
Gastrointestinal
  Hemorrhage
  Nausea, vomiting
  Malnutrition
Neurological
  Mental status changes and seizures from uremia, un-
    derlying disease, hypertension or electrolyte disorders
Metabolic
  Acidosis
  Hypocalcemia
  Hyperkalemia
  Uremia
  Hypermagnesmia
  Hyperphosphatemia
  Hyperuricemia
Hematological
  Anemia
  Coagulopathy
Infectious
  Catheter-related infection
  Septicemia
  Pneumonia
  Urinary tract infection

of exogenous K sources. The pathophysiological effects of hyperkalemia are assessed by electrocardiogram. Intervention is required when serum K exceeds 6.5 mEq/L and urgent therapy is needed when electrocardiographic findings other than peak T-waves are noted. Although hyperkalemia is a well-recognized complication of ARF, 5 to 10% of adults and up to 25% of newborns can still die as a direct consequence of this disorder (5,22) (see Chapter 12).

Metabolic acidosis typically occurs during the course of ARF and can exacerbate hyperkalemia. Loss of renal excretory capacity coupled with continued acid production from cellular metabolism leads to the accumulation of sulfuric, phosphoric and other organic acids and causes a high anion gap metabolic acidosis. Specific intervention is usually not required because of respiratory compensation. Treatment should be considered if hyperkalemia is present or when blood pH or bicarbonate (HCO_3^-) concentration are persistently less than 7.20 and 10 mEq/L, respectively. Hypertonic $NaHCO_3$ solutions can cause abrupt changes in plasma volume and tonicity and should always be infused slowly.

Hyperphosphatemia and associated hypocalcemia are also frequently encountered. Dietary phosphorus (P) restriction or enteral phosphate binders are usually sufficient to lower serum phosphorus levels. Prolonged use of aluminum- or magnesium-containing antacids should be avoided (see Chapter 15). Calcium should not be administered until the serum P level is relatively normal, unless symptomatic hypocalcemia is present.

C. Uremia

Azotemia can progress to produce the clinical syndrome of uremia. This disorder involves a variety of organ system abnormalities, including encephalopathy, nausea and vomiting, coagulopathy and rarely pericarditis and pleuritis. The level of azotemia needed to cause uremia is unpredictable. In general, BUN levels over 100–150 mg/dL are associated with this complication.

D. Cardiovascular Disorders

High blood pressure in ARF usually indicates hypervolemia or some form of glomerular-vascular disease, e.g. acute glomerulonephritis, hemolytic uremic syndrome or neonatal aortic thrombosis. Evaluation should consider both of these etiologies. After excluding hypervolemia as a cause, children with moderate to severe hypertension should be treated in a step-wise approach with either beta adrenergic blocking drugs, alpha adrenergic blockers, central sympatholytic agents, direct vasodilators or calcium-entry blockers. The presence of encephalopathy, congestive heart failure or other manifestations or a hypertensive crisis requires immediate intravenous therapy which traditionally has included the administration of either diazoxide or sodium nitroprusside.

E. Infection

This complication is the leading cause of morbidity and death in adults with ARF (22). Similar statistics are not available for children. Renal failure, associated underlying diseases and iatrogenic complications all contribute to this problem. The lung and the urinary tract appear to be the most common sites of infection. Intravascular, bladder and peritoneal catheters are also important sources of infection. Careful clinical assessment, maintenance of pulmonary toilet and close monitoring or removal of indwelling catheters will help prevent this potentially devastating problem.

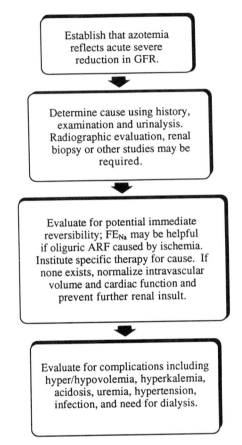

FIGURE 14-3. Approach to the child with acute renal failure.

F. Dialysis

Evaluation for complications in ARF should also include periodic assessment of a need for hemo or peritoneal dialysis. Indications for emergent dialysis in ARF include uremia and hypervolemia, hyperkalemia or acidosis refractory to other forms of management. Ideally, dialysis should be instituted before these life-threatening complications develop. Considerable clinical judgment is required for this decision. Dialysis may also be required to treat certain diseases associated with ARF, such as acute tumor lysis syndrome or ethylene glycol poisoning, to allow administration of medications, blood products or to facilitate parenteral nutrition.

Other management considerations include the use of medications and the need for nutritional supplementation. Information about nephrotoxicity and adverse effects and changes in pharmacokinetics induced by renal failure and/or dialysis should be obtained before prescribing any drug in ARF. The exact role and the appropriate composition of nutritional supplements during ARF remain unclear. The possibility that amino acid administration may cause further renal damage is a complicating factor (23). In our opinion, aggressive nutritional support is indicated when ARF is prolonged, requires frequent dialysis or is associated with illnesses, in which severe protein catabolism occurs. Detailed discussions of this important aspect of renal failure care are available elsewhere (24,25).

VII. Summary

Acute renal failure is a potentially fatal, but often reversible disorder defined by an abrupt severe decline in GFR. Proper evaluation depends on the interpretation of readily available laboratory studies in the context of an accurate history and physical examination. This evaluation should establish the diagnosis of ARF and determine its cause, recognize immediately reversible cases and identify complications. Our approach to this evaluation is summarized in Figure 14-3.

References

1. Gaudio KM, Siegel NJ (1987) Pathogenesis and treatment of acute renal failure. Pediatr Clin North Am 34:771–787
2. Maxwell LG, Fivush BA, McLean RH (1987) Renal failure. In: Rogers MC (ed) Textbook of Pediatric Intensive Care. Williams & Wilkins, Baltimore, pp 1001–1055
3. Feld LG, Springate JE, Fildes RD (1986) Acute renal failure. I. Pathophysiology and diagnosis. J Pediatr 109:401–408
4. Fildes RD, Springate JE, Feld LG (1986) Acute renal failure. II. Management of suspected and established disease. J Pediatr 109:567–571
5. Stapleton FB, Jones DP, Green RS (1987) Acute renal failure in neonates: Incidence, etiology and outcome. Pediatr Nephrol 1:314–320
6. Wilkes BM, Mailloux LU (1986) Acute renal failure: Pathogenesis and prevention. Am J Med 80:1129–1136
7. Siegel NJ (1984) Acute renal failure. In: Tune BM, Mendoza SA (eds) Contemporary Issues in Nephrology, Vol 12, Pediatric Nephrology. Churchill-Livingstone, New York, pp 297–320
8. Ellis D, Gartner JC, Galvis AG (1981) Acute renal failure in infants and children: Diagnosis, complications and treatment. Crit Care Med 9:607–614
9. Anderson RJ, Gabow PA, Gross PA (1984) Urinary chloride concentration in acute renal failure. Miner Electrolyte Metab 10:92–97
10. Steiner RW (1984) Interpreting the fractional excretion of sodium. Am J Med 77:699–702
11. Zarich S, Fang LST, Diamond JR (1985) Fractional excretion of sodium: Exceptions to its diagnostic value. Arch Intern Med 145:108–112

12. Badr KF, Ichikawa I (1988) Prerenal failure: A deleterious shift from renal compensation to decompensation. N Engl J Med 319:623–629
13. Materson BJ, Preston RA (1988) Myoglobinuria versus hemoglobinuria. Hosp Pract 23:29–38
14. Nolan CR, Anger MS, Kelleher SP (1986) Eosinophiluria—a new method of detection and definition of the clinical spectrum. N Engl J Med 315:1516–1519
15. Reinberg Y, Gonzalez R (1987) Upper urinary tract obstruction in children: current controversies in diagnosis. Pediatr Clin North Am 34:1291–1304
16. Barratt TM, Dillon MJ, Gordon I, et al (1987) Clinical quiz. Pediatr Nephrol 1:379–380
17. Warren DJ (1987) Acute renal failure: diagnosis of cause needed within hours. Br Med J 294:1569
18. Tolkoff-Rubin NE (1986) Monoclonal antibodies in the diagnosis of renal disease: A preliminary report. Kidney Int 29:142–152
19. Brosius FC, Lau K (1986) Low fractional excretion of sodium in acute renal failure: Role of timing of the test and ischemia. Am J Nephrol 6:450–457
20. Levinsky NG, Bernard DB (1988) Mannitol and loop diuretics in acute renal failure. In: Brenner BM, Lazarus JM (eds) Acute Renal Failure. Churchill-Livingstone, New York, pp 841–856
21. Gaudio KM, Siegel NJ (1987) New approaches to the treatment of acute renal failure. Pediatr Nephrol 1:339–347
22. Knochel JP, Steinman TI, Lazarus JM (1988) The metabolic consequences of acute renal failure. In: Brenner BM, Lazarus JM (eda) Acute Renal Failure. Churchill-Livingstone, New York, pp 677–742
23. Zager RA (1987) Aminoacid hyperalimentation in acute renal failure: a potential therapeutic paradox. Kidney Int 32:S72–S75
24. Feld LG (1986) Total parenteral nutrition in children with renal insufficiency. In: Lebenthal E (ed) Total Parenteral Nutrition. Raven Press, New York, pp 385–410
25. Mitch WE, Wilmore DW (1988) Nutritional considerations in the treatment of acute renal failure. In: Brenner BM, Lazarus JM (eds) Acute Renal Failure. Churchill Livingstone, New York, pp 743–765

15
Chronic Renal Failure

ZOE L. PAPADOPOULOU

I. Introduction

Chronic renal failure (CRF) is defined as the stage at which the irreversibly damaged kidneys are unable to maintain the homeostasis of the body. Patients with established CRF do not recover but instead experience a continuous loss of function, even when the original disease that damaged the kidneys is no longer active, as for example, obstructive uropathy.

When nephrons are progressively damaged, the first clinical sign of functional deterioration is a diminution of renal reserve and a decrease of the glomerular filtration rate (GFR). Before this becomes clinically evident, and during the initial phase of loss of renal function, the body uses various physiological mechanisms to maintain homeostasis so that there is a clinically normal interval. The approach to the child during this early phase is to limit any further injury to the kidney; during the latter phase, the aim is to prevent the metabolic consequences that follow from the progressive loss of renal function (1).

II. Criteria for Staging Progressive Renal Disease

The staging of disease based on the percent of residual renal function following the progressive loss of nephrons constitutes the most comprehensive approach to the diagnosis of CRF (1). It must be pointed out, however, that the GFR usually indicates a residual renal function that is inappropriately high when compared with the actual residual potential based on the number of functioning nephrons that remain in the renal ablation model. With that in mind, the progressive loss of renal function can be divided into four stages:

1. Early stage of impaired renal function. This is characterized by a moderate reduction in nephron number and residual renal function between 80 to 50% of normal. The various adaptive renal and metabolic responses that follow compensate for the loss of renal function, hence, no clinical signs are evident.
2. Chronic renal insufficiency. In this stage, the residual renal function is between 50 and 25% of normal. The patient becomes symptomatic with evidence of electrolyte disturbances, poor growth potential and calcium-phosphorus imbalance. Following a major stress such as an intercurrent illness, the patient's condition may deteriorate and acute renal failure is likely to develop as a result of dehydration. The major emphasis of any therapeutic intervention in this stage is preservation of renal function.
3. Chronic renal failure. This is the stage in which the residual renal function is less than 25% of normal and metabolic abnormalities related to marked reduction in nephron number, such as metabolic acidosis, renal osteodystrophy, anemia, hypertension and others, appear. Ther-

apeutic intervention here is aimed at the prevention of various metabolic complications.
4. End-stage renal disease (ESRD). The residual renal function in patients with ESRD may range between 12 to less than 5% of normal. The major emphasis in this stage is directed at maintaining the metabolic status as near to normal as possible. Patients with ESRD are treated with chronic dialysis and transplantation.

Some clinicians use the term *uremia,* which refers to a syndrome or a constellation of symptoms that encompass all the overt consequences of renal failure, interchangeably with ESRD. It is characterized by nausea, fatigue, irritability, gastrointestinal bleeding, somnolence, convulsions and coma. It may occur in a well-stabilized patient following an acute insult, such as an intercurrent illness that induces a catabolic response. This in turn will precipitate the above symptoms, which can be reversed with either conservative or dialysis therapy.

III. Incidence of Chronic Renal Failure

The incidence of progressive renal disease leading to chronic renal failure in children varies between 1.5 to 3.0 children per million total population in patients less than 16 years of age.

According to the EDTA registry, during 1981, 3.0 new cases per million child population (pmcp) were started on dialysis in Europe, with a range of 0.2 to 12.0 new cases reported by the 33 participating countries (2); during 1984, there were 4.1 new cases pmcp, with a range of zero to 15.9 new cases (3). Figures of eight new cases per year pmcp in northern California (4), and twenty pmcp in Virginia (5), are most likely overestimates because of the mobility of the population in the United States. Incidence also varies with age (Table 15-1).

IV. Causes of End-Stage Renal Disease in Children

The etiology of ESRD in children is listed in Table 15-2, which represents data from five different centers (6–10). It is very important to establish the exact etiology of ESRD in a child, since different disorders may require a different approach to treatment. Furthermore, the establishment of a precise diagnosis may possibly alter the timing of renal transplantation, especially in those cases associated with a high incidence of recurrence of the primary renal disease in the transplanted kidney.

Data from the EDTA pediatric registry (6) indicate that glomerulonephritis and pyelonephritis/interstitial nephritis are the most common

TABLE 15-1. Proportional Distribution of Children Commencing Renal Replacement Therapy in Europe According to Age at Start of Therapy[a]

Time period	Age Group		
	0–5 years (%)	5–10 years (%)	10–15 years (%)
1978	5	25	70
1980	8	25	67
1982	13	29	58
1984	15	25	60

[a]Proceedings of the European Dialysis and Transplant Association (EDTA).

TABLE 15-2. Proportional Distribution of Causes of End-stage Renal Disease in Children[a]

Cause of ESRD	EDTA(6) (%)	France(7) (%)	Sweden(8) (%)	Canada(9) (%)	California(10) (%)
Glomerulonephritis	24	26	24	29	37
Hereditary diseases	15	26	44	13	13
Pyelonephritis and malformations of the urinary tract	24	20	10	14	23
Hypoplasia/dysplasia	7.5	13	7	23	13
Systemic diseases	10.5	10	7	} 8	9
Vascular diseases	3	1	5		2
Miscellaneous and unclassified	16	4	3	13	3

[a]EDTA: Analysis of EDTA registry from 1980–1983 (6); France: Data analysis from 1969–1981 (391 children) (7); Sweden: Data analysis from 1974–1977 (41 children) (8); Canada: Data analysis from 1981–1983 (87 children) (9); and California: Data analysis (276 children) (10)

cause of ESRD in children (24% of cases each), followed by hereditary diseases (15%), systemic diseases (10.5%), renal hypoplasia (7.5%), vascular diseases (3%), other diseases (9%) and illnesses of unknown etiology (7%). Within the pyelonephritis/interstitial nephritis group, congenital obstructive uropathy and reflux nephropathy accounted for more than 60% of the affected children; congenital renal dysplasia with or without urinary tract malformation was the next most frequent disease entity. The differences observed among various centers may be related to differences in genetic or ecological factors, in diagnostic practice or even in the actual prevalence of disease. The low incidence of pyelonephritis and urinary tract malformations observed in Sweden, for example, has been attributed to better diagnostic and treatment practices.

V. Pathophysiology of Chronic Renal Failure: Renal Adaptive Mechanisms

Renal parenchyma destruction occurs as a result of immunological, ischemic, toxic, or infectious insults, or nonspecific causes such as hypertension. Regardless of the cause of the initial nephron injury, a progressive loss of functional nephrons follows.

A. Glomerular Adaptation

The initial adaptation of the kidney to a reduction in nephron number, as a result of renal parenchymal disease or surgical ablation, consists of nephron hypertrophy and such hemodynamic changes as a decrease in arteriolar resistance and an increase in capillary blood flow and pressure. This in turn leads to hyperfiltration of the remaining nephrons, which eventually leads to a progressive glomerular sclerosis and the total loss of renal function (11). Hypertension often develops during the course of progressive renal injury and contributes to further increase of glomerular capillary pressure which leads to further glomerular damage. This phenomenon of progressive glomerular injury that is hemodynamically mediated and which progresses to renal failure is observed in certain diseases in humans despite adequate control of the original disease process.

B. Tubular Adaptation

With the progressive loss of nephron number and the reduction in the GFR, the kidney is able to adjust sodium (Na) excretion appropriately to maintain a zero Na balance. This is accomplished by an adaptive decrease in the proximal tubular reabsorption and an exponential rise in distal tubular excretion of Na. The Na balance is maintained over a large range of Na intake and with a residual renal function of less than 25 and even 10% of normal. With further deterioration of renal function, renal adaptation becomes more limited and the kidney is unable to increase Na excretion much beyond 150 to 200 mEq/day. This explains the poor tolerance of patients with advanced chronic renal failure to an acute Na load. Conversely, such patients cannot adjust to a sudden reduction in Na intake, due to their continuous obligatory urinary Na loss. The above findings have direct relevance to patient care. Sodium restriction should be reserved only for those patients with such clinical evidence of Na excess as edema, congestive heart failure and hypertension.

The fractional excretion of water increases progressively as the number of nephrons decreases. This is accompanied by solute diuresis, which explains the development of isosthenuria and the inability to respond quickly to an excess or lack of water so characteristic of these patients. The inability to concentrate the urine maximally occurs early in renal insufficiency, whereas the capacity to dilute the urine is severely limited only at very low levels of renal function (12). Because of the isosthenuria the rate of urine formation remains constant throughout the 24-hour period and results in nocturia, which is one of the earlier manifestations of chronic renal disease. Under these circumstances, the disappearance of nocturia in a patient with chronic renal insufficiency may signify a further reduction in renal function. The concentrating defect has other clinical implications as well, the most serious one being the rapid development of hypovolemia and/or hypernatremia as a result of fluid loss or decreased fluid intake.

With the progressive decrease in nephron number, the fractional reabsorption of potassium (K) decreases and the rate of secretion of K by the distal nephron segments increases. When the GFR falls below 30% of normal the capacity to excrete a load of K becomes limited and hyperkalemia may develop. At this point, there is an adaptive increase in the fecal excretion of K, which may be as much as 35% of the total.

The renal adaptive mechanisms to effect hydrogen ion (H^+) excretion remain intact until the GFR falls below 25 to 20% of normal, at which point a high anion gap acidosis develops. The major factor in the development of acidosis is a decrease in the ammonia excretion, which is proportional to the decline in GFR and is directly related to the reduction in nephron number. Bicarbonate reabsorption and titratable acid excretion remain intact and may be enhanced. Because of the increased excretion of Na per nephron with the progressive reduction in nephron number, the amount of Na that reaches the collecting tubule is increased, thus favoring a Na for H^+ exchange. The H^+ is excreted as titratable acid, since there is also an enhanced excretion of phosphate. With a more severe reduction in nephron number, the total acid excretion becomes progressively limited and patients develop acidemia.

The ability of the body to affect the acidemia by extrarenal buffering has important clinical implications, particularly in children, since the most important source of the buffer is bone; consequently, this contributes to the development of renal osteodystrophy. It is, therefore, mandatory to correct the acidosis by alkali administration.

Phosphate (PO_4^{-2}) excretion is adjusted by the kidney in a way similar to that for Na. An external balance of PO_4^{-2} is maintained by a reduction of tubular PO_4^{-2} reabsorption, which results in the maintenance of a normal serum PO_4^{-2} concentration up to a GFR of approximately 30 to 25% of normal. Further reduction in nephron number will result in hyperphosphatemia. Inhibition of tubular PO_4^{-2} reabsorption observed in early renal insufficiency is mediated by the parathyroid hormone (PTH). The secretion of PTH is stimulated by both the hypocalcemia that results from decreased intestinal absorption of calcium (Ca) and by dietary phosphorus (P). In response to increased PTH secretion, Ca is mobilized from bone so that plasma Ca levels are normal; meanwhile, tubular reabsorption of PO_4^{-2} is decreased, resulting in normal plasma PO_4^{-2} levels. These adaptive mechanisms help maintain a normal PO_4^{-2} balance, but the price for this is hyperparathyroidism and renal osteodystrophy.

C. Overt Consequences of Chronic Renal Failure

With progressive deterioration of renal function to less than 30 or 25% of normal, the adaptive mechanisms eventually become limited, and overt clinical signs develop. Nitrogen retention and the appearance of uremia start to affect ion transport and cellular metabolism. In addition, metabolic abnormalities, biochemical changes—including impaired energy utilization and abnormal metabolism of carbohydrate, fat and protein—advancing anemia due to bone marrow failure and endocrine disturbances become evident. At this stage, therapeutic measures are directed to restoring and maintaining the functional state of the child and preventing the development of complications associated with CRF.

VI. Workup of the Child with Chronic Renal Failure

Certain manifestations of the uremic syndrome, such as growth failure and metabolic bone disease, may result in long-term morbidity in spite of adequate treatment with hemodialysis or even a successful renal transplant. The initial and subsequent assessment of a child with chronic renal insufficiency serves as a point of reference for subsequent evaluation of the various measures taken that are designed to slow or halt the progression of certain pathological processes of uremia. A plan to investigate children with CRF is presented in Table 15-3.

A. Evaluation of Residual Renal Function

The accurate measurement of the GFR is quite important in monitoring the progression of renal disease as well as the response to treatment.

Various experimental studies have shown that in most glomerular diseases there is an impairment of the ultrafiltration capacity of the glomerular capillary wall. This, however, is accompanied by an elevation of the net ultrafiltration pressure so that the GFR does not decrease significantly. Under these circumstances, measurement of the GFR underestimates the extent of the glomerular capillary wall injury, that is, the measured GFR indicates a residual renal function that is inappropriately

TABLE 15-3. Plan to Investigate Children with Chronic Renal Failure

I. Establish the chronic nature of the disease
   A. Past history (long standing proteinuria or hypertension, growth failure, recurrent urinary tract infections, etc.)
   B. Family history (Alport's syndrome, polycystic kidney disease, etc.)
   C. Physical examination (anemia, hypertensive vascular or eye changes, small stature, rickets)
   D. Kidney size (contracted kidneys confirm chronicity; normal or large kidneys do not exclude it)
   E. Radiological evidence of osteodystrophy
   F. Severity of renal failure (see section II)
II. Identify the etiology of renal failure (imaging, biopsy, other studies)
III. Determine the clinical and biochemical consequences of CRF
IV. Identify factors that increase the rate of deterioration of renal function (hypertension, pyelonephritis, nephrotoxic drugs, obstruction, dehydration, extracellular volume depletion)

high when compared to the actual number of normal nephrons present. This problem is further compounded when the technique used to measure renal function overestimates the true GFR, and may therefore underestimate the rate of deterioration of renal function. The various methods that are usually employed for follow-up of the residual renal function in children with chronic renal insufficiency are discussed in Chapter 5.

B. Growth Assessment

Growth and the potential for growth are extremely important in the assessment and future management strategies of children with CRF, particularly those with congenital renal disease. Growth retardation has been reported to occur in 50 to 70% of children with congenital renal disease, and in 10 to 40% of children with acquired disease (13,14).

The purpose of growth assessment is a) to determine the status of the child's present size and development and the effect of the underlying renal disease on growth, b) to define the variables of disease most affecting growth and c) to plan and evaluate the efficacy of various therapeutic interventions on growth potential.

Measurements should be taken at intervals of six months from the first observation of the child, as well as at each change of mode of treatment (at the time of first dialysis, prior to transplantation, etc.) (15,16). A detailed description of these measurements is given by Roche (16).

1. Chronological Age

This should be given in years and expressed in decimals to the nearest one-hundredth, rather than fractions of the month, weeks or days.

2. Weight, Height, Height Velocity and Standard Deviation Scores for Height and Height Velocity

Infants should be weighed in the nude, while older children can wear underclothing or light gowns. Weight is measured in the fasting state; in dialysis patients it is measured at the end of the dialysis treatment.

In children under two years of age, a recumbent length is obtained and recorded to the nearest millimeter. In older children, stature can be measured, preferably by using an apparatus in which a counter-weighted headboard moves in the correct plane, as for example, by using a Harpenden stadiometer or one of the newer stadiometers with solid state electronic circuitry. In children with leg deformities, it is preferable to obtain a sitting height.

The values obtained for height and weight are plotted using the standard growth curves (see Appendix III). The weight-for-height ratio, according to Waterlow (17), can also be used as an index of nutrition. It expresses the actual weight as a percentage of the weight expected on the basis of the patient's height. Values of over 90% are considered normal. However, a fluid overload with an expansion of the ECF volume may obscure a low index value.

In order to determine whether the rate of growth in a given child is within normal limits, established standard and standard deviations for height velocity are used (18,19). Height velocity is the change in height expressed as centimeters per year. It is considered particularly useful because it depicts the growth process accurately and, consequently, may reveal significant changes in growth during disease. The increment and standards are expressed in terms of yearly increments because this is the minimum period over which seasonal differences between children are eliminated. For that reason, growth velocities should be interpreted with caution when they are based upon periods of less than one year.

In analyzing growth data in children whose growth is retarded, and which lies below the fifth percentile, it is best to express their height in standard deviation scores (SDS) (18,19). The SDS for height is calculated by using the published tables for mean heights and standard deviations for the United States and by utilizing the following formula:

Height SDS

$$= \frac{\text{Actual height (cm)} - \text{Mean expected height for age (cm)}}{\text{Standard deviation for age}}$$

For example, the height SDS for an eight-year-old boy who has a height of 110 cm can be calculated as follows:

$$\text{Height SDS} = \frac{110 - 127}{5.35} = (-)\,3.18$$

Thus, growth rate over time can be measured in terms of change in SDS for height (16,18,20). With severe growth retardation (Height SDS > -2 SD) the use of SDS for height velocity is preferable, especially when one needs to determine growth throughout a specific treatment regimen. In this case, the above formula is used, substituting height for height velocity, and the published tables are used for mean height velocity and standard deviations. It must be remembered, however, that for accurate interpretation of results, the specific treatment regimen must be followed for periods of six to twelve months and the age of the patient should be between three and ten years, in order to minimize the variability in growth observed during puberty.

3. Head Circumference

This parameter should be obtained for all children under three years of age, using a tape measure that does not stretch.

4. Skinfold Thickness and Upper Arm Circumference

These measurements are used to estimate body fat and to obtain an index of muscle mass, respectively (21–22). Skinfold thickness should be measured at the triceps and subscapular sides on the left side of the body, using a standard calibrated caliper (Lange or Harpenden).

The above measurements are expressed both as absolute measurement and as percent normal for age (millimeters measured/normal mean millimeters for age) (21–22). They can be used to determine nutritional state and body composition. Standards for skinfold thickness in U.S. children are given by Johnston et al (21).

5. Pubertal Stage

The stage of puberty should be determined initially and thereafter at yearly intervals, according to Tanner's grades (23). Similarly, testicular size should be measured and graded (24). The onset of menarche should be recorded accurately, indicating the exact age expressed in decimals.

6. Dental Age

This can be obtained by grading the degree of development of either four or seven permanent teeth (25).

C. General Evaluation

This involves an initial assessment and a subsequent close monitoring of the clinical status relative to the severity of the underlying renal disease, as well as laboratory, radiological and nutritional assessments.

1. Clinical Status

A complete history and physical examination including a fundoscopic examination (especially in children on corticosteroid therapy), as well as assessment of ECF volume status (overload or depletion) should be performed initially and at regular intervals thereafter, preferably every one to three months, depending on the patient's condition. All prescribed medications should be thoroughly reviewed, and the dosage modified according to the degree of GFR reduction. Guidelines for prescribing drugs in children with renal insufficiency have been reviewed recently (26).

The impact of the disease and its treatment on the child's psychological status, school attendance, intellectual performance and social activities should be thoroughly evaluated. This is important, since renal disease can affect specific areas of development in infants and young children, as well as cognitive functioning in older children (27–29). Such evaluations can best be performed by a child psychologist and should include the Bayley scales for infant development and the Gesell developmental schedules for infants and young children, and intelligence and achievement tests for older children. Special conferences should then be scheduled with the family to discuss findings and recommendations. In addition, the psychological effects of the child's illness on the siblings and the parents should also be addressed. Regular conferences with the family should be scheduled at frequent intervals, preferably every three months, to discuss problems and ways to cope with them (30). Plans should be made for certain members of the nephrology team to visit the child's school and discuss with the teachers the nature of the child's underlying disease as well as his or her special needs.

2. Laboratory Assessment

The initial and subsequent laboratory evaluations should be designed to assess the status of the renal function as well as the presence and/or severity of various metabolic abnormalities associated with chronic renal disease such as electrolyte disturbances, metabolic acidosis, anemia, hyperparathyroidism and lipid abnormalities.

Serum urea nitrogen, creatinine, electrolytes (including CO_2), Ca, P, alkaline phosphatase and proteins should be determined initially and thereafter at monthly intervals. Electrolyte disorders should be recognized promptly and treated appropriately. Hypokalemia may result from judicious diuretic therapy. Metabolic acidosis should be recognized and treated promptly, since it may further demineralize bone. Particular attention should be given to the status of Ca and P homeostasis and appropriate steps should be taken early in the course of renal insufficiency to maintain plasma levels within normal limits to prevent secondary hyperparathyroidism. Parathyroid hormone levels should be determined

as soon as radiological signs of bone disease become evident and thereafter every three months to assess the effect of therapeutic intervention.
Similarly, serial measurements of alkaline phosphatase are useful to monitor therapy, particularly vitamin D therapy.

The determination of electrolyte excretion, as well as Ca, P and creatinine, on a 24-hour urine should be performed during the initial patient
evaluation and subsequently at three- to six-month intervals, depending
on the patient's condition. Based on the urine volume and electrolyte
excretion, fluids and dietary Na should be tailored to the needs of the
individual patient, since it would be inappropriate to restrict them ar-
bitrarily. The amount of Na excreted in the urine will provide information
on Na intake and will identify children who are salt wasters, such as those
with tubulointerstitial disease. The Na replacement therapy should be
frequently monitored to prevent hypervolemia and congestive heart failure, especially in those patients with rapid deterioration of renal function.

A complete blood count with evaluation of peripheral smear, red blood
cell indices and serum ferritin should be assessed initially and thereafter
at monthly intervals. Serum ferritin concentration is now regarded as a
better indicator of body iron (Fe) stores than the estimation of serum
Fe, Fe binding capacity or bone marrow Fe deposition. A more complete
discussion on the assessment of the hematological abnormalities seen in
CRF is given later in this chapter.

Fasting triglycerides, cholesterol and uric acid should be assessed initially and thereafter at three-month intervals. Evaluation of lipid metabolism in patients with renal insufficiency has received intense attention
recently because of the high incidence of cardiovascular disease and ath-
erosclerosis in adult patients with CRF. Other special tests, such as evaluation of thyroid function, especially in patients with heavy proteinuria,
as well as in certain patients with renal failure, should be performed when
indicated.

3. Radiological Evaluation

All patients should have a chest X-ray during the initial assessment and
at yearly intervals thereafter. Renal ultrasound may be used in the initial
evaluation of children with CRF, especially for measuring the kidney size
and detecting hydronephrosis, posterior urethral valves, calculi and cystic
or solid lesions of the kidney. Recommendations for the use of dynamic
or static radioisotope scans, intravenous pyelography (IVP), micturating
cystourethrogram and radionuclide cystogram are presented in Chapter
6. The use of bone radiography for monitoring renal osteodystrophy, as
well as special procedures to detect cardiovascular abnormalities, are discussed later in this chapter.

4. Nutritional Assessment

As discussed previously, the nutritional status is assessed by anthropometric measurements, which include weight, skinfold thickness and mid-arm muscle circumference. Some investigators use the weight-to-height ratio of Waterlow (see section VI.B.2).

The above findings should be related to the patient's total calorie intake, as well as such nutrients as protein (especially of high biological value), Na, K, Ca and P. This is achieved by obtaining a prospective record of the weight or volume of all items consumed during a three-day period. The total intake of each of the above-mentioned nutrients can be calculated from standard tables of food composition and compared to the recommended daily allowances (RDA) for children with chronic renal insufficiency (31).

D. Assessment of Metabolic Consequences

1. Renal Osteodystrophy

a. Clinical Evaluation

Renal osteodystrophy occurs in approximately 60 to 80% of uremic children. It is particularly important in children because they have open epiphyses and their growth affects mineralization and remodeling of bone, which proceeds at a rate eight to ten times higher than that of adults. Significant reduction of mean plasma concentration of 1, 25 dihydroxy-vitamin D3 has been observed in children with moderate renal insufficiency (32). As a consequence of vitamin D deficiency and high circulating PTH levels, severe clinical and orthopedic problems may develop within a very short period of time (Table 15-4).

The main forms of bone disease that may develop in children with renal osteodystrophy include osteitis fibrosa and osteomalacia. Osteitis fibrosa occurs as a result of secondary hyperparathyroidism and is characterized by fibroosteoclastic lesions that represent a high turnover state. Osteomalacia is the result of delayed or defective primary mineralization of the osteoid matrix, which is due to a relative deficiency of vitamin D. To the extent that either mechanism predominates, the patient may have one or the other form of bone disease, although one usually finds a mixture of both lesions. Norman et al found histological evidence of osteomalacia, hyperparathyroidism or both, in children with a GFR of less than 45 ml/1.73 m^2 per minute, in spite of the fact that 25% of them had normal serum levels of Ca, P and alkaline phosphatase, as well as normal bone radiographs (33).

A very careful history and physical examination should be performed in an attempt to evaluate the extent of involvement. Myopathy is a com-

TABLE 15-4. Clinical and Orthopedic Problems Associated with Renal Osteodystrophy

Myopathy
Bone pain
Stunted growth
Metaphyseal fractures
Slippage of the epiphyses
  Preschool children
    Upper and lower femoral epiphyses
    Distal tibial epiphyses
  Older children
    Upper femoral epiphyses
    Distal radial and ulnar epiphyses
  Puberty
    Distal radial and ulnar epiphyses
Impairment of gait
Gross deformities of skeleton
  Ulnar deviation of hand
  Pes (talipes) varus
  "Swelling" of wrists, ankles or medial end of clavicles
  Pseudo-drumstick fingers (pseudo-clubbing)
  Very young children
    Rachitic rosary
    Harrison groove
    Enlargement of wrists and ankles
    Severe bowing and sharp angulation of bones

mon feature of renal bone disease, but it is often overlooked or its manifestations may be interpreted as malaise or generalized weakness. Similarly, children with renal osteodystrophy do not complain of bone pain but rather tend to restrict their physical activity in an attempt to protect the painful extremity. Specific inquiry should therefore be made regarding the occurrence of pain during long walks or exercise. When children do complain of severe bone pain, it is usually a sign of serious bone disease such as epiphyseal slippage or fracture of the metaphyses. The diagnosis of epiphyseal slipping of the femoral head is often missed during routine physical examination unless special attention is paid to subtle abnormalities in the patient's gait. Enamel defects in the form of white or brown discoloration of the teeth are frequently observed in children with congenital renal disease.

b. Radiological Evaluation

Skeletal roentgenograms help to distinguish between lesions of cortical bone (subperiosteal, intracortical and endosteal bone resorption), and lesions of cancellous bone (osteomalacia or osteosclerosis). An X-ray of the hand, wrist and long bones should be performed at six-month intervals to evaluate renal osteodystrophy and the effect of specific therapy, and to determine bone age.

Resorptive defects of the outer contour of the cortical bones with the characteristic "spicular" appearance are the main characteristic features of secondary hyperparathyroidism. The classic site of subperiosteal resorption is in the inner side of the middle phalanges II and III. In infants and preschool children, subperiosteal resorption zones are best depicted at the lateral aspect of the distal radius and ulna as well as at the inner side of the upper tibia. Erosions may also be observed at the metaphyseal shaft junction of long bones, as well as at the tufts of the terminal phalanges. Healing of these lesions is achieved by the administration of vitamin D. The radiological findings in cases of osteomalacia are not as distinct as those of secondary hyperparathyroidism. The typical picture is a radiolucent zone at the distal end of long bones. Occasionally, pseudofractures may be the only characteristic finding.

Certain patients with severe renal osteodystrophy have cyst formation or brown tumors located primarily in the metacarpals, distal femur, proximal tibia and distal radius. The manner of their formation is not well understood. Slipping of the upper femoral epiphysis can occur either in the medial or in the dorsolateral direction. The diagnosis can therefore be made by obtaining two views, namely an anterior posterior view for medial slipping and an oblique view for dorsolateral displacement. Distal radial and ulnar epiphyses slip to the dorsolateral side.

c. Aluminum Osteomalacia

The accumulation of aluminum in uremic children is the result of enhanced gastrointestinal absorption, reduced ability to excrete aluminum and the ingestion of large amounts of aluminum-containing, phosphate-binding gels. Aluminum concentration levels in normal subjects are depicted in Table 15-5 (34–38). Since aluminum is tightly bound to tissue, its levels in the plasma do not correlate directly with the amount of tissue loading. Tissue levels of aluminum are related to multiple factors such as the GFR, duration of therapy, total dose of aluminum and tissue turnover rate. In one study, most children whose plasma aluminum levels were more than 100 mg/L showed signs of aluminum toxicity and were receiving more than 75 mg/kg a day of elemental aluminum orally (39).

TABLE 15-5. Aluminum Concentration Levels in Normal Subjects

Source	Aluminum concentration	Reference
Plasma level	10 μg/L	34
Bone level	3.3 mg/kg	35
Total body aluminum	35 mg	36
Urine aluminum excretion	13 $\pm$ 7 to 65 $\pm$ 85 μg/day	34,37,38

Plasma aluminum levels should be monitored in all children who require more than 30 mg/kg a day of elemental aluminum.

Aluminum osteomalacia is characterized by proximal muscular weakness, progressive skeletal pain, bone pain, low plasma alkaline phosphatase and PTH levels and resistance to vitamin D. It is postulated that increased plasma aluminum levels may damage the osteoblasts, with a concomitant loss of bone mass, as well as the microtubular system of the parathyroid cells, with a concomitant suppression of parathyroid function. As a result, the PTH level in these patients is usually low and unresponsive to stimulation by hypocalcemia.

d. Bone Mineral Content

The measurement of skeletal bone mineral content can be of great value, since it reflects the Ca balance. It is used clinically to assess the response of renal osteodystrophy to various therapeutic interventions. An accurate and precise measurement of bone mineral content can be performed by photon absorptiometry. Sequential studies performed by this method can be used to assess the effect of therapy on bone mineral status (40).

e. Bone Biopsy

Bone biopsy, usually of the iliac crest, is not usually required for the routine workup of children with chronic renal failure. Quantitative histological studies can be performed in certain situations, such as quantitative evaluation of renal osteodystrophy and verification of aluminum osteomalacia, and in patients being considered for a parathyroidectomy.

2. Hematological Disorders

Anemia develops gradually during the course of CRF as a result of 1) decreased red blood cell (RBC) production due to diminished production and release of erythropoietin and 2) decreased RBC survival in the presence of some degree of hemolysis. Factors that may further aggravate the decrease in erythropoietin production include infection, malnutrition and nephrectomy. Hemolysis may be further exacerbated by an acquired defect of the pentose-phosphate shunt, which in the majority of the patients may be due to a glucose 6-phosphate-dehydrogenase (G6PD) deficiency. Iron deficiency anemia is not part of the basic anemia but may often be found as a result of gastrointestinal blood loss or in patients on hemodialysis due to the adherence of RBCs to the dialysis membranes. Folic acid deficiency is also common in patients with ESRD.

The anemia of CRF is characteristically normocytic and normochromic and is associated with a low or "normal" reticulocyte index (% reticulocytes $\times$ hematocrit/45). The presence of a Fe or folic acid deficiency may alter the above findings and cause a microcytic or megaloblastic anemia, respectively. Various degrees of poikilocytosis, as well as Burr cells, may be frequently detected on a peripheral blood smear. In the absence of Fe or folic acid deficiency, the bone marrow is normocellular, but the degree of erythropoiesis is markedly decreased, relative to the severity of the anemia. The serum Fe is usually high, and the Fe-binding capacity is normal to high.

In evaluating a child with CRF, the first step should be to detect the presence of anemia and determine its etiology. A decrease or increase in the mean corpuscular volume (MCV) may signify the presence of a Fe or folic acid deficiency, respectively. A significant increase in the reticulocyte index may occur as a result of an increase in the rate of hemolysis or of severe hypoxia. The presence of Burr cells correlate better with the severity of the uremia than with either anemia or hemolysis. The presence of schistocytes may signify microangiopathy, whereas the presence of spherocytes may indicate hypersplenism. The diagnosis of hypersplenism should be confirmed by demonstrating an increase in the rate of sequestration of chromium-51 labeled RBCs, as well as high transfusion requirements.

The serum ferritin level determination is most accurate in assessing body Fe stores and should be performed at monthly intervals. The ascorbate-cyanide test can be used to detect malfunction of the pentose-phosphate shunt and should be performed in patients suspected to have a Heinz body type of hemolysis. Once identified, these patients should not be given medications with a high oxidative potential (sulfonamides, nitrofurantoin, antimalarials), and if on hemodialysis, they should be dialyzed only with distilled or deionized water.

3. Cardiovascular Disorders

Children with CRF have an abnormal cardiac function attributable to hypertension, anemia and uremia. Left ventricular function is impaired and the cardiac load is increased, which in turn may lead to cardiomegaly. The presence of anemia and a large vascular access in patients on hemodialysis may further increase the cardiac work load and may contribute to the development of congestive heart failure. Heart murmurs, which are quite common in children with CRF, are attributed to a combination of anemia, hypertension and volume overload. Electrocardiographic abnormalities are not as frequent in children as in adults and, when present, they indicate left ventricular hypertrophy, particularly in hypertensive patients, as well as characteristic K and Ca disturbances and alterations of cardiac conduction and dysrrhythmias associated with drug therapy.

Hypertension is quite common in children with moderate to severe CRF and is the result of an increase in peripheral vascular resistance relative to the normal or high cardiac output, as well as to volume overload associated with ESRD. Pericarditis is a later manifestation of CRF and, although its incidence and death rate have declined in recent years, its early recognition is imperative. The clinical manifestations of pericarditis are shown in Table 15-6.

The status of the cardiovascular system should be assessed in all children with CRF at the time of their first visit. A chest X-ray and a baseline electrocardiogram should be performed initially and at six-month intervals thereafter. Echocardiography should be performed in all patients with ESRD. It is valuable not only for the evaluation of cardiac chamber size, ventricular performance and cardiac output but also for the detection of pericardial effusion, which is a relatively common finding in adults with advanced CRF (41).

4. Neurological Disorders

The main neurological disturbances observed in children with advanced renal failure include uremic neuropathy and encephalopathy. Uremic neuropathy is primarily a distal symmetrical polyneuropathy in which the lower limbs are most frequently involved. It is a mixed polyneuropathy and involves impairment of both motor and sensory function. In addition, autonomic dysfunction has been frequently demonstrated, especially in patients on dialysis. The clinical manifestations of uremic neuropathy are shown in Table 15-7.

TABLE 15-6. Clinical Manifestations of Uremic Pericarditis

Fever	Sudden drop of hemoglobin
Precordial pain	Leukocytosis
Friction rub	Cardiomegaly
Cardiac failure	Cardiac arrhythmias

TABLE 15-7. Clinical Manifestations of Uremic Neuropathy

Impaired motor function
  Muscle weakness
  Loss of deep tendon reflexes (especially knee, ankle)
  "Restless leg syndrome"
    Prickling sensation
    Pruritus
Impaired sensory function ("stocking-glove anesthesia")
  Loss of pain, light touch, vibratory sensation, and pressure
Autonomic dysfunction
  Postural hypotension
  Impaired sweating
  Dialysis-related hypotension

Uremic encephalopathy is initially characterized by nonspecific symptoms of cerebral dysfunction, which become progressively more pronounced as renal function deteriorates. The earlier symptoms of encephalopathy are observed in the majority of the children with CRF and include headache, fatigue and listlessness. As kidney function deteriorates, symptoms may include memory loss, decreased attention span, drowsiness and speech impairment. With advanced renal failure, symptoms may include psychosis, ataxia, tremors, seizures and coma. In the very young child, encephalopathy is difficult to assess. Recent observations in young children with onset of CRF in infancy have demonstrated the presence of severe developmental delay in all areas—gross motor, language, cognitive, fine motor skills and psychosocial skills; these skills did not improve with dialysis-transplantation therapy.

Based on the above findings, and in view of the fact that increasingly more young children are being accepted into dialysis-transplantation programs, it is imperative that careful assessment of the neurological status be performed more systematically in this young age group. Head circumference should be accurately recorded at three- to six-month intervals. It has been demonstrated that in nonrenal failure patients, a head circumference more than 2 SD below the mean is associated with a high incidence of mental retardation. The status of the cranial sutures and the presence of craniosynostosis should be noted. Computed tomography should be performed, since generalized cerebral atrophy has been demonstrated to occur in patients with CRF and to correlate inversely with age. Electroencephalograms are not helpful, since the findings are nonspecific, with evidence of diffuse slow-wave activity. Developmental assessment using the Revised Yale Developmental Schedules should be performed in all children with onset of CRF in infancy and should be repeated at six- to nine-month intervals. Other tests may include the Denver Developmental Screen and Bayley Scales of infant development, or the Stanford Binet or the Wechsler Intelligence scale for older children. Every attempt should be made to avoid the use of aluminum hydroxide gels, since a syndrome similar to dialysis dementia, and postulated to be due to aluminum therapy, has been described in young children not receiving dialysis (42).

References

1. Chantler C, Holliday M (1987) Progressive loss of renal function. In: Pediatric Nephrology, 2nd edition. Holliday MA, Barratt TM, Vernier RL (eds). Williams and Wilkins, Baltimore, pp 773–798
2. Donckerwolcke RA, Broyer M, Brunner FP, et al (1982) Combined report on regular dialysis and transplantation of children in Europe, XI, 1981. Proc Eur Dial Transplant Assoc 19:61–91

3. Broyer M, Brunner FP, Brynger H, Fassbinder W, et al (1986) Demography of dialysis and transplantation in children in Europe, 1984. Nephrol Dial Transplant 1:9

4. Potter DE, Holliday MA, Piel CF, et al (1980) Treatment of end stage renal disease in children: a 15 year experience. Kidney Int 18:103–109

5. Chan JC, Mendez-Picon GJ, Landwehr DM (1981) A 3-year survey of referral pattern and case material in pediatric nephrology. Int J Pediatr Nephrol 2:109–113

6. Broyer M, Rizzoni G, Brunner FP, et al (1985) Combined report on regular dialysis and transplantation of children in Europe, 1984. Proceedings of EDTA-ERA 22:55

7. Donckerwolcke RA, Chantler C, Broyer MJ (1983) Pediatric dialysis. In: Drukker W, Parsons FM, Maher JF (eds) Replacement of Renal Function by Dialysis, 2nd edition. Martinus Nijhoff, Boston, pp 514–535

8. Helin I, Winberg J (1980) Chronic renal failure in Swedish children. Acta Paediatr Scand 69:607–611

9. Arbus GS, Geary DF, McLorie GA, et al (1986) Pediatric renal transplants: A Canadian perspective. Kidney Int 30:S31-S34

10. Fine RN (1982) Renal transplantatoin in children. In: Chaterjee SN (ed) Organ Transplantation. John Wright, Boston, p 243

11. Klahr S, Schreiner G, Ichikawa I (1988) The progression of renal disease. New Engl J Med 318:1657–1666

12. Rodriquez-Soriano J, Arant BS, et al (1986) Fluid and electrolyte imbalances in children with chronic renal failure. Am J Kidney Dis 7:268–274

13. Betts PR, Magrath G (1974) Growth pattern and dietary intake of children with chronic renal insufficiency. Br Med J 2:189–193

14. Potter DE, Greifer I (1978) Statural growth of children with renal disease. Kidney Int 14:334–339

15. Potter DE, Broyer M, Chantler C, et al (1978) Measurement of growth in children with renal insufficiency. Kidney Int 14:378–382

16. Roche AF (1978) Growth assessment in abnormal children. Kidney Int 14:369–377

17. Waterlow JC (1976) Classification and definition of protein energy malnutrition. In: Beaton GH, Bergen JM (eds) Nutrition in Preventive Medicine. World Health Organization, Geneva, pp 530–555

18. Roche AF, Himes JH (1980) Incremental growth charts. Am J Clin Nutr 33:2041–2052

19. Tanner JM, Davies PW (1985) Clinical longitudinal standards for height and height velocity for North American children. J Pediatr 107:317–329

20. Barrett TM, Broyer M, Chantler C, et al (1986) Assessment of growth. Am J Kidney Dis 7:340–346

21. Johnston FE, Hamill PVV, Lemeshow S (1972) Skinfold thickness of children 6–11 years, United States Department of Health, Education and Welfare, National Center for Health Statistics, Publication, No. (HSM) 73-1602, series 11, No. 120, U.S. Government Printing Office, Washington, D.C., pp 20–24. Also Publication No. (HPA) 74-1614, Series 11, No. 132 (1974) U.S. Government Printing Office, Washington, D.C., p 20

22. Frisancho AR (1974) Triceps skin fold and upper arm muscle size norms for assessment of nutritional status. Am J Clin Nutr 27:1052–1058

23. Tanner JM (1962) Growth at adolescence, 2nd edition, Blackwell Scientific Publications, Oxford, pp 32–38
24. Burr IM, Sizonenko PC, Kaplan SL, et al (1970) Hormonal changes in puberty: I. Correlation of serum luteinizing hormone and follicle stimulating hormone with stages of puberty, testicular size, and bone age in normal boys. Pediatr Res 4:25–35
25. Demirjian A, Godstein H (1976) New systems for dental maturity based on seven and four teeth. Ann Hum Biol 3:411–421
26. Trompeter RS (1987) A review of drug prescribing in children with end-stage renal failure. Pediatr Nephrol 1:183–194
27. Rasbury WC, Fennell RS, Morris MK (1983) Cognitive functioning of children with end-stage renal disease before and after successful transplantation. J Pediatr 102:589–592
28. Crittenden MR, Holliday MA, Piel CF, et al (1985) Intellectual development of children with renal insufficiency and end-stage disease. Int J Pediatr Nephrol 6:275–280
29. Polinsky MS, Kaiser BA, Stover JB, et al (1987) Neurologic development of children with severe chronic renal failure from infancy. Pediatr Nephrol 1:157–165
30. Fielding D, Moore B, Dewey M, et al (1985) Children with end-stage renal failure: psychological effects on patients, siblings and parents. J Psychosom Res 29:457–465
31. National Research Council, Food and Nutrition Board (1980) Recommended Dietary Allowances, 9th edition. National Academy of Sciences, Washington, D.C.
32. Portale AA, Booth BE, Tsai HC, et al (1982) Reduced plasma concentration of 1,25 dihydroxyvitamin D in children with moderate renal insufficiency. Kidney Int 21:627–632
33. Norman ME, Mazur AT, Borden S, et al (1980) Early diagnosis of juvenile renal osteodystrophy. J Pediatr 97:226–232
34. Kaehny WD, Hegg AP, Alfrey AC (1977) Gastrointestinal absorption of aluminum from aluminum containing antacids. N Engl J Med 296:1389–1390
35. Alfrey AC (1980) Aluminum metabolism in uremia. Neurotoxicology 1:43–53
36. Alfrey AC (1983) Aluminum. Adv Clin Chem 23:69–91
37. Recker RR, Blotcky AJ, Leffler JA, et al (1977) Evidence for aluminum absorption from the gastrointestinal tract and bone deposition by aluminum carbonate ingestion with normal renal function. J Lab Clin Med 90:810–815
38. Gorsky JE, Dietz AA (1978) Determination of aluminum in biological samples by atomic absorption spectrophotometry with a graphite furnace. Clin Chem 24:1485–1490
39. Sedman AB, Miller NL, Warady BA, et al (1984) Aluminum loading in children with chronic renal failure. Kidney Int 26:201–204
40. Chesney RW, Rose P, Mazess RB, DeLuca HF (1988) Long term follow-up of bone mineral status in children with renal disease. Pediatr Nephrol 2:22–26
41. Luft FC, Gilman IK, Weyman AE (1980) Pericarditis in the patient with uremia: clinical and echocardiographic evaluation. Nephron 25:160–166
42. Rotundo A, Nevins TE, Lipton M, et al (1982) Progressive encephalopathy in children with chronic renal insufficiency in infancy. Kidney Int 21:486–491

16
Hypertension

Mouin G. Seikaly and Billy S. Arant, Jr.

I. Documentation

A. Definition

In children, blood pressure (BP) is a continuous variable, dependent on age, sex, body size and genetic and environmental factors, but no single comparison is considered ideal. Traditionally, BP has been compared most commonly to chronological age and sex (1). Curves showing age-specific distributions of systolic and diastolic BP for boys and girls are presented in Figure 16-1). These data represent BP in children who are awake; 7 mm Hg should be added to the systolic, and 5 mm Hg to the diastolic BP obtained when the child is sleeping. Similar data for newborn and premature babies are scarce (2). Figure 16-2 shows the predicted mean systolic and diastolic BP in healthy newborns; and Figure 16-3 shows the BP in the critically ill neonate. Children of the same age may vary in size, with heavier and taller children having higher BPs than smaller children of the same age (3). Hence, in a child or adolescent who has a BP above the 90th percentile for his or her age and is not tall or heavy, there is a greater probability that the BP elevation is pathological (1). So far, there is no universal agreement with regard to the upper limits far, there is no universal agreement with regard to the upper limits of normal BP in children, and the task of defining hypertension remains a challenge to the pediatrician. An operant, but arbitrary definition is the persistence of BP, measured using a standardized approach, above the 95th percentile for a matched population on at least three different occasions (Table 16-1).

B. Measurement

The relative difficulty of measuring BP in the young pediatric patient poses a nearly insurmountable problem with regard to establishing normal values for this age group. In infants, BP can be measured most reproducibly either directly from an intraarterial catheter connected to a pressure transducer or indirectly by Doppler ultrasound or automatic oscillometry (4). When the appropriate cuff size is used, indirect systolic BP measurements correlates well with intraarterial BP determinations (5). Infants in whom hypertension is suspected ought to be referred to a facility where the appropriate equipment is available for monitoring BP. The BP at any given moment depends upon the degree of the infant's agitation, position, time since feeding, state of alertness and body mass, as well as gestational or postnatal age (6). The BP in the crying infant can vary by as much as 17 to 25 mm Hg (7).

Beyond infancy, BP by sphygmomanometry becomes more reproducible and should be an integral part of the routine physical examination, with measurement at least once a year. Several types of instruments are available for home and office BP monitoring (8). These devices have variable accuracy, reliability, durability, ease of operation, and expense (9). Regardless of the type of instrument used, it is recommended that the accuracy of a particular gadget be validated periodically against a mercury-gravity manometer. Erroneous BP measurement due to improper technique is not an uncommon cause of unnecessary workups for hypertension in children. The use of a properly sized cuff is of critical importance in the pediatric patient. This very small, but important detail cannot be over-emphasized for the health care worker measuring BP in

--►

FIGURE 16-1. Age-specific percentiles of blood pressure measurement in children. From Task Force on Blood Pressure Control in Children (1987) Report of the Second Task Force on Blood Pressure Control in Children—1987. Reproduced by permission of Pediatrics 79:1–25, copyright 1987.

    16–1-A: Boys, birth to 12 months of age
    16–1-B: Girls, birth to 12 months of age
    16–1-C: Boys, 1–13 years of age
    16–1-D: Girls, 1–13 years of age
    16–1-E: Boys, 13–18 years of age
    16–1-F: Girls, 13–18 years of age

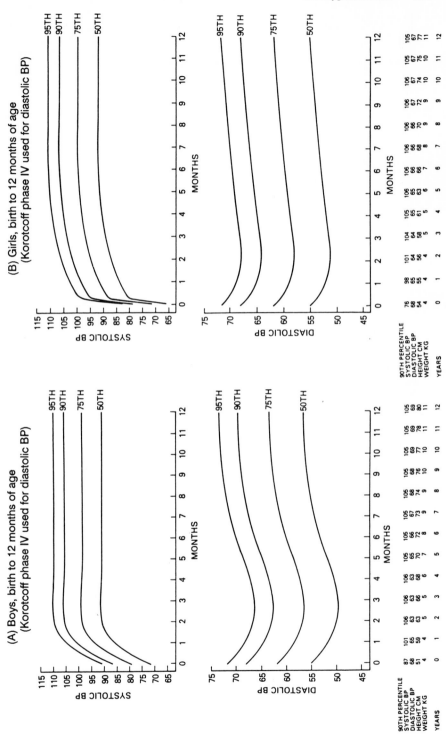

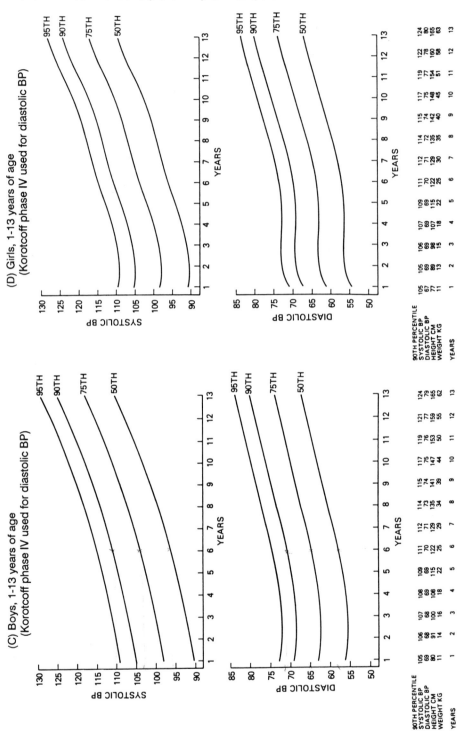

(D) Girls, 1-13 years of age
(Korotcoff phase IV used for diastolic BP)

(C) Boys, 1-13 years of age
(Korotcoff phase IV used for diastolic BP)

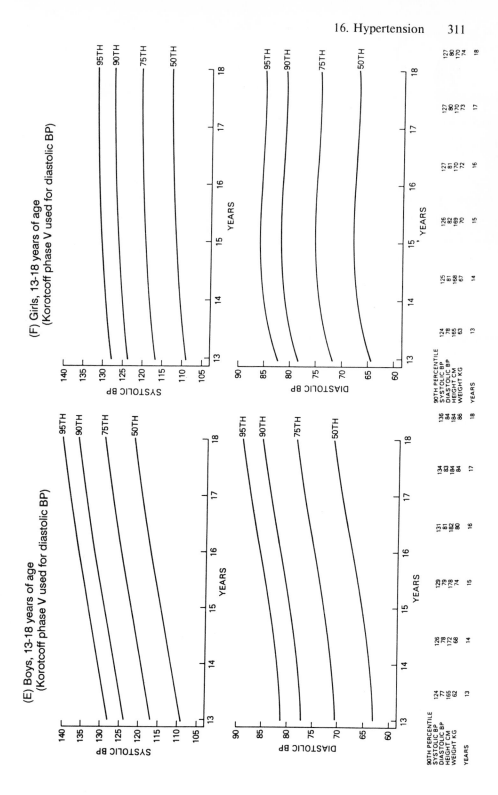

(E) Boys, 13-18 years of age
(Korotcoff phase V used for diastolic BP)

(F) Girls, 13-18 years of age
(Korotcoff phase V used for diastolic BP)

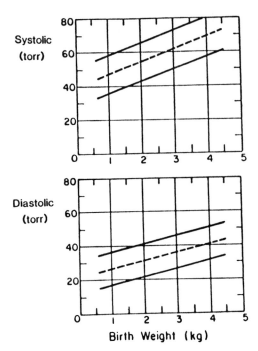

FIGURE 16-2. Predicted mean systolic and diastolic blood pressure (dotted lines) and 95th percentile confidence limits for healthy newborns in the first 12 hours of life. From Versmold HT, Kitterman JA, Phibbs RH, Gregory GA, Tooley WH (1981) Aortic blood pressure during the first 12 hours of life in infants with birth weight 610–4220 gm. Reproduced by permission of Pediatrics 67: 607–613, copyright 1981.

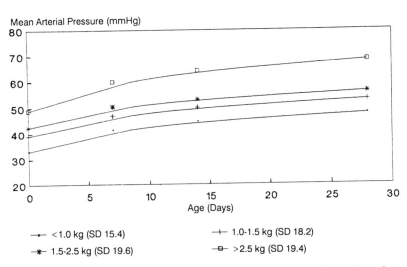

FIGURE 16-3. Blood pressure in the critically ill neonate. Curve drawn from figures in Stork EK, Carlo WA, Kliegman RM, Fanaroff AA (1984) Hypertension redefined for critically ill neonates. Pediatr Res 18:321A

TABLE 16-1. Classification of Hypertension by Age Group

Age group	Significant hypertension (mm Hg)[a]	Severe hypertension (mm Hg)[a]
Newborns		
7 days	SBP ≥ 96	SBP ≥ 106
8–30 days	SBP ≥ 104	SBP ≥ 110
Infants (≤2 yr)	SBP ≥ 112	SBP ≥ 118
	DBP ≥ 74	DBP ≥ 82
Children (3–5 yr)	SBP ≥ 116	SBP ≥ 124
	DBP ≥ 76	DBP ≥ 84
Children (6–9 yr)	SBP ≥ 122	SBP ≥ 130
	DBP ≥ 78	DBP ≥ 86
Children (10–12 yr)	SBP ≥ 126	SBP ≥ 134
	DBP ≥ 82	DBP ≥ 90
Adolescents (13–15 yr)	SBP ≥ 136	SBP ≥ 144
	DBP ≥ 86	DBP ≥ 92
Adolescents (16–18 yr)	SBP ≥ 142	SBP ≥ 150
	DBP ≥ 92	DBP ≥ 98

[a]SBP: systolic blood pressure; DBP: diastolic blood pressure.
Adapted with permission. Task Force on Blood Pressure Control in Children (1987) Report of the Second Task Force on Blood Pressure Control in Children—1987. Reproduced by permission of Pediatrics 79:1–25, copyright 1987.

children. Every medical facility treating children should have on hand a graded assortment of cuffs, and use of the correct bladder size for each patient should be emphasized. The American Heart Association recommends that the width of the inflatable part of the cuff (the bladder) should be approximately 40% of the limb circumference and cover 75% of the length of the humerus or femur, depending upon the limb examined. Moreover, the lower margin of the bladder should not impinge on the diaphragm of the stethoscope placed over the brachial artery. Other causes of error in BP determination are listed in Table 16-2.

Blood pressure should be recorded in both upper extremities and at least one lower extremity to exclude the possibility of coarctation of the aorta. The examiner listens with the stethoscope positioned over the artery distal to the cuff, no sound is heard when the artery is completely occluded. When the pressure is released, vascular sounds in seperate phases are heard (Korotkoff sounds):

I.   Sudden appearance of first sound
II. Sound is prolonged to a murmur
III. Sound intensity increases
IV. Sound becomes muffled
V.   Sound Disappears

TABLE 16-2. Common Errors in Blood Pressure Measurement

Technical errors
  Failure to select proper cuff size
  Failure to apply cuff properly (too loose, uncentered)
  Instrument errors
  Failure to use the proper technique
    Excessive stethoscope pressure over artery
    Failure to estimate systolic BP by palpation
    Failure to inflate to 20 mm Hg above systolic BP
    Too rapid deflation
    Failure to keep arm at the level of the heart
    Failure to relax extremity before and between BP measurements
    Reliance on single BP measurement
    Failure to record BP in both arms or, preferably, all four extremities
Observer-related errors
  Hearing problems
  Subjective differences in interpretation
  Memory errors between measuring and recording
  Reliance on previous recording "bias"
  Improper documentation
Patient-related error
  Anxiety and apprehension
  Poorly audible Korotkoff sound
  Hypotension
  Arrhythmias (atrial fibrillation, pulsus alternas) Obese or conically shaped arms
  Distended urinary bladder

Although there is agreement that sound I corresponds to systolic pressure, there is no universal agreement whether sound IV or sound V represent the diastolic blood pressure. The nomograms published by the Task Force on Blood Pressure Control in Children specifies the sound used at different ages (Figure 16-1).

At times, sound IV is used in conjunction with sound V to indicate diastolic BP (10). When the stethoscope compresses the artery, which happens more often in struggling infants and young children, the bruit may be heard even when the cuff has been deflated completely. The BP is recorded frequently as systolic pressure (sound III)/*P*, which traditionally has meant that systolic pressure was estimated by palpation rather than auscultation; however, BP expressed in this manner more recently has meant that the bruit persisted to a cuff pressure of zero. These two quite different ways of recording BP must be acknowledged, lest an erroneous diagnosis of an absent aortic valve be made. If the bruit does persist to zero pressure, diastolic pressure can be recorded as the cuff pressure at which the character of the bruit changes. Usually, a second attempt at lowering the cuff pressure with less pressure against the artery will permit a clear disappearance of the bruit or Korotkoff sound V, even in neonates. Although a good systolic reading is a satisfactory estimate for screening infants and children for hypertension, it is this pressure that is most often increased in anxious or uncooperative patients so that the diagnosis of hypertension is too often made. If systolic pressure is normal for age and sex, an elevated diastolic pressure will rarely be encountered. The extra effort to obtain diastolic BP, however, can alleviate undue concern for normal patients and identify those patients who should undergo further observation for hypertension. Elevation of both systolic and diastolic pressures is more significant than elevation of the systolic pressure alone. Recently, systolic and diastolic BP reading have been reliably measured by oscillometry in the young infant and older child.

In children, BP can be labile. Many surveys have shown that BP elevation noted during the first office visit could not be confirmed on subsequent visits. The importance of taking more than one BP measurement cannot be overemphasized. One screening study in Dallas (11) observed that the initial incidence of abnormal BP of 8.9%, estimated from the first reading during an outpaient visit, decreased to 1% when only the third reading was used. It is advisable to evaluate patients for hypertension by measuring BP three separate times during the examination—at the outset of the visit, midway through the examination and, finally, at the completion of the examination; discarding the first value and averaging the second and third recorded pressures is a standardized way of following BP in children. Instruments for continuous ambulatory BP monitoring are available, but their use in pediatrics remains investigational and is not warranted for routine evaluation of hypertension (8). The role of echocardiography in detecting early cardiac changes as evidence of BP elevation in labile or borderline hypertension is yet to be determined.

The BP measurements should be documented, indicating the cuff size, the patient's posture, side and limb used and a brief description of the clinical status of the patient during the examination (e.g. anxiety, apprehension, crying, pain and muscle tension). These outlined difficulties in obtaining reliable and meaningful BP values are the major reasons why routine screening of BP in school children has not been encouraged.

After establishing the existence of hypertension, it is advantageous to characterize the nature of BP elevation as borderline or sustained. Borderline or high normal BP is defined as an average systolic or diastolic BP between the 90th and 95th percentile for age and sex; these patients often represent a dilemma for clinical management, since they are at highest risk for developing hypertension and its sequalae at a later time; however, the risk to the patient, as it is perceived currently, does not warrant antihypertensive medication (12). An unequivocally high BP is defined as BP above the 95th percentile for age and sex.

A thorough physical examination should be performed in every child with elevated blood pressure (see Chapter 2). Special attention should be given to the cardiovascular system, fundi and stigmata of syndromes that are associated with hypertension.

II. Prevalence

With so many variables affecting BP measurements, it is not surprising that the incidence of hypertension, between birth and adulthood, is difficult to determine. The incidence in adults and, perhaps, in adolescents is quite different from that reported in infants and children, which has been reported to be as low as 1.2% and as high as 13%. This variability could be explained, in part, by differences in techniques of measuring BP (13). On the basis of clinical experience alone, it is accepted generally that the prevalence of hypertension is far less in children than in adults. One difference could be the much higher incidence of essential hypertension in adults, which has not been identified with certainty in children. This may be explained by our failure to know what the "normal" BP should be in various conditions or to follow serial BP measurements in the same child plotted on individual graphs or chronological age and sex just as with height, weight and head circumference. Although a child's BP may always be found to fall between ±2 standard deviations of (SD) mean normal values, values may be at the 25th percentile at 3 years of age, at the 50th percentile at 5 years of age and at the 90th percentile at 7 years of age. Thus, this pattern of change in BP with age in any child deserves equal attention to a BP recorded at or above the 95th percentile. Longitudinal data from several surveys indicate that movement into and out of the upper quintile of BP is not uncommon (11). The long-term outcome for the child with hypertension is uncertain; hence, the role for BP monitoring in this subpopulation of hypertensives cannot be overemphasized.

III. Clinical Presentation

The presenting symptoms of children with hypertension vary and may either be subtle or absent, even when hypertension is pronounced. This fact explains why, despite the recent awareness of hypertension, patients still present with severe symptoms. Presenting symptoms also vary with age, and may be either nonspecific (Table 16-3) or part of the spectrum of symptoms of a specific disease entity.

IV. Etiology

When classifying the causes of hypertension, it is often advantageous to differentiate its etiology according to age at onset, severity and duration. Most of the causes of hypertension reported in neonates are secondary, the majority of them being renovascular. The rather dramatic rise in the incidence of renal artery thrombosis in the newborn is associated clearly

TABLE 16-3. Nonspecific Symptoms in Patients
with Moderate to Severe Hypertension

Infancy
   Irritability
   Vomiting
   Failure to thrive
   Respiratory distress
   Congestive heart failure
Beyond infancy
   Irritability
   Easy fatigability
   Vomiting
   Polyuria, polydipsia
   Growth failure
   Headache
   Epistaxis
   Neurological deficit (Bell's palsy, visual impairment)
   Chest pain

with the more widespread use of indwelling aortic catheters placed either through an umbilical or femoral artery (3). Catheter insertion may produce intimal injury resulting in a nidus that can develop into a mural thrombus and propagate cephalically or caudally. When blood flow into one or both renal arteries is compromised, the renin-angiotensin-aldosterone axis is stimulated, and hypertension develops. Renal vein thrombosis, renal cortical or medullary necrosis, asphyxia neonatorum, obstructive uropathy, congenital nephrosis and autosomal recessive polycystic kidney disease are also causes of hypertension in neonates.

Conditions associated with childhood hypertension are listed in Tables 16-4 and 16-5. Renal scarring accounts for nearly 35% of all causes of sustained hypertension in children (14). A transient rise in BP is seen typically with acute nephritic syndromes, Henoch-Schönlein purpura, hemolyticuremic syndrome, acute renal failure and in certain instances of idiopathic nephrotic syndrome either because of the activation of endogenous vasopressor systems when effective arterial blood volume is decreased or as a result of corticosteroid therapy (15). The diagnosis of these conditions are presented elsewhere in this text. Other causes of transient hypertension include increased intracranial pressure, Guillain-Barré syndrome, drugs, infections, pain and leg traction.

V. Investigation

The extent to which elevated BP should be investigated will depend upon the age of onset, persistence, duration and degree of hypertension. Usually, the younger the child and the higher the BP, the more extensive is

TABLE 16-4. Some Causes of Hypertension in Infants and Children

Renal
   Acute glomerulonephritis
   Other forms of nephritis (Alport's syndrome, Henoch-Schönlein purpura, collagen
      disease)
   Obstructive uropathy
   Congenital abnormalities (polycystic kidney disease, segmental hypoplasia)
   Chronic renal insufficiency
   Renal tumors (Wilms', tumor, tuberous sclerosis)
   Hemolytic-uremic syndrome
   Renal cortical or medullary necrosis
   Acute renal failure
   Following renal transplantation (rejection)
   Unilateral renal disease (parenchymal disease, perirenal masses)
Vascular
   Aortic thrombosis
   Renal artery thrombosis
   Renal vein thrombosis
   Coarctation of the aorta
   Renal artery stenosis
   Hypoplastic aorta
   Arteriovenous fistula (systolic)
   Radiation aortitis and renal arteritis
   Cardiac disease (aortic insufficiency, subacute bacterial endocarditis)
   Takayasu's arteritis
Endocrine
   Pheochromocytoma
   Congenital adrenal hyperplasia
   Hyperthyroidism
   Aldosteronism, primary
   Neuroblastoma
   Cushing's disease
   Hyperparathyroidism
   Ovarian tumors
Neurological
   Dysautonomia (Riley-Day syndrome)
   Neurofibromatosis
   Increased intracranial pressure
   Poliomyelitis
   Guillain-Barré syndrome
   Anxiety

the evaluation required. A major question facing the primary care physician is what to do when a child is discovered to have a BP within the 90th to 95th centile for age or size? Borderline elevations of BP, not associated with evidence of end-organ involvement such as cardiomegaly or renal insufficiency, would require little more than a detailed medical history, physical examination, urinalysis, complete blood count, serum electrolytes, calcium, phosphorus, creatinine clearance and chest X-ray. Any abnormality identified will require further evaluation. A preliminary

TABLE 16-4. *Continued*

Others
  Essential hypertension
  Anemia (systolic)
  Fluid overload, blood transfusion
  Asphyxia
  Pneumothorax
  Hypercalcemia
  Genitourinary tract surgery
  Drugs
    Ocular phenelephrine
    Corticosteroids
    Theophylline
    Sympathomimetics (DOP) drugs
    Nonsteroidal antiinflammatory drugs
    Birth control pills
    Recreational drugs
  Heavy metals
  Leg traction
  Burns
  Ventilator therapy

TABLE 16-5. Causes of Severe Sustained Hypertension in Children at the Hospital for Sick Children

Diagnosis		%
Renal scarring	52% reflux nephropathy obstructive uropathy 48% neuropathic bladder	35
Glomerulonephritis		23
Renovascular disease		10
Aortic coarctation (thoracic, abdominal)		9
Polycystic kidney disease (infantile, adult)		6
Hemolytic uremic syndrome		4
Idiopathic (essential)		3
Catecholamine-excess states (pheochromocytoma, neuroblastoma)		3
Nephroblastoma		2
Miscellaneous		5
Total		100

Modified with permission from Dillon MJ (1986) Hypertension. In: Postle-thwaite RJ (ed) Clinical Pediatric Neohrology. Wright, Bristol, pp 1–23.

investigation of moderate elevation of BP is outlined in Table 16-6; a more detailed evaluation in Table 16-7. The more severe the hypertension, the greater the importance of completing the investigation in a timely fashion. Although essential hypertension is presently diagnosed by exclusion, red blood cell electrolyte transport studies may be performed if facilities are available.

TABLE 16-6. Primary Investigation of Children and Adolescents With Moderate to Severe Hypertension

Urinalysis, urine culture
Complete blood count
Serum creatinine, urea, electrolytes, uric acid, calcium, phosphorus
Plasma renin activity
Urine sodium, chloride, vanillylmandelic acid/metanephrine
Abdominal ultrasound
[99m]Tc-dimercaptosuccinic acid (DMSA) (static) scan of kidneys, excretory urogram
Chest X-ray
Echocardiogram
Fundoscopy

Modified with permission from Second International Symposium on Hypertension in Children and Adolescents, Heidelberg, Federal Republic of Germany (1987) Recommendations for the management of hypertension in children and adolescents. Pediatr Nephrol 1:56–58.

A. Renal Imaging

The intravenous pyelogram (IVP) has been, for decades, the standard imaging technique used in evaluating renal structure and, to some extent, the differential function of the kidneys (see Chapter 6). However, the risk of contrast nephropathy and the availability of other superior diagnostic tests has reduced the use of IVP in the evaluation of children with hypertension. A static ^{99m}Tc-dimercaptosuccinic acid (DMSA) renal scan to evaluate renal morphology and scarring may be a part of the initial screening for evidence of renovascular disorders responsible for hypertension (15).

Renal scintigraphic perfusion (dynamic) scan using ^{99m}Tc-diethylene-triamine-penta acetic acid (DTPA) as a tracer offers an alternative procedure to evaluate the role of the kidney in hypertension. Analysis of the uptake phase allows the examiner to assess differential renal blood flow, and coupled with 20-minute blood sampling, the glomerular filtration rate (16). Recently, assessing uptake phases before and after the administration of angiotensin-converting enzyme (ACE) inhibitors has proven to be a promising diagnostic tool for investigating renovascular hypertension (17). The excretory phase, especially when combined with furosemide use, provides information about urinary tract obstruction, such as ureteropelvic junction stenosis, which may cause hypertension (18,19).

Many physicians consider selective renal arteriography as the only definitive method to evaluate renovascular hypertension and predict the surgical outcome of renal artery stenosis or unilateral reduction in renal parenchymal mass. This test, however, is invasive and may be complicated by femoral artery puncture and contrast nephropathy (20). The most common renal vascular pathology is medial fibromuscular hyperplasia. Although it is often considered in the differential diagnosis of pediatric renovascular hypertension, the adult-type medial fibroplasia is

TABLE 16-7. Supplementary Investigations in Hypertensive Children and Adolescents

Suspected renal etiology
  Glomerular filtration rate
  Excretory urogram
  ^{99m}Tc-diethylenetriaminepentaacetic acid (DTPA) renal scan
  Voiding cystourethrogram
  Renal angiography or digital substraction angiography
  Renin sampling from renal veins and vena cava
  Saralasin/ACE inhibitor test
  CT scan of kidneys and adrenals
  Renal biopsy
Suspected endocrine etiology
  Plasma catecholamines:
  If high
    Urinary catecholamines
    ^{131}I-meta-iodobenzylguanidine (MIBG) scan
    CT scan and/or MRI of abdomen, pelvis, chest, neck
    Vena cava sampling for catecholamines
  Plasma aldosterone:
    If high
    Urine mineralocorticoids
    Dexamethasone suppression test
    Adrenal scintigraphy
    If low
    Urine mineralocorticoids
    Other mineralocorticoids
    Cortisol response to ACTH or dexamethasone
Suspected cardiovascular etiology
  Echocardiography
  Angiography or digital subtraction angiography

Modified with permission from Second International Symposium on Hypertension in Children and Adolescents, Heidelberg, Federal Republic of Germany (1987) Recommendations for the management of hypertension in children and adolescents. Pediatr Nephrol 1:56–58

found only in less than 10% of children with renovascular disease. Neurofibromatosis is the second most common cause for renal artery stenosis, the tipoff to which is the presence, on physical examination, of café-au-lait spots. Other less common causes of renal vascular disease include Takayasu's arteritis, localized postirradiation damage to the renal artery and Williams syndrome (21).

Digital vascular imaging permits the visualization of the arterial vessels and, because of better contrast resolution, relatively smaller amounts of contrast material are used. Venous digital subtraction angiography (DSA) is relatively innocuous; however, experience in children is still limited (22). In adults, this method fails to outline intrarenal arterial vasculature. More recently, DSA with intraarterial injection is being evaluated in diagnosing pathology in the arterial distal branches of the renal artery; the risks of this procedure are nearly equivalent to that of the more conventional renal angiography. The use of voiding cystourethrography, and computerized axial tomography are discussed in Chapter 6.

B. Echocardiography

The Task Force on Blood Pressure Control in Children recommends the use of the echocardiogram for establishing base-line left ventricular mass, detecting possible target organ damage and determining the reversibility of these changes with appropriate therapy (1,23,24). Studies in pediatric populations have demonstrated the precision of m-mode echocardiogram in assessing the left ventricular chambers and their dimensions (25). Concentric left ventricular hypertrophy is among the earliest cardiac changes in hypertension. Moreover, echocardiography is a valuable tool in diagnosing coarctation of the aorta, which is responsible for up to 27% of hypertension in children during the first year of life (26).

C. Plasma Renin Activity

Measurement of plasma renin activity (PRA) in a peripheral blood sample is recommended in the initial workup of children with hypertension. In the pediatric population, and in contradistinction to adults, peripheral PRA could be of some value, since children with reflux nephropathy have increased PRA before hypertension is recognized as a clinical problem (27,28). Renin, an enzyme synthesized by and stored primarily in the juxtaglomerular cells, is released by several different mechanisms including decreased renal perfusion pressure, increased sympathetic nerve activity and vasodilator prostaglandins. Activity is measured most commonly by radioimmunoassay technique, expressed in nanograms of angiotensin I generated in 1 ml of plasma incubated at 37 °C with angiotensinogen for 1 hour.

Some laboratories take a shortcut, measuring angiotensin I generation only at 37 °C; here, the result would include the angiotensin I present in the stored plasma plus that formed during incubation for 1 hour at 37 °C. The precise method is to divide the plasma sample and run it in duplicate: One aliquot is incubated at 4 °C, the other at 37 °C. The difference in angiotensin I levels between the two is PRA. Single sample assays at 37 °C only tend to overestimate the actual PRA. Morever, PRA can appear elevated in hypertensive children without the renal disease if it is compared to the adult range of normal values provided by the reference laboratory. For this reason, the age-related differences in normal values for PRA in children must either be either learned or kept on file. The hourly PRA decreases from over 27 ng/ml during the first week of life to about 5 ng/ml at 3 years of age, with a continued gradual decrease with chronological age, until around the time of puberty when normal values are comparable to the adult of ≤ 2 ng/ml an hour (Figure 16-4) (29,30).

Circulating concentrations of angiotensin II follow a similar developmental pattern after birth; normal plasma angiotensin II concentrations in human adults are under 25 pg/ml, but such measurements are available only in research laboratories. Since PRA and plasma angiotensin II concentrations in the same blood sample vary directly at all ages, and since PRA is available in most clinical laboratories, PRA, and not angiotensin I, is measured to evaluate hypertension. Normal values for PRA are stated usually for blood samples obtained after overnight resting in a supine position or upon assuming an upright posture. The PRA measured under these conditions is impractical as a screening test for renovascular hypertension. However, if a peripheral PRA obtained during an outpatient evaluation for hypertension is within the range for "upright" normal values, the diagnosis of angiotensin-mediated hypertension is unlikely. When peripheral PRA is elevated above normal or when diagnostic imaging studies suggest a renovascular abnormality, then PRA from both renal veins, or even a segmental renal vein when a solitary parenchymal scar is noted, can be helpful in identifying the site of increased renin secretion. Although a ratio of over 1.5:1 is considered generally to be 80% sensitive in lateralizing the cause of renovascular hypertension (28,30),

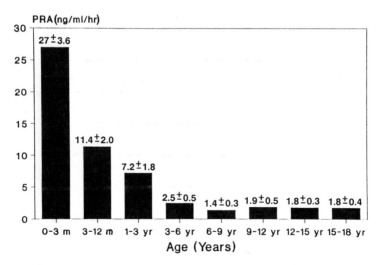

FIGURE 16-4. Mean plasma renin activity (PRA) in children. Curve derived from Stalker HP, Holland NH, Kotchen JM, Kotchen TA (1976) Plasma renin activity in healthy children. J Pediatr 89:256–258, and Sassard J, Sann L, Vincent M, Francois R, Cier JF (1975) Plasma renin activity in normal subjects from infancy to puberty. J Clin Endocrinol Metab 40: 524–525

one must consider whether the PRA in the contralateral renal vein is normal or elevated but not as high as the elevated value measured in the ipsilateral renal vein. Renal vein PRA can be normal in unilateral renovascular although renin secretion is increased in a single cortical segment; the false reading is due to a dilution effect as blood from that segment is added to renal vein blood draining all other parenchymal areas (30). Renal vein blood samples obtained after angiographic studies may show suppressed PRA because the hypertonic solutions used in these studies expand the blood volume. Moreover, diuresis due to furosemide administration, prior to or during the study, will increase renin release from a normal kidney by stimulating renal prostaglandin synthesis and by reducing blood volume. Prior use of ACE inhibitor, which blocks the feedback loop of angiotensin II to suppress further renin release, and any sedation given prior to blood sampling that lowers BP, may stimulate renin release through a baroreceptor-mediated mechanism. Inhibitors of prostaglandin synthesis, such as nonsteroidal antiinflammatory agents that act through the cyclooxygenase pathway, or by inhibiting phospholipase activity to make arachidonic acid available from membrane phospholipid, such as corticosteroids, may reduce renin secretion and lower PRA to within the range of normal values in a patient with renovascular or angiotensin-mediated hypertension. Other factors affecting PRA include changes in extracellular fluid volume, catecholamine levels, serum potassium levels and renal perfusion pressure.

There are some instances when PRA in peripheral and renal vein blood is normal or even low in patients with renovascular hypertension. If no other cause can be identified, and the examiner wishes to go one step further in the evaluation of any possible role of angiotensin II in hypertension, saralasin, a competitive antagonist of angiotensin II, can be infused. Because the test is difficult to do and because of the potential of serious side effects, its routine use is not recommended. A more practical approach to answer the same question, however, is a therapeutic trial with an ACE inhibitor. If BP is lowered by this treatment, angiotensin II may be considered to play a role in the pathogenesis of hypertension in the patient, regardless of measured values of PRA.

D. Adrenal Corticoids

Hypertensive children with excessive cortisol production usually have the typical features of such production on physical examination. However, hypertension without cushingoid features or hypokalemia and with normal PRA may be associated with excess production of mineralocorticoid—the most potent of which is aldosterone secreted by the zona glomerulosa of the adrenal cortex in response to either angiotensin II or potassium excess. The basis for hypertension in either kind of adrenal hypercorticism is excess extracellular fluid volume and, perhaps, some vasoconstriction. Plasma aldosterone concentrations must be interpreted according to either acute and a chronic sodium chloride balance, with which aldosterone secretion varies indirectly. Aldosterone secretion rate is more useful than a single plasma measurement. Adrenocortical disorders that can be associated with hypertension are listed in Table 16-8.

Hyperaldosteronism may be associated with a solitary aldosterone-secreting tumor (Conn's syndrome) or bilateral adrenal hyperplasia. An additional diagnostic feature of primary hyperaldosteronism is the failure of dexamethasone to suppress aldosterone to undetectable levels. The dexamethasone suppression test is also used to assess the adrenal-hypothalamic axis. After a base-line, 24-hour urine collection for 17-ketosteroids, 17-hydroxycortico- steroids, aldosterone and pregnanetriol, dexamethasone is administered for 5 days, and another 24-hour urine collection is obtained (31). An elevated base-line 17-hydroxycorticosteroid excretion suppressed by dexamethasone suggests the diagnosis of adrenocortical hyperplasia due to excessive pituitary secretion, and thus, elevated plasma adrenocorticotropic hormone (ACTH) levels. Suppression of urinary aldosterone secretion by dexasamethasone suggests a rare autosomal dominant disorder of hyperaldosteronism, which is clinically similar to primary hyperaldosteronism. Hypertension associated with this entity responds to steroid therapy (32).

Cushing's syndrome is another cause of low-renin hypertension. The diagnosis of hypercortisolism is made on a 24-hour urine collection for 17-hydroxycorticosteroids, which measures approximately one third of the end-products of cortisol metabolism, and urinary 17-ketosteroids, which measures the endproducts of androgen metabolism. To assess the autonomy of adrenocortical tumors, the adrenal cortex is stimulated with intravenous synthetic ACTH (0.1 mg, <1 yr; 0.15 mg, 1–5 yr; 0.25 mg,

TABLE 16-8. Adrenocortical Disorders Associated with Hypertension

Disease	Oversecreted hormones	Source of Hormone
Congenital adrenal hyperplasia	DOC (low aldo)	Fasciculata
Cushing's syndrome	Cortisol	Fasciculata or tumor
Low-renin hyperaldosteronism (Conn's syndrome)	Aldosterone	Glomerulosa tumor
Idiopathic	Aldosterone	Nodular hyperplasis
Dexamethasone suppressible	Aldosterone	Fasciculata (?)
High-renin hyperaldosteronism (renovascular hypertension)	Aldosterone	Glomerulosa
Primary hyperreninism (juxtaglomerular tumor)	Aldosterone	Glomerulosa

>5 yr). Plasma cortisol concentrations is determined before, and at several time intervals, for two hours following ACTH administration. An increment equal to or greater than 10 mcg/dl indicates a normal response (31); a lack of response, adrenal carcinoma; hyperresponsiveness, bilateral adrenal hyperplasia (32).

E. Catecholamines

Neuroblastoma and pheochromocytoma occur in approximately 3% of children with hypertension. Antihypertensive therapy must be instituted in children with neuroblastoma until the tumor mass is reduced or ablated by surgery or chemotherapy. The diagnosis of pheochromocytoma is more difficult, since the tumor can be located in the vicinity of any sympathetic ganglion. Some, but not all patients will have typical clinical symptoms of a catecholamine "rush"—flushing, tachycardia and hypertension. The measurement of plasma catecholamine concentrations are helpful only when values are elevated above normal, which occurs in 23% of patients with surgically proven pheochromocytoma even during the normotensive, symptom-free interval (33). Urinary metanephrine excretion is elevated in 96% of these patients (34).

Clonidine suppression is a safe, simple adjunctive test, which has been used in adult patients with suggestive symptoms and borderline catecholamine values (35). Clonidine suppresses plasma norepinephrine levels in normal human beings by stimulating central α-adrenergic receptors. Following an overnight fast and the determination of two control plasma catecholamine levels, oral clonidine (300 μg/ 1.73 m²) is administered. Plasma catecholamines are then determined at hourly intervals for three hours, with the patient in the supine position. Following clonidine administration, plasma catecholamines are usually unchanged in patients with pheochromocytoma, but they fall significantly in tumor-free patients.

The radiolabeled epinephrine analog metaiodo-benzylguanidine (^{131}I-MIBG), has been used in patients suspected of having a pheochromocytoma, either to confirm the diagnosis or to localize the lesion. Compared to the CT scan, scintigraphy is as sensitive, and has more specificity in making the preoperative diagnosis of pheochromacytoma (21). Multiple vena caval sampling for plasma catecholamine determination is another technique used to localize the tumor when other methods fail.

References

1. Task Force on Blood Pressure Control in Children (1987) Report of the Second Task Force on Blood Pressure Control in Children—1987. Pediatrics 79:1–25
2. Tan KL (1988) Blood pressure in very low birth weight infants in the first 70 days of life. J Pediatr 112:266–270

3. Voor AW, Webber LS, Berenson GS (1978) Epidemiology of essential hypertension in youth—implications for clinical practice. Pediatr Clin North Am 25:15–27

4. Adelman RD (1983) Neonatal hypertension. In: National Heart Lung and Blood Institute. Proceedings from a symposium. Bethesda, MD, May 26–27, pp 267–282

5. Lum LG, Jones MD Jr (1977) The effect of cuff width on systolic blood pressure measurements in neonates. J Pediatr 91:963–966

6. Stork EK, Carlo WA, Kliegman RM, et al (1984) Hypertension redefined for critically ill neonates. Pediatr Res 18:321A

7. Moss AJ, Duffie ER, Emmanouilides G (1963) Blood pressure and vasomotor reflexes in the newborn infant. Pediatrics 32:175–179

8. Daniels SR, Loggie JMH, Burton T, et al (1987) Difficulties with ambulatory blood pressure monitoring in children and adolescents. J Pediatr 111:397–400

9. Rocchini AP (1987) New blood pressure instruments for office and home. Cont Pediatr 39:22–39

10. Nelson WP, Egbert AM (1984) How to measure blood pressure—accurately. Primary Cardiol 50:14–26

11. Fixler DE, Kautz JA, Dana K (1980) Systolic blood pressure differences among pediatric epidemiological studies. Hypertension 2 (Suppl I):3–12

12. Julius S (1978) Clinical and physiological significance of borderline hypertension at youth. Pediatr Clin North Am 25:35–45

13. Portman RJ, Robson AM (1980) Controversies in pediatric hypertension. In: Tune et al (eds) Contemporary Issues in Nephroloqy. Churchill- Livingstone, New York pp 265–296

14. Scharer K (1987) Hypertension in children and adolescents—1986. Pediatr Nephrol 1:50–58

15. Dillon MJ (1987) Investigation and management of hypertension in children: a personal perspective. Pediatr Nephrol 1:59–68

16. Fine EJ, Scharf SC, Blavfox MD (1984) The role of nuclear medicine in evaluating the hypertensive patient. Nuclear Med Ann 1984:23–79

17. Fommei E, Ghione S, Palla L, et al (1987) Renal scintigraphic captopril test in the diagnosis of renovascular hypertension. Hypertension 10:212–220

18. Howman-Giles R, Uren R, Roy PL, et al (1987) Volume expansion diuretic renal scan in urinary tract obstruction. J Nucl Med 28:824–828

19. Grossman IC, Cromie WJ, Wein AJ, et al (1981) Renal hypertension secsondary to ureteropelvic junction obstruction. Urology 17:69–72

20. Taliercio CP, Burneh JC (1988) Contrast nephropathy cardiology and the newer radiocontrast agents. Int J Cardiol 19:145–151

21. Siegel MJ, St. Amour TE, Siegel BA (1987) Imaging techniques in the evaluation of pediatric hypertension. Pediatr Nephrol 1:76–88

22. Amundson GM, Wesenberg RL, Mueller DL, et al (1984) Pediatric digital subtraction angiography. Radiology 153:649–654

23. Laird WP, Fixler DE (1981). Left ventricular hypertrophy in adolescents with elevated blood pressure: Assessment by chest roentgenography, electrocardiography, and echocardiography. Pediatrics 67:255–259

24. Fouad FM, Liebson PR (1987) Echocardiographic studies of regression of left ventricular hypertrophy in hypertension. Hypertension 9 (Suppl II):65–68

25. Schieken RM (1987) Measurement of left ventricular wall mass in pediatric population. Hypertension 9 (Suppl II):47–52
26. Uhari M, Koskimies O (1979) A survey of 164 Finish children and adolescents with hypertension. Acta Pediatr Scand 68:193–198
27. Gerdts KG, Shah V, Savage JM, et al (1979) Renal vein renin measurement in normotensive children. J Pediatr 95:953–958
28. Dillon MJ (1981) Application of study of the renin-angiotensin system to pediatric pathology. In: Giovannelli G, New MI, Gorini S (eds) Hypertension in Children and Adolescents. Raven Press, New York, pp 137–146
29. Dillon MJ, Gillin MEA, Ryness JM, et al (1976) Plasma renin activity and aldosterone concentration in the human newborn. Arch Dis Child 51: 537–540
30. Stalker HP, Holland NH, Kotchen JM, et al (1976) Plasma renin activity in healthy children. J Pediatr 89:256–258
31. Bacon GE, Spencer ML, Hopwood NJ, et al (1982) Abnormal adrenal function. In: Bacon GE, Spencer ML, Hopwood NJ, Kelch RP (eds) A Practical Approach to Pediatric Endocrinology, 2nd edition. Year Book Medical Publishers, Chicago, pp 152–178
32. Wallach J (1983) Endocrine diseases. In: Wallach J (ed) Interpretation of Pediatric Tests. Little, Brown and Co, Boston, pp 447–507
33. Bravo EL, Tarazi RC, Gifford RW, et al (1979) Circulating and urinary catecholamines in pheochromocytoma. Diagnostic and pathophysiologic implications. New Engl J Med 301: 682–686
34. Rudnick MR, Bastl CP, Navins RG (1981) Diagnostic approaches to hypertension. In: Brener BM, Stein JH (eds) Hypertension. Contemporary Issues in Nephrology, vol 8. Churchill-Livingstone, New York, pp 270–338
35. Bravo EL, Tarazi RC, Fouad FM, et al (1981) Clonidine-suppression test. A useful aid in the diagnosis of pheochromocytoma. New Engl J Med 305: 623–626

17
Urological Workup of the Child with Renal and Urinary Tract Disease

BRENT F. TREIGER and ROBERT D. JEFFS

I. Introduction

Screening for and workup of urinary tract problems is an important aspect of both office and hospital practice. A large majority of patients found to have abnormalities of the kidney, bladder and genital system do not look sick and on examination have few symptoms or physical findings. The detection of disease or abnormality depends on an established routine of history taking, physical examination and basic laboratory tests (Chapters 2 and 4).

The microscopic examination of the urine is so important in the diagnosis of urological disease that it should not be replaced by dipstick tests, which only tell part of the story. Identification of bacteria, white blood cells, red blood cells (RBCs), renal casts and crystals must be considered part of the routine evaluation of every patient (Chapter 3). When RBCs are seen, their morphology must be characterized. Dysmorphic RBCs (in contrast to the usual biconcave round or crenated RBCs) are pathognomonic of hematuria of glomerular origin (Chapter 8).

Midstream voided urine in properly prepared older boys and in cooperative older girls can be reliable. However, bag specimens in young children of both sexes and midstream specimens in boys who are unable to retract the foreskin or in girls who are unable, or unwilling, to hold the labia apart are suspect. In these children, urine should be collected by catheter or needle aspiration from the bladder or kidney. Careful technique is required in both methods to avoid contamination from skin, vulva or vagina in the case of the catheter or from skin or large bowel in the case of the suprapubic tap (Chapter 9).

II. Imaging and Endoscopy

Investigation of the urinary tract can be precise in regard to anatomy, pressure, flow and function. With little or no invasion, a diagnosis of the exact nature of a problem can be made and the operative approach, when surgery is necessary, can be designed in advance of surgical exploration.

The intravenous pyelogram (IVP), a standard test in urology for many decades, has been supplemented by the newer imaging techniques of ultrasound, nuclear scanning, computed tomography (CT) and magnetic resonance imaging (MRI) (Chapter 6). The IVP is now used less frequently as the initial examination due to concern about radiation and the need for intravenous access. However, the anatomical detail afforded by the IVP is still very important in many situations.

Ultrasonography, which is noninvasive, has proved to be of great value in initial screening, in prenatal examination, in differentiating between cystic and solid masses, in estimating renal parenchymal size and texture and in evaluating ureteropelvic dilation and bladder drainage.

Computed tomography has proved most useful in evaluating solid tumors and their extent and possible spread. Inflammatory lesions, trauma and unusual anatomy in congenital anomalies may best be evaluated by this modality.

Magnetic resonance imaging is used infrequently in pediatric urology because of the long imaging time, during which the patient must be still. However, MRI can identify tissue planes and organ anatomy and can be very useful in reconstructive surgery. It is also very valuable in investigating the spinal cord and canal in patients with a neurological deficit in the bladder or lower limbs and has largely replaced myelography.

Because the anatomy of the renal vasculature can be defined by digital intravenous angiography and Doppler flow studies, arteriography is seldom necessary. However, when precise definition of the vascular anatomy is required, as in certain cases of partial nephrectomy, renovascular hypertension and renal aneurysms, arteriography is indicated.

Cystoscopy, once the only investigative tool of the urologist, is now used infrequently in evaluating children. The voiding cystourethrogram (VCUG) gives excellent anatomical detail of the bladder and urethra, and evaluates reflux at the same time. The nuclear cystogram lacks the detail of the VCUG but is useful in following patients with reflux.

Cystoscopy in children may be performed to confirm a developmental abnormality and to exclude vesical obstruction. It is unnecessary in the investigation of the child with infection that responds to treatment or as an initial procedure in the investigation of incontinence. However, patients with chronic or recurring infections unresponsive to medication may benefit from endoscopy, even when radiological examinations have revealed no abnormality. Routine dilation of the urethra beyond the normal size for age has no place in the modern management of urinary tract infection or reflux.

Urothelial tumors are uncommon in children and therefore cystoscopy and retrograde pyelography are not routinely performed in the evaluation of hematuria. Cystoscopy and retrograde pyelography are necessary in children with ureteropelvic junction (UPJ) obstruction to assess the patency of the ureter distal to the level of the UPJ obstruction. Similarly, children with an ectopic ureteral orifice or vesicoureteral reflux requiring ureteral reimplantation require cystoscopy prior to surgical repair. In these cases, the cystoscopic examination should be done immediately before the surgical repair to avoid anesthetizing the patient twice. The cystoscope may also be used to perform surgery such as resection of posterior urethral valves.

Antegrade pyelography by percutaneous puncture may be useful when retrograde pyelography is impossible and the results obtained weith other imaging techniques are unclear. The *Whitaker test,* used to evaluate obstruction between the renal pelvis and the bladder, is performed by percutaneous access to the renal pelvis to provide a constant flow of fluid and continuous monitoring of renal pressure. Renal pelvic pressures above 20 cm of water at a flow of 10 cc/minute indicate obstruction, pressures below 15 cm indicate free flow and pressures between 15 and 20 cm are equivocal. The Lasix washout IVP and the Lasix washout ^{99m}Tc-DTPA (diethylenetriamine pentaacetic acid) renal scan can usually identify most cases of obstruction, leaving the Whitaker test for a few cases in which direct measurement is needed. These patients usually have reduced renal function and markedly dilated collecting systems, which are difficult to evaluate by noninvasive means.

Evaluation of renal function is covered in Chapter 5 and will not be dealt with in this chapter, other than to emphasize that the glomerular filtration rate obtained by sampling the clearance of DTPA or other radionuclide from the blood can be particularly useful when urine collection is difficult, as in the very young child, the incontinent child or the patient with urinary diversion.

Urodynamics can be helpful in evaluating the function of the lower urinary tract. Bladder and bladder outlet function can be estimated by careful history and physical examination. The age at which day and night urinary continence was achieved, the quality of the urinary stream, the dry interval, the ability to delay voiding and to interrupt the stream and bowel function all give information about bladder and urethral function and cerebral control. Information can also be obtained from the radiologist's description of detrusor activity, residual urine and urethral response during fluoroscopy for the VCUG. Urodynamics can confirm suspicions by measurement of flow rate, urethral resistance, leak pressure and bladder sensation, capacity and contractions. Sphincter activity can be further evaluated by electromyography of the anal or urethral sphincters. It should be remembered that invasion by catheter may mask or induce bladder activity. Thus, the recorded urodynamic tracings must be compared with the findings arising from the history and physical examination. The child with urge or precipitant incontinence while squatting in Vincent's curtsy has bladder instability regardless of what the urodynamic tracing shows. This instability is but a sign for which there are many causes, ranging from infection and obstruction to neurogenic or psychological causes.

In the above general outline of investigation of the urinary tract in children, many options are given. The specific tests needed in a given situation will be outlined in the following paragraphs. The choice between ultrasound, nuclear scans and IVP to image the kidneys will depend in part on their availability and the experience of the clinician.

III. Urinary Tract Infection

When the child suspected of having urinary tract infection is febrile, the urine for culture should in most instances be obtained by catheter to avoid contamination and subsequent uncertainty in treatment. Suprapubic puncture is acceptable but, in our experience, too often unsuccessful. Carefully collected midstream urines are acceptable in the afebrile child.

The frequency with which structural abnormalities will be uncovered in the workup of the child with infection varies with the presentation. To avoid unrewarding testing, the investigation should be directed by the clinical setting. Febrile urinary tract infections are more apt to be associated with reflux or renal abnormality; afebrile infections are more likely to be confined to the bladder. The damage from renal infection is most severe in infants, and all infants should be investigated after the first urinary infection. The frequency of urinary tract abnormalities in boys with urinary tract infection is as high as 50% (1); therefore, boys at any age should be investigated after the first infection. Girls beyond infancy with a first infection without fever can be treated without imaging provided careful follow-up can be expected; however, all girls should be investigated after the second documented infection.

When reflux, hydronephrosis, obstruction or renal scarring is detected on initial investigation, further evaluation with IVP, nuclear renal scan or cystoscopy may be necessary.

IV. Incontinence

The types of incontinence and their etiology are listed in Table 17-1. These types can be easily differentiated by history and physical examination in the office. The child with *urge incontinence* has a dry interval but frequently fails to reach the bathroom in time. The child may pause while attempting to stop the bladder from contracting (heel sitting, Vincent's curtsy), lose a few drops of urine and then be temporarily unable to void on reaching the bathroom.

Stress incontinence indicates that the bladder leaks with increased intraabdominal pressure. In the child, this can usually be easily demonstrated in the office by applying pressure over the bladder while observing the urethra. In the extreme case, there may be no dry interval, indicating "total" incontinence.

Overflow incontinence implies outlet resistance such as obstruction or neurogenic dysfunction. The bladder becomes overfilled to the point at which vesical pressure exceeds outlet resistance.

In the female, the ectopic ureter emptying at the urethral meatus, distal urethra or vagina may continually leak; however, children with this condition referred to as *paradoxical incontinence,* will void at intervals in the normal fashion. The paradox is due to the incontinence in the face of apparent mature bladder function. Post-micturitional dribbling due to vaginal voiding might also be included in this category.

Giggle incontinence is a specific entity and should not be confused with stress incontinence. This is a rare entity seen in young girls who experience a spontaneous bladder contraction during a fit of giggling, with complete bladder emptying. They do not have stress incontinence and do not leak with coughing, sneezing or other physical activity (2,3).

Enuresis is the involuntary loss of urine beyond the age by which control should be present. Diurnal enuresis encompasses the entities described above, including the child with delayed maturation whose urinary tract is structurally and neurologically normal. However, the term enuresis is usually reserved for nocturnal enuresis or bedwetting, which is a functional complaint occurring in the structurally normal urinary tract.

TABLE 17-1. Types of Incontinence

Type	Etiology
Urge	Infection, obstruction, neurogenic, psychological, immaturity
Stress	Structural defects, epispadias, urethral injury, neurogenic
Overflow	Obstruction, neurogenic
Paradoxical	Ectopic ureter
Giggle	Temporal lobe defect
Nocturnal enuresis	Maturation lag, genetic factors, sleep disorders, psychological

Nocturnal enuresis, the commonest wetting problem, and giggle incontinence seldom require renal imaging or urodynamic evaluation. Normal micturition in the daytime or between episodes of giggling suggest normal structure and innervation. The recognition of a full urinary stream, and a clear morning urine with a high specific gravity will tend to confirm this impression. Improvement with time and treatment will be further reassurance.

Secondary nocturnal enuresis, occurring after a period of dry nights, needs to be explained. Evaluation, both physical and psychological, will be important.

The causes of the other types of incontinence shown in Table 17-1 indicate that upper and lower tract imaging should follow the history, careful physical examination and urinalysis. Renal ultrasound and VCUG are required as the initial examination, except when paradoxical incontinence is suspected, in which case the initial imaging study should be an IVP.

A neurological assessment is important to evaluate for the presence of spinal dysraphism, which can cause neurogenic bladder. Spinal MRI is most helpful in looking for the cause of a neurogenic bladder. Detailed examination of the genitalia is also required to detect anomalies such as mild epispadias and ectopic ureter.

V. Vesicoureteral Reflux

Reflux should be suspected in the child with urinary tract infection. The initial evaluation should be done by a VCUG to make the diagnosis and to give visual detail of the bladder and ureteral anatomy. Follow-up evaluation can be done by nuclear cystogram which reduces radiation exposure yet adequately determines the presence or absence of reflux. Renal imaging either by IVP or nuclear scan is necessary to detect and monitor renal scars and renal growth during management.

The 32% incidence of reflux in siblings of children who have reflux suggests the need for screening family members by VCUG or nuclear cystogram (4,5).

VI. Hematuria

The most common causes of hematuria in children are glomerular diseases and infection. Other causes include hematological conditions, drugs, tumors, obstruction, trauma and stones (Chapter 8). When caused by infection, pyuria and bacilluria may be present and infection may be confirmed by culture. Bacterial infections should be investigated as described above. In the initial stages of viral infection, the urine will be sterile but secondary infection may occur. Clear urine usually returns in 10 to 14 days and recurrence is unlikely. This clinical course can usually be recognized even in the absence of viral cultures, but an IVP is usually performed to exclude other problems.

In the absence of infection or findings to suggest glomerular disease, an IVP should be performed. Gross hematuria is seen in 25% of children with ureteropelvic junction obstruction (6). Other obstructive lesions and rare polyps of the ureter or posterior urethra may also cause hematuria. Hematuria may arise from tumors, which are rare in children and usually present in other ways. An IVP is usually sufficient to detect these tumors and cystoscopy is rarely indicated in the evaluation of hematuria.

Gross or microscopic hematuria may be due to hypercalciuria. In one series, nine of twenty-three children with hematuria secondary to hypercalciuria subsequently developed renal calculi (7). The investigation of renal calculi is described in Chapter 18. Hematuria due to renal vein thrombosis usually occurs in the sick and dehydrated infant. The kidney may be palpably enlarged and the diagnosis can be confirmed by ultrasound and Doppler flow study. Renal artery occlusion is usually secondary to umbilical artery catheterization in neonates and the diagnosis can be made by ultrasound and nuclear scan.

VII. Trauma

Trauma may be due to penetrating or blunt injury. Penetrating trauma is uncommon in children but requires prompt surgical intervention after radiological evaluation (Chapter 6).

Blunt trauma may cause kidney, bladder or urethral injury. It should be remembered that 20% of renal injuries occur in kidneys with preexisting abnormalities (8). Hematuria is an indication that the urinary tract has been injured. If there is blood at the meatus a retrograde urethrogram to detect extravasation of urine must be performed before attempting catheterization.

In the absence of blood at the meatus, both gross and microscopic hematuria should be evaluated by a cystogram with a post-drainage film to detect extra- or intraperitoneal bladder rupture. Upper tract evaluation may be performed by an intravenous pyelogram, but a CT scan with contrast is preferable, since the liver, spleen and retroperitoneum are evaluated simultaneously.

It must be remembered that significant renal injury (i.e. injury to the renal pedicle) can be present in the absence of hematuria. The injured child must be evaluated with a high index of suspicion.

VIII. Perinatal Urology

The diagnosis of many obstructive and cystic lesions of the urinary tract may be achieved by fetal ultrasound. In the fetus with a severely obstructed urinary tract, prenatal intervention may be considered, but there is little evidence that this results in better renal function when compared with treatment undertaken at birth (9) (Chapter 21).

An approach to the fetus with renal anomalies is presented in Figure 21-6; and the postnatal evaluation of urinary tract abnormalities discovered prenatally is shown in Figure 17-1. Initial ultrasound will indicate the presence of unilateral or bilateral disease, and the VCUG will identify infants with posterior urethral valves or bilateral vesicoureteral reflux. Bilateral ureteral dilation without reflux or bladder outlet obstruction suggests bilateral primary megaureter. The degree of obstruction and the need for treatment can be assessed by DTPA scan with Lasix washout. In some cases, the Whitaker test (see section II) may be necessary. The unilateral primary megaureter should be managed in a similar fashion.

Hydronephrosis due to an ectopic ureteral orifice or an ectopic ureterocele may be diagnosed by ultrasound and DTPA scan. However, preoperatively, an IVP may be required for anatomical definition.

Multicystic dysplastic kidney can usually be diagnosed on sonogram by the nature of the noncommunicating cysts and the lack of parenchyma.

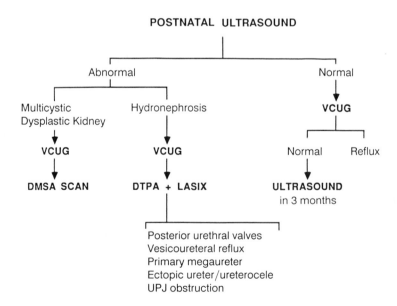

FIGURE 17-1. Postnatal evaluation of urinary tract abnormalities discovered prenatally.

Nonfunction on the ^{99m}Tc-DMSA (dimercaptosuccinic acid) scan will confirm this diagnosis. A VCUG should be performed to exclude reflux, which may occur on the ipsilateral or contralateral side.

The Lasix washout DTPA scan, performed for suspected UPJ obstruction, may clearly indicate obstruction by the prolonged $t_{1/2}$ time and decreased function. When function is good even with prolonged $t_{1/2}$ time, the patient may be followed with a scan at three months and six months of age, since some cases of apparent obstruction will improve. Should function decrease or obstruction increase at the three- or six-month examination, surgical repair is indicated.

At birth, anomalies that affect the urinary tract may be visible on physical examination. Anorectal anomalies such as imperforate anus and cloacal outlet obstruction may cause or be associated with urinary tract problems. Ultrasound, VCUG, nuclear renal scan and IVP may be indicated to determine the best management. Similarly, the child with prune belly syndrome must have a full urological assessment, since urinary tract abnormalities vary widely from one case to another. The cystourethrogram, renal scan and IVP will indicate 1) whether upper tract obstruction is present, 2) whether reflux exists and to what extent, 3) whether the urethra is patent, 4) there is smooth muscle activity in the ureters and bladder, and 5) the differential and total glomerular filtration rate. Drainage procedures, prognosis and progress will be determined on the basis of these tests.

Hypospadias, epispadias, exstrophy of the bladder and ambiguous genitalia are infrequently associated with obstruction. However, renal imaging is required to determine the presence and position of the kidneys. In cases of ambiguous genitalia, evaluation of the posterior urethra may be important for management. Children with epispadias, closed exstrophy and severe hypospadias should be evaluated for vesicoureteral reflux.

IX. Abdominal Masses

Nearly two-thirds of abdominal masses in neonates are renal in origin; one-half of all abdominal masses in neonates are due to ureteropelvic junction abnormality causing hydronephrosis or multicystic kidney (9). In older children, neoplasms account for 40 to 70% of abdominal masses (10).

An abdominal mass in a child should be evaluated first with ultrasonography, which can determine the location of the mass and distinguish between solid and cystic masses. Table 17-2 lists the common types of masses that arise in the retroperitoneum (also see Figure 6-14).

Wilms' tumor and neuroblastoma occur with approximately equal frequency in children, but the peak incidence of Wilms' tumor is 3.5 years (11), and of neuroblastoma, 1.5 years (12). Both usually present as an abdominal mass. Classically, Wilms' tumor has a smooth surface and is

TABLE 17-2. Common Masses Arising in the
Retroperitoneum

Cystic masses
  Hydronephrosis
  Multicystic dysplastic kidney
  Adrenal hematoma

Solid masses
  Benign
    Renal vein thrombosis
    Horseshoe kidney
    Ectopic kidney
    Autosomal recessive polycystic kidney disease
  Malignant
    Wilms' tumor
    Neuroblastoma
    Mesoblastic nephroma

confined to one side of the abdomen; in neuroblastoma, the edge of the tumor is usually irregular and extends across the midline. On plain film, calcifications are unusual in Wilms' tumor, occurring in less than 10% of patients. On IVP, Wilms' tumor distorts the calyceal system and may displace the pelvis medially. In contrast, neuroblastoma shows calcification in 50 to 65% of patients and the tumor displaces the kidney inferiorly and laterally but does not otherwise distort the calyceal systems. Urine levels of vanillylmandelic or homovanillic acid may be useful, since they are elevated in 80 to 95% of neuroblastomas, and normal in Wilms' tumor (13).

Adequate staging of these patients prior to surgery includes CT scan of the abdomen and chest. As many as 70% of patients with neuroblastoma may have bone marrow involvement at the time of diagnosis (14). Since differentiating between neuroblastoma and Wilms' tumor is often difficult, bone marrow aspirate and biopsy should be examined in both conditions. Venacaval extension is evaluated by ultrasonography and CT scan. However, in equivocal cases, inferior venacavography and MRI may be necessary.

Wilms' tumor is bilateral in 4 to 7% of cases (11,15), making the evaluation of the opposite kidney by IVP and CAT scan important. Visual inspection of the opposite kidney at surgery is imperative, since one-third of bilateral Wilms' tumors are not detected before surgical exploration.

Mesoblastic nephroma is indistinguishable from Wilms' tumor during the preoperative evaluation. Masses are discovered within the first few months of life and only a few have been known to invade or metastasize. The diagnosis is made pathologically after surgical removal of the abdominal mass.

References

1. Burbige KA, Retik AB, Colodny A, Bauer SB, Lebowitz R (1984) Urinary tract infections in boys. J Urol 132: 541–542
2. Glahn BE (1979) Giggle incontinence (enuresis risoria). A study and an aetiological hypothesis. Br J Urol 51: 363–366
3. Rogers MP, Gittes RF, Dawson DM (1982) Giggle incontinence. JAMA 247: 1446–1448
4. Dwoskin JY (1976) Sibling uropathology. J Urol 115: 726–727
5. Jerkins GR, Noe HN (1982) Familial vesicoureteral reflux: a prospective study. J Urol 128: 774–778
6. Perlmutter AD, Retick AB, Bauer, SB (1986) Anomalies of the upper urinary tract. In: Walsh PC, Gittes RF, Perlmutter AD, Stamey TA (eds) Campbell's Urology, 5th edition. WB Saunders, Philadelphia, pp 1665–1759
7. Noe HN, Stapleton FB, Roy S III (1984) Potential surgical implications of unexplained hematuria in children. J Urol 132: 737–738
8. Mertz JHO, Wishard WN, Nourse MH, et al (1963) Injury of the kidney in children. JAMA 183:730–733
9. Elder JS, Duckett JW (1987) Perinatal urology. In: Gillenwater JY, Grayhack JT, Howards SS, et al (eds) Adult and Pediatric Urology. Yearbook Medical Publishers, Chicago, pp 1512–1603
10. Kaplan GW, Brock WA (1985) Abdominal masses. In: Kelalis PP, King LR, Belman AB (eds) Clinical Pediatric Urology, 2nd edition. WB Saunders, Philadelphia, pp 57–75
11. Breslow NE, Beckwith JB (1982) Epidemiological features of Wilms' tumor: results of the National Wilms' Tumor Study. US Natl Cancer Inst J 68: 429–436
12. Kramer SA, Kelalis PP (1987) Pediatric urologic oncology. In: Gillenwater JY, Grayhack JT, Howards SS, et al (eds) Adult and Pediatric Urology. Yearbook Medical Publishers, Chicago, pp 2001–2042
13. Williams CM, Greer M (1963) Homovanillic acid and vanillylmandelic acid in diagnosis of neuroblastoma. JAMA 183: 836–840
14. Finkelstein JZ, Ekert H, Isaacs H, Jr, et al (1970) Bone marrow metastases in children with solid tumors. Am J Dis Child 119: 49–52
15. Wasiljew BK, Besser A, Roffensperger J (1982) Treatment of bilateral Wilms' tumor—a 22 year experience. J Pediatr Surg 17: 265–268

18
Renal Calculi

MITSURO NAKANO, GAD KAINER, JOHN W. FOREMAN
and JAMES C.M. CHAN

I. Introduction: Incidence and Epidemiology

Nephrolithiasis is an uncommon disorder in childhood; however, in view of the sometimes dramatic clinical presentations, the likelihood of recurrence and the possibility of damage to the kidneys, the clinician should be conversant with renal stones and associated disorders.

The incidence of renal calculi in adults in the United States is estimated to be 140 per 100,000 (1); in children the incidence is about 1/50th that of adults (2). The incidence of pediatric hospital admissions due to renal calculi varies from 1 per 6,400 (3) to as high as 1 in 1,066 (4) in some southeastern (stone belt) states of America. There is a male predominance with a sex ratio of 2:1 and a positive family history in up to 50% of patients (5–10). Approximately 94% of children with renal calculi are white, 5% are black and 1% are of other racial origin (11). A report from Japan shows a relatively high incidence of pediatric renal calculi (1 per 420 hospital admissions) (12). The incidence and type of renal stones varies with environmental and socioeconomic factors. Water availability, diet, climate, and region of habitation, are clearly associated with the incidence and type of urolithiasis. Bladder stones and so-called endemic stones are more commonly seen in developing countries (5,8). Nephrolithiasis should be considered as a symptom, and a systematic approach to investigation and management of possible underlying conditions should be the aim of the practicing pediatrician.

II. Clinical Features

Pain, hematuria and fever are the most common presentations in children with renal calculi; however, 50% of children with renal stones are asymptomatic, and in many cases stones are diagnosed as incidental findings on x-ray of the abdomen. "Renal colic," which is present in 40 to 50% of children with calculi, is often atypical. The pain begins gradually, building up to a crescendo over several minutes, and remaining at peak of intensity for up to several hours. The pain may radiate along the flanks into the groin or to the lower back, especially if the stone is in the lower portions of the ureter. Bladder or urethral calculi may be accompanied by symptoms of urgency, frequency and dysuria. Young children localize pain poorly and may manifest only inconsolable behavior or severe agitation.

Hematuria, microscopic or macroscopic, is an extremely common finding in patients with renal calculi. Fever and other symptoms of urinary tract infection are present in 15% of affected children. Over 95% of renal calculi are radio-opaque and may be identified on a plain radiograph of the abdomen.

III. Types of Calculi: Composition and Formation

Renal calculi may be classified into four major categories by chemical composition: calcium (oxalate and phosphate), infection related or struvite, cystine, and uric acid stones (Table 18-1). Many stones, however, are a mixture of the above components, and occasionally other types of stones associated with inherited disorders of purine metabolism may be found (Table 18-2).

A. Calcium Oxalate and Calcium Phosphate Stones

Approximately 50 to 70% of stones in the urinary tract are composed of calcium oxalate, calcium phosphate or mixtures of these substances (13). Calcium oxalate or mixed calcium stones are the most common stones found in Western societies. The formation of monosodium urate or uric

TABLE 18-1. Types of stones.

Composition	North America $n = 340$	Europe $n = 315$
Calcium	57.6%	37.1%
Struvite	25.3%	54.0%
Cystine	6.2%	2.9%
Uric acid/urate	9.4%	2.2%
Others	1.5%	3.8%

Modified from Polinsky MS, Kaiser BA, Baluarte HJ (1987) Urolithiasis in childhood. Pediatr Clin North Am 34:683–710, with permission.

TABLE 18-2. Clinical disorders associated with types of urolithiasis.

I. Calcium stones
  A. Normocalcemic hypercalciuria
    1. Idiopathic hypercalciuria (absorptive, renal)
    2. Distal renal tubular acidosis
    3. Drug induced (furosemide)
  B. Hypercalcemic hypercalciuria
    1. Immobilization
    2. Idiopathic hypercalcemia of infancy
    3. Hypervitaminosis D
    4. Adrenocorticosteroid excess (Cushing syndrome, exogenous)
    5. Primary hyperparathyroidism
    6. Hyperthyroidism
    7. Adrenal insufficiency
    8. Milk–alkali syndrome
  C. Hyperoxaluria
    1. Enteric hyperoxaluria
    2. Hereditary hyperoxaluria (Types I and II)
    3. Pyridoxine deficiency
  D. Other causes
    1. Idiopathic calcium urolithiasis
    2. Hyperuricosuria
    3. Hypocitraturia
II. Urate stones
  A. Leukemia, lymphoma
  B. Lesch–Nyhan syndrome
  C. Glycogen storage disease (Type I)
  D. Polycythemia
  E. Chronic volume contraction
III. Infection related stones
IV. Cystinuria
V. Uncommon diseases
  A. Hereditary xanthinuria
  B. Orotic aciduria

acid micro-crystals may provide a nidus upon which calcium oxalate stones grow.

Pure calcium phosphate stones are rare. They are less soluble in alkaline urine and, therefore, may occur in distal renal tubular acidosis or in association with infections caused by urea splitting organisms. The consistency of phosphate stones varies from soft and crumbly to hard; their size ranges from small to staghorn calculi filling the renal pelvis.

1. Factors Influencing Calcium Stone Formation

Hypercalciuria is by far the most common cause of renal stone formation (11). Less common causes include hyperoxaluria, hyperuricosuria, elevated urinary pH, hypocitraturia, and excessive dietary intake of calcium and vitamins A, D and C. Dehydration, immobilization, positive family history, malformations of the urinary tract and reduced urinary concentrations of inhibitory substances are risk factors for stone formation.

2. Hypercalciuria

Daily urinary calcium excretion greater than 4 mg/kg and a fasting urinary calcium to creatinine ratio of greater than 0.21 (14) are suggestive of hypercalciuria and should be followed up with further investigations. Although hypercalciuria may occur as a result of hypercalcemia, this is unusual in children. Hypercalciuria may be divided into five major subtypes: 1) excessive dietary calcium intake, 2) absorptive hypercalciuria caused by excessive calcium absorption by the gut, 3) resorptive hypercalciuria in which calcium is derived from bone, 4) renal hypercalciuria in which an idiopathic defect in calcium reabsorption by the renal tubule is present and 5) idiopathic hypercalciuria in which the hypercalciuria cannot be strictly categorized into one of the aforementioned groups. This occurs in 30 to 40% of stone formers.

Patients with absorptive hypercalciuria have a normal fasting urinary calcium to creatinine ratio of less than 0.21, which rises to over 0.28 after an oral calcium load of 1g/1.73 m² (15). Parathyroid hormone concentration in this type is normal or decreased. Renal hypercalciuria is defined by a fasting urinary calcium to creatinine ratio over 0.21. The most common form of resorptive hypercalciuria in children is due to immobilization, accounting for 16 to 18% of pediatric renal stones (16).

Furosemide may cause hypercalciuria and nephrolithiasis, especially in the neonate (17). Nephrocalcinosis and nephrolithiasis may be encountered in untreated patients with renal tubular acidosis Type 1 which is associated also with hypocitraturia (Figure 18-1). Citrate is an important inhibitor of calcium stone formation.

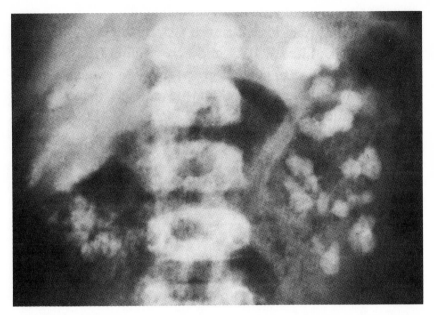

FIGURE 18-1. Medullary nephrocalcinosis in distal renal tubular acidosis. From: Chan JCM (1979) Acid-base, calcium, potassium and aldosterone metabolism in renal tubular acidosis. Nephron 23:153–159, with permission.

3. Hyperoxaluria

Oxalic acid is an end product of ascorbic acid and glyoxylate metabolism. Oxalate is relatively insoluble in body fluids and is an important anion in the formation of calcium stones. Small increases in urinary oxalate concentration can markedly enhance the tendency to form a stone. The normal daily excretion of oxalate ranges between 20 and 50 mg/1.73 m² (18). Approximately 15% of urinary oxalate is derived from dietary sources, while the remainder is an end product of endogenous metabolism. Foods high in oxalate content include tea, cocoa, spinach, rhubarb, beets and nuts. Excessive intake of vitamin C, a precursor of oxalate, may also lead to hyperoxaluria. Ingestion of ethylene glycol or the use of methoxyflurane anesthetic have been associated with hyperoxaluria.

Hyperoxaluria may occur if bile salts and unsaturated fatty acids are incompletely absorbed in the distal small intestine and reach the colon in abnormally high quantities. These compounds enhance oxalate absorption by the colon, resulting in hyperoxaluria. This has been noted in patients with ileal bypass or conditions affecting the terminal ileum such as Crohn's disease (10). Two rare autosomal recessive inborn errors of metabolism cause hyperoxaluria or oxalosis: Type I caused by 2-oxoglutarate: glyoxylate carboligase deficiency, and Type II caused by D-glycerate dehydrogenase deficiency. Both are associated with nephrolithiasis and recurrent stone formation, leading to early renal failure (19).

4. Hyperuricosuria and Uric Acid Calculi

Approximately two thirds of the uric acid formed each day as an end product of purine metabolism is excreted by the kidney. Uric acid is poorly soluble in biological fluids and precipitates under conditions of low urine flow, low urinary pH and supersaturation of urine by urate. By creating a nidus for calcium oxalate and other calcium stones and also by adsorbing inhibitors of calcium oxalate crystal growth, hyperuricosuria creates a situation favorable to stone formation (14). The normal urinary excretion of urate in adults is less than 750 mg/24 hours; in children, it varies with age and weight. In children over 2 years of age, the amount of uric acid excreted in a fasting early morning collection is usually < 0.56 mg/dl of glomerular filtrate calculated by the following formula (11):

$$\frac{\text{Urine uric acid (mg/dl)} \times \text{Serum creatinine (mg/dl)}}{\text{Urine creatinine (mg/dl)}}$$

Uric acid excretion is extremely high in the neonate, and it is not uncommon to find precipitation of orange crystals in the diaper in the first days of life.

Uric acid calculi constitute 2 to 5% of pediatric urolithiases. These stones, which are generally multiple and radiolucent, are hard and yellowish-brown and have a smooth surface and a round contour.

Uric acid stones in children may be due to primary disorders resulting in hyperuricosuria such as the Lesch–Nyhan syndrome and Type 1 glycogen storage disease, or secondary causes found mostly during the course of leukemia and chemotherapy (20).

Prevention of uric acid stones by inhibiting uric acid formation with the xanthine oxidase inhibitor allopurinol, adequate hydration and urinary alkalinization is very effective. In some children with hypercalciuria, there is concurrent hyperuricosuria. In parts of Asia and in the Mediterranean region, there is a familial tendency for uric acid stones. Alleviation of the situation may be achieved if exogenous purine intake is reduced by decreasing dietary protein.

5. Hypocitraturia

Citrate in the urine inhibits formation of stones by binding to calcium and magnesium ions. Citrate excretion is higher in girls than in boys; the lower limit of citrate excretion in girls is approximately 300 mg/g of creatinine per day and in boys, 128 mg/g of creatinine per day. The lower citrate excretion in boys may explain the increased male incidence of renal calculi as compared to females. Hypocitraturia is also encountered in distal renal tubular acidosis and in patients with intestinal malabsorption (21,22).

B. Infection-Related Stones

Struvite/carbonate-apatite calculi are associated with stasis and urinary infections. The majority of pediatric patients are males under 5 years of age, with congenital abnormalities of the urinary tract including foreign bodies, vesicoureteral reflux, neurogenic bladder, posterior urethral valves and other congenital malformations.

Infection with such urea-splitting organisms as *Proteus, Pseudomonas* and *Klebsiella* elevates urinary pH secondary to ammonia and carbon dioxide production. This results in supersaturation of the urine with magnesium ammonium phosphate, calcium phosphate and carbonate–apatite crystals predisposing to stone formation. Struvite stones usually occur in the upper urinary tract and may form staghorns in up to 8% of children with nephrolithiasis (4,23). More often, the stones are gelatinous or friable, containing Tamm-Horsfall glycoprotein and inorganic constituents, mainly magnesium ammonium phosphate ($MgNH_4PO_4$) and carbonate apatite {$Ca_{10}(PO_4)6CO_3$}.

C. Cystine Calculi (Cystinuria)

Cystinuria is an autosomal recessive disease with an approximate incidence of 1 in 15,000 for the homozygous condition, leading to a defect in dibasic amino acid transport in the renal tubule. Cystine stones account for 1 to 4% of pediatric urolithiasis (24). Urine chromatography reveals high quantities of cystine, lysine, arginine and ornithine. A presumptive diagnosis can be made on the basis of the cyanide–nitroprusside test. The urine turns purple in the presence of excess cystine (25).

Cystine stones may occur in children of any age, and there is a cumulative increase in the risk of stone formation with age such that by adulthood the majority of cystinuric patients will suffer from nephrolithiasis.

Cystine stones are usually radio-opaque because of their high sulfur content. Cystine crystals in the urine are always abnormal and can be easily identified by their flat hexagonal shape (Figure 18-2). Cystine is relatively insoluble at pH <7.5; therefore, crystalluria may be absent in dilute or alkaline urine and is best looked for in a morning specimen after an overnight fast.

D. Crystalluria

Crystal formation from solution is a complex process involving precipitation and growth of crystals from the various stone forming constituents.

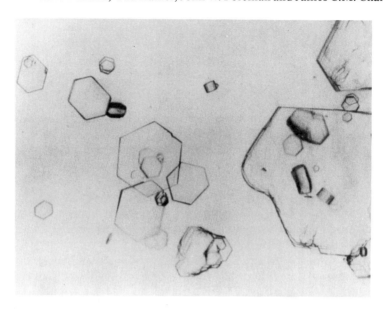

FIGURE 18-2. Hexagonal cystine crystals in urine. From: Foreman JW, Segal S (1985) Aminoaciduria. In: Gonick HC, Buckalew VM (eds) Renal Tubular Disorders, Marcel Dekker, New York, pp 131–157. Reprinted by courtesy of Marcel Dekker, Inc.

In the case of calcium oxalate stones, for example (Figure 18-3), as the concentration of the ions in solution rises, a critical point is reached at which the product of the ions is in equilibrium with the solid phase (solubility product). When the solubility product is exceeded by the product of the ions, the solution is said to be supersaturated. However, de novo crystal formation does not occur until the ion product is much higher (formation product). The range of log relative supersaturation between the solubility product and the formation product is called the metastable zone. In the metastable zone, the presence of heterogeneous nuclei can induce precipitation of the de novo solid phase. Inhibitors of crystal growth, such as inorganic pyrophosphate and glycosaminoglycans, can influence the degree of supersaturation required for precipitation (26).

Office microscopy of urine for crystalluria as a means of identifying at risk patients is not satisfactory. However, the finding on microscopy of numerous cystine crystals is diagnostic of cystinuria. Calcium oxalate crystals are commonly seen in urine of normal children (Figure 18-4). Other constituents will crystallize when the temperature of the urine falls.

Correlation between propensity to stone formation and crystalluria has been reported by specialized research units using a technique whereby freshly collected urine is concentrated to a standard osmolality of 1250 mOsm/liter, then incubated for a standard time before examination on

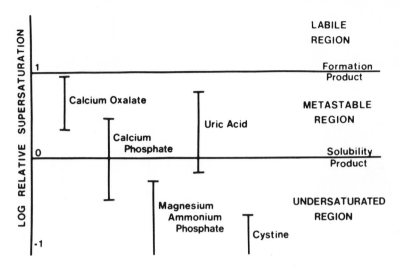

FIGURE 18-3. The three zones of saturation, on a log scale. The vertical bars represent the range of values in normal urine. From: Nordin BEC, Horseman A, Aaron J (1976) Diagnostic procedures. In: Nordin BEC (ed) Calcium, Phosphate and Magnesium Metabolism, Churchill Livingstone, Edinburgh, pp 469–524, with permission.

warm-stage microscopes (27). However, such facilities are not regularly available, and the reliability of these methods in children has not been established.

IV. Evaluation of Patients with Nephrolithiasis

The clinical evaluation of a child with proven nephrolithiasis, or of a child who is at risk for nephrolithiasis, involves a detailed history with particular attention to the social, environmental, family and dietary factors implicated in lithogenesis. Carefully planned laboratory studies are the key to diagnosis and management (Figure 18-5).

The history should include questions regarding age at onset of symptoms, episodes of unexplained pyrexias, passage of cloudy or overtly crystalline urine, localization of pain and abnormal micturition patterns.

Thorough physical examination should be followed by obtaining a clean catch mid-stream urine for bacteriological culture and microscopy. Radiological studies are essential, since 95% of stones are radio-opaque. Renal ultrasound, together with plain abdominal films of the kidneys, ureters and bladder (KUB), will detect the majority of stones. An excretory urogram (IVP), when indicated, may demonstrate some radiolucent stones as filling defects. Renal scans may be performed in patients with suspected obstruction and radiographic contrast sensitivity.

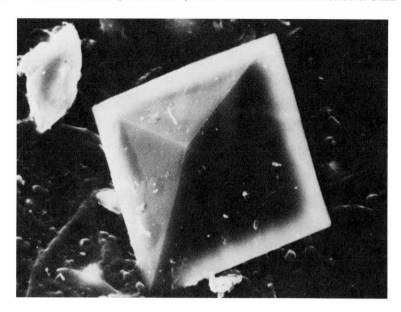

FIGURE 18-4. High-power magnification of calcium oxalate crystal. From: Rogers AL, Spector M (1987) Crystallographic analysis of urinary calculi. In: Rous SN (ed) Stone Disease: Diagnosis and Management. W.B. Saunders Company, Philadelphia, pp 41–55, with permission.

Stones that are passed or removed surgically should be sent to a recognized calculus laboratory for analysis. Attempts to collect stones should be made until a definitive diagnosis is available. This may be done by filtering the urine or collecting it before discarding it into the toilet.

Children with urolithiasis should be investigated as outpatients whenever possible. Variations in diet, fluid intake and environmental factors are thus minimized. Collections of urine during representative days of the week will help in the interpretation of test results. Because of the day-to-day variability in excretion of minerals, it is prudent to repeat urine tests on at least two occasions. Blood tests should be coordinated with urine collections and processed without delay.

Two sets of 24-hour urine collections, each set on two consecutive days while on the same diet, but a week apart, are needed for accurate evaluation of mineral excretion. The parents are supplied with two clearly marked bottles: one containing thymol or toluene (citrate and uric acid collection), and the other containing 10 ml of 6 N hydrochloric acid (for calcium, oxalate, magnesium, phosphorus and cystine). The 24-hour urinary creatinine, proteins and net acid excretion should also be measured. In a child who is not toilet trained, or as a screening test for hypercalciuria, a fasting morning urine specimen for calcium/creatinine ratio is a useful compromise.

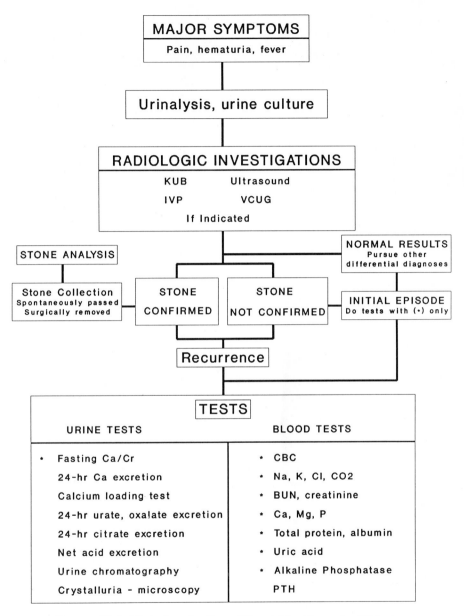

FIGURE 18-5. Clinical evaluation of the child with nephrolithiasis.

Blood tests should be drawn during urine collections for complete blood count, electrolytes, CO_2 content, blood urea nitrogen, creatinine, calcium, magnesium, phosphorus, total protein, albumin, uric acid, alkaline phosphatase and parathyroid hormone.

Interpretation of screening tests requires confidence in both the accuracy and the completeness of the collections and the laboratory quality control and precision. Abnormal values in blood or urine should be repeated. Provocation tests such as calcium loading, renal acidification testing and metabolic balance studies are best carried out in pediatric clinical research centers, with experienced nurses dedicated to run such complex studies.

A. Stone Analysis

Stone analysis should include an accurate morphological evaluation with binocular magnifying apparatus (operating microscope 10× power) and chemical and physicochemical techniques for component quantitation.

Most urinary calculi are mixtures of crystalline and organic and/or inorganic noncrystalline materials. Constituent analysis is helpful in the characterization of the chemical "scenario" that leads to stone formation. Stone analysis may help to identify the initiating conditions in stone formation and thus provides the basis for a more rational treatment

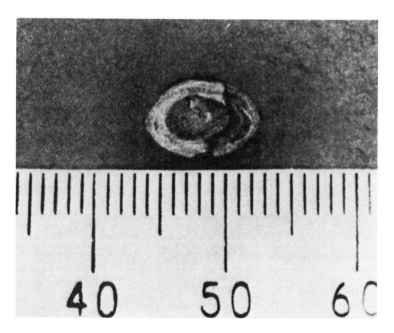

FIGURE 18-6. Mixed calcium oxalate/uric acid stone. Calcium oxalate core would indicate investigation for conditions that resulted in deposition of calcium oxalate. From: Rogers AL, Spector M (1987) Crystallographic analysis of urinary calculi. In: Rous NS (ed) Stone Disease: Diagnosis and Management. W.B. Saunders Company, Philadelphia, pp 41–55, with permission.

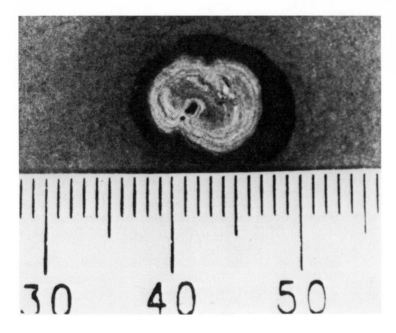

FIGURE 18-7. Mixed calcium oxalate/uric acid stone. Uric acid core would indicate that conditions associated with uricosuria be investigated. From: Rogers AL, Spector M (1987) Crystallographic analysis of urinary calculi. In: Rous SN (ed) Stone Disease: Diagnosis and Management. W.B. Saunders Company, Philadelphia, pp 41–55, with permission.

approach. For example, in a stone with a calcium oxalate core, hypercalciuria and/or hyperoxaluria may be suspected as the initiating events, even if the major component of the stone is urate (Figure 18-6); the converse may also apply (Figure 18-7).

X-Ray diffraction studies of stones are regarded by some as the method of choice in stone analysis. The technique allows accurate analysis of constituents without sample destruction and the ability to choose a representative specimen from the entire sample. Disadvantages of the technique include lack of sensitivity for minor constituents and the inability to differentiate apatite in struvite stones because of common reflections in the diffraction pattern.

Chemical stone analysis is based on standard chemical techniques after stone dissolution in acid (H_2SO_4), or alkali solutions (NaOH or KOH) (28).

The understanding of stone pathophysiology has advanced considerably in recent years with the introduction of sophisticated testing laboratories. But even with the most meticulous and arduous techniques, 20% of stones have unexplained etiologies and are therefore idiopathic. Management of patients with unexplained recurrent stone disease relies on general measures to reduce calcium excretion and on potential inhibitors of lithiasis such as citrates, orthophosphates and pyridoxine. More specific treatment depends on the results of systematic investigations.

Acknowledgements. Supported in part by NIH grants RO1 DK 31370 and RO1 DK 522736. The authors wish to thank Martha D. Wellons and Faith S.Boyle for research assistance and Virginia Murrell for secretarial assistance.

References

1. National Center for Health Statistics, Dennison CF (1985) 1984 Summary: National Hospital Discharge Survey. Advance data from Vital and Health Statistics. No. 112. DHHS Publication No. (PHS)85–1250. Public Health Service, Hyattsville, MD, September 27
2. Gill WB (1984) Renal calculus disease: Classification, demographic and etiologic considerations. Semin Urol 2:1–11
3. Bass HN, Emanuel B (1966) Nephrolithiasis in childhood. J Urol 95: 749–753
4. Walther PC, Lamm D, Kaplan GW (1980) Pediatric urolithiasis: A ten-year review. Pediatrics 65:1068–1072
5. Eckstein HB (1961) Endemic urinary lithiasis in Turkish children—a clinical study of 119 cases. Arch Dis Child 36:137–145
6. Ghazali S, Barratt TM, Williams DI (1973) Childhood urolithiasis in Britain. Arch Dis Child 48:291–295
7. Malek RS, Kelalis PP (1975) Pediatric nephrolithiasis. J Urol 113:545–551
8. Chutikorn C, Valyasevi A, Halstead SB (1967) Studies of bladder stone disease in Thailand. II. Hospital experience. Urolithiasis at Ubol Provincial Hospital, 1956–62. Am J Clin Nutr 20:1320–1328
9. Androulakakis PA, Barratt TM, Ransley PG, et al (1982) Urinary calculi in children: a 5 to 15-year follow-up with particular reference to recurrent and residual stones. Br J Urol 54:176–180
10. Polinsky MS, Kaiser BA, Baluarte HJ (1987) Urolithiasis in childhood. Pediatr Clin North Am 34:683–710
11. Noe HN, Stapleton FB (1987) Pediatric stone disease. In: Rous SN (ed) Stone Disease. Grune & Stratton, Orlando, FL, pp 347–379
12. Kawamura T, Ogawa O, Hoshinaga K, et al (1987) Clinical experience with pediatric urolithiasis. In: Murakami K (ed) Recent Advances in Pediatric Nephrology. Elsevier Science Publishers BV, pp 539–542
13. Coe FL, Parks JH (1988) Nephrolithiasis: Pathogenesis and Treatment, 2nd edition, Year Book Medical Publishers, Inc., Chicago
14. Stapleton FB, Noe N, Jerkins G, et al (1982) Urinary excretion of calcium following an oral calcium loading test in healthy children. Pediatrics 69:594–597
15. Stapleton FB, Noe N, Roy S, III, et al (1982) Hypercalciuria in children with urolithiasis. Am J Dis Child 136:675–678
16. Bennett AH, Colodny AH (1973) Urinary tract calculi in children. J Urol 109:318–320

17. Hufnagle KG, Khan SN, Penn D, et al (1982) Renal calcifications: A complication of long-term furosemide therapy in preterm infants. Pediatrics 70:360–363
18. Barratt TM (1987) Urolithiasis and nephrocalcinosis. In: Holliday MA, Barratt TM, Vernier RL (eds) Pediatric Nephrology. Williams & Wilkins, Baltimore, MD, pp 700–708
19. Morris MC, Chambers TL, Evans PWG, et al (1982) Oxalosis in infancy. Arch Dis Child 57:224–228
20. Chan JCM (1979) Hyperuricemic nephropathy: A complication of acute leukemia in children. Med Coll Virg Quart 15:68–70
21. Norman ME, Feldman NI, Cohn RM, et al (1978) Urinary citrate excretion in the diagnosis of distal renal tubular acidosis. J Pediatr 92:394–400
22. Rudman D, Dedonis JL, Fountain MT, et al (1980) Hypocitraturia in patients with gastrointestinal malabsorption. N Engl J Med 303:657–661
23. Sinno K, Boyce WH, Resnick MI (1979) Childhood urolithiasis. J Urol 121:662–664
24. Evans WP, Resnick MI, Boyce WH (1982) Homozygous cystinuria—evaluation of 35 patients. J Urol 127:707–709
25. Foreman JW, Segal S (1985) Aminoaciduria. In: Gonick HC, Buckalew VM (eds) Renal Tubular Disorders, Marcel Dekker Inc, New York, pp 131–157
26. Nordin BEC, Horsman A, Aaron J (1976) Diagnostic Procedures. In: Nordin BEC (ed) Calcium, Phosphate and Magnesium Metabolism, Churchill Livingstone, Edinburgh, pp 469–524
27. Rous SN (1987) Determining the success of medical therapy. In: Rous SN (ed) Stone Disease Diagnosis and Management. Grune & Stratton, Orlando, FL, pp 207–210
28. Daudon M, Reveilland R-J (1986) Methods of urinary calculus analysis: A critical review. In: Grunfeld JP, Maxwell MH, Back JF, Crosnier J, Funck-Brentano JL (eds) Advances in Nephrology, Year Book Medical Publishers, Inc, Chicago, pp 219–244

19
Clinical Evaluation of the Kidney in Systemic and Collagen Diseases

ROBERT E. LYNCH and ELLEN G. WOOD

I. Introduction

The specialized nature of the renal vasculature and the relatively large renal blood flow make kidney damage particularly likely whenever systemic illness threatens the patient's vascular integrity. Involvement may be minor, or kidney failure and homeostatic catastrophe may result.

The prognosis will depend in part on the clinician's recognition of and response to the renal sequelae of the illness. Under these and less dramatic circumstances, renal abnormality may be the initial sign of systemic illness. An accurate renal diagnosis, often requiring renal biopsy, will reveal the underlying systemic pathology (Chapter 7).

In the following discussion, it is assumed that the diagnosis of renal involvement in systemic disease is based on general clinical findings and a basic knowledge of renal pathophysiology. We hope to provide assistance at that point in further discriminating among diagnoses and in identifying critical factors for detailed evaluation.

Table 19-1 presents the renal features of some common systemic diseases. For a more detailed presentation of renal involvement under different conditions and in specific syndromes, the reader is referred to Appendix IV. Primary glomerular diseases are discussed in Chapter 10.

II. Henoch-Schönlein Purpura

Vasculitic injury to very small vessels can produce the Henoch-Schönlein purpura syndrome (HSP) (1,2). Typical clinical findings include a petechial and often purpuric, rash, predominately on the lower extremities; abdominal distress with crampy pain; anorexia and vomiting; and ar-

TABLE 19-1. Systemic Diseases Commonly Associated with Renal Involvement in Children

Disease	Main features	Renal features	Reference
Henoch-Schönlein purpura	Petechial rash, abdominal pain, arthralgia	Hematuria, proteinuria, nephrotic syndrome, hypertension, renal insufficiency	1
Systemic lupus erythematosus	Fever, rash, arthritis	Hematuria, proteinuria, nephrotic syndrome, hypertension, renal insufficiency	5,6,7,8
Rheumatoid arthritis	Fever, arthritis, arthropathy	Mild proteinuria, microhematuria, hypertension, amyloidosis, nephrosclerosis	9
Acute glomerulonephritis	Antecedent streptococcal phrayngitis or impetigo	Hematuria >> proteinuria, hypertension, edema, renal insufficiency	13
Subacute bacterial endocarditis	Bacteremia	Hematuria, proteinuria, azotemia	14
Hemolytic uremic syndrome	Antecedent gastroenteritis, microangiopathic hemolysis	Acute renal failure	16,17
Diabetes mellitus	Glucose intolerance	Microalbuminuria progressing to proteinuria and mesangial sclerosis, end-stage renal disease	18, 19
Lymphoid malignancy	Fever, lymphadenopathy, hepatosplenomegaly	Proteinuria, nephrotic syndrome, acute renal failure, obstructive uropathy, tumor lysis syndrome	20

thralgia, frequently in lower extremity joints and accompanied by periarticular soft tissue edema. This syndrome is variable and often presents with one major symptom, while other symptoms are either absent or delayed in onset.

Renal involvement occurs in about 80% of the patients, although nephritis is clinically manifest in 20 to 30% of unselected children. Older children and children with recurrent purpura seem to have a higher incidence of renal involvement. The nephritis associated with HSP occurs as a usually mild, transient focal proliferative lesion, which is first suspected when urinalysis reveals proteinuria and microscopic hematuria. Identifying patients who are at high risk of more serious disease is the main goal of the initial evaluation and follow-up. Historical evaluation should search for a past illness suggestive of a previous HSP episode, current complaints of periorbital or dependent edema, or symptoms or risk factors suggestive of HSP-like presentations of other illnesses to be discussed later.

Physical examination of an HSP patient may be quite complex. Vasculitic edema may be present near joints, large purpura, and over the forehead and scalp, and can be confusing. Thus, the presence of a nephrotic syndrome must be confirmed in the laboratory.

Initial blood tests should include a complete blood cell and platelet count and the determination of electrolyte, creatinine, albumin and total protein levels. A generous aliquot of serum (5 to 10 ml) should be frozen for possible later analysis. In HSP, one expects mild anemia, a mild to moderate granulocytosis and, of course, a normal platelet count despite the presence of petechiae. More marked anemia may occur as a consequence of unusual gastrointestinal (GI) blood loss, sequestration or prolonged renal failure. A marked leukocytic left shift suggests infection, and a low platelet count requires diagnostic reconsideration. Electrolyte disturbances reflect GI deficits or acute renal insufficiency. Hyperkalemia and hyponatremia, in particular, may be immediately life threatening. The serum creatinine level should be determined to assess renal function; however, repeated determinations are necessary in an individual in whom renal function is rapidly changing. Such changes may occur early in HSP due to dehydration or a worsening nephritis.

True nephrotic syndrome in HSP is a serious finding. Hypoalbuminemia is usually associated with heavy proteinuria, but enteral protein loss can also be very significant. Proteinuria over 1 g/m^2, decreased renal function or hypertension may suggest the presence of crescentic glomerulonephritis and a renal biopsy should be considered.

Individual presentations may dictate such additional blood studies as blood culture; screening for hepatitis B, or liver function tests may be required. Coagulation studies are in order if an early biopsy is anticipated or if injury due to child abuse is suspected. An elevated IgA level or a characteristic skin biopsy may be diagnostically helpful in certain patients. Of occasional value are ANA and complement studies. In HSP, the anti-nuclear antibody screen should be negative and the C_3 or CH_{50} values are normal or mildly elevated. Recent studies have demonstrated elevated levels of circulating IgA immune complexes in patients with HSP.

Laboratory studies of urine include urinalysis, urine culture and quantitative protein determinations. After initial evaluation and follow-up of one to three months, most mild HSP nephritis cases will have largely resolved by themselves. However, patients with hypertension, significant renal insufficiency or nephrotic syndrome should generally undergo a renal biopsy; patients with chronic changes on biopsy will need very close follow-up. Many milder cases with normal kidney function but persistent hematuria or proteinuria should be kept under observation. Recurrence of HSP nephritis is rare but may have a more serious prognosis.

III. Necrotizing Vasculitis with Nephritis: Henoch-Schönlein Purpura-Like Presentations

The petechial, pupuric rash and other common symptoms characteristic of HSP may occasionally be the presenting signs of other, very serious vasculitic illness including polyarteritis nodosa, Wegener's granulomatosis, cryoglobulinemia with persistent hepatitis B antigenemia and systemic lupus erythematosus (SLE).

Large artery vasculitis, or polyarteritis nodosa, should be considered when an HSP-like illness presents with unusual systemic severity, particularly with muscle tenderness without large creatinine kinase elevations, persistent fever, severe abdominal symptoms, central or peripheral nervous system involvement, or palpable inflammatory lesions in the scrotum or peripheral arteries (3). Diagnosis is difficult and depends upon a fortuitous biopsy or angiography that demonstrates renal, celiac or arterial aneurysms. If intravenous pyelography suggests ureteral vascuitis, renal and celiac angiography should be undertaken, unless serological tests for systemic lupus erythematosus (SLE) are positive.

The renal disease seen in large vessel vasculitis may be that of proliferative glomerulonephritis or may alternatively be that of segmental arterial thrombosis and renal cortical infarction. Moderate proteinuria, microscopic hematuria and variable degrees of azotemia are common in patients with glomerulonephritis. Patients with infarctions but little glomerulopathy tend to have marked hypertension, with minimal urinary abnormalities. Renal biopsy is not diagnostically reliable and probably adds little to the initial management. The biopsy, however, may help guide therapy in patients with persistent glomerulonephritis. These patients generally require immunosuppression and should be followed for renal function, hypertension and control of systemic symptoms, particularly of the central nervous system. This process appears to arise in idiopathic, drug-induced, post-infectious and genetic forms.

Rare patients with Wegener's granulomatosis may present with HSP-like findings but may also have or develop pulmonary and upper respiratory granulomatous disease (4). Confirmation of this diagnosis allows effective therapy and should be sought through biopsy of accessible inflammatory lesions and the kidney. A chronic glomerulonephritis is frequently involved; its management is aided by base-line biopsy and serial renal function determinations.

A suspicious history of hypocomplementemia, membranoproliferative glomerulonephritis on biopsy or a prolonged HSP-like course with minimal abdominal symptoms should prompt screening for mixed cryoglobulinemia and the variably associated hepatitis B antigenemia. If cryoglobulinemia is suspected clinically and serologically, and if abnormalities are present on urinalysis, a biopsy is indicated to exclude other histological types of glomerulonephritis that may be present with similar clinical and laboratory findings.

Anti-nuclear antibodies should also be sought in an atypical or prolonged HSP-like illness, since SLE may occasionally produce a petechial, purpuric rash with other compatible clinical signs. Suspicion should be high in the presence of hypocomplementemia, small joint arthritis, and blanching skin rashes. Further evaluation of the SLE patient is discussed below.

IV. Systemic Lupus Erythematosus

Patients presenting with SLE most often complain of combinations of arthritis, rash and fever (5,6). Commonly affected joints include knees, wrists and the PIP and MP joints of the hand. Symptoms may be mild or severe, but evidence of renal disease should be sought in the initial evaluation of any patient in whom SLE is suspected (7,8). At a minimum, a serum creatinine and a urinalysis should be quickly obtained, since advanced renal failure may present with minimal systemic symptoms and an abnormal urinalysis will require further investigation.

Compatible history, physical findings and an ANA $\geq$1:80 with a rim or diffuse pattern make the overall diagnosis of SLE very probable, subject to confirmation by the demonstration of circulating antibody to double-stranded DNA. Early evaluation should also include a complete blood cell and platelet count, electrolyte determinations, liver function tests, PT, PTT, albumin and total protein, and creatinine. Also appropriate are complement values for C_3, C_4, and CH_{50} and additional studies related to organ systems as suggested by presenting symptoms or findings. Patients with urinary abnormalities should have GFR and quantitative urinary protein determinations.

Some subcategories of SLE patients can be identified by further serological or genetic tests. Further definition of renal involvement is possible with renal biopsy.

Most nephrologists believe that an initial biopsy and often serial renal biopsies are essential in the care of SLE patients, since renal histology is useful in the design of therapeutic regimens, when the risks of immunosuppression are weighed, and in prognostic counseling. Thus our SLE patients with urinary abnormalities and hypertension, hypocomplementemia, reduced clearance or moderate to marked proteinuria are evaluated by biopsy.

The histology of the kidney can be categorized as minimal abnormality or mesangial proliferation, generally responsive to therapy; membranous glomerulopathy, frequently rather quiescent but also relatively resistant to therapy; focal proliferative glomerulonephritis, usually responsive to therapy, with transformation to a milder lesion, but focal glomerulonephritis can deteriorate or diffuse proliferative glomerulonephritis, often at least partially responsive to therapy, although it remains an ominous finding. Additional prognostic factors include glomerular crescents, necrosis or sclerosis, interstitial fibrosis or inflammation, and vascular inflammation and hypertrophy, sclerosis and thrombosis.

Renal disease in SLE frequently responds to therapy but renal exacerbation with or without chronic deterioration tends to occur with generalized flares in disease activity. Monitoring nephritis activity, then, involves a follow-up of the general clinical condition, serum complement, ANA and anti-double stranded DNA antibody, quantitative proteinuria and GFR estimated by the best available method.

Other collagen-vascular disorders of concern include juvenile rheumatoid arthritis (JRA), mixed connective tissue disease (MCTD), scleroderma and dermatomyositis. Juvenile rheumatoid arthritis is rarely the direct cause of serious renal disease, although hypertension and mild hematuria or proteinuria may be observed more commonly (9). Urinalysis and renal function should be periodically evaluated in these patients, however, since renal amyloidosis is an occasional but ominous development. Of more frequent concern is the nephrotoxicity produced by therapy in JRA, particularly the nonsteroidal anti-inflammatory agents gold and penicillamine. Again, proteinuria and mild functional compromise may be presenting signs.

Mixed connective tissue disease (MCTD) in children is associated with a significant incidence of renal disease that may progress to chronic renal failure (10). Patients should be monitored for development of proteinuria and hematuria, deterioration of renal function and hypocomplementemia with development of antibody to double-stranded DNA.

Childhood scleroderma may evolve into an SLE serological and clinical picture, but serious renal vascular disease, which presents with proteinuria, hypertension or azotemia, is rare (11). Glomerulonephritis associated with childhood dermatomyositis is also unlikely (12).

V. Renal Injury from Remote Infection

Postinfectious acute glomerulonephritis (AGN) follows streptococcal pharyngitis or impetigo, with a latent period of 4 to 21 days, and generally has a brief, mild course (13). The long-term prognosis in the pediatric age range is excellent. This relatively benign typical course must never be assumed, however, because the exceptions are not rare and may be fatal. Severe hypertension is a common complication.

Hypertensive patients should be hospitalized, treated aggressively and observed closely until the blood pressure is stable and well controlled. Acute renal failure may progress rapidly, with pulmonary edema, acidosis, hyperkalemia, hypocalcemia, anemia and advanced uremia.

The initial evaluation of suspected AGN must include history for antecedent illness; physical examination for impetigo, pharyngitis, edema, fluid overload, blood pressure and general findings; the laboratory evaluation must include electrolytes, azotemia, CBC, and throat or lesion culture.

In addition, laboratory and clinical support for the basic diagnosis of AGN must be gathered because other forms of acute and chronic nephritis, for which therapy is quite different, are easily confused with AGN. Therefore, an ASO titer, Streptozyme® (Wampole Laboratories, Division of Carter Wallace; Cranberry, NJ), and a serum C_3 complement level should be obtained. Anti-streptolysin titer is not strongly stimulated after impetigo, and all three tests may return to normal only a few weeks after presentation. In the case of inconclusive results, an anti-DNase B titer determination may be useful. This streptococcal antibody is seen with either pharyngitis or impetigo and remains elevated for up to six months. Elevated titers establish a recent streptococcal infection; hypocomplementemia suggests that the infection and nephritis are related. Neither test is foolproof, however, and a consistent clinical course must also be sought in the evaluation of suspected cases. Characteristic features include a predominance of hematuria (gross in 40% of the cases) over proteinuria, resolution of gross hematuria and improvement in cases with mild to moderate azotemia within two weeks, improvement in hypertension within two months and resolution of proteinuria and mioroscopic hematuria within six months and twelve months, respectively. Some patients may have gross hematuria with intercurrent infection up to six months after presentation. These episodes occur without azotemia or hypocomplementemia, and the hematuria revolves in a few days. Exceptions occur, but should be viewed with suspicion and considered for biopsy. Finally, patients with evidence of a rapidly progressive glomerulonephritis and advanced renal failure should generally be biopsied to be certain other treatable forms are not present.

When other remote or systemic infections including bacterial endocarditis (14), persistent intravascular (IV) catheter infection, chronic abcesses, syphilis and malaria, are identified urinalysis and serum creatinine determination should be performed. Persistent antigenemia associated with bacterial endocarditis, IV catheter infection, or chronic abscesses frequently leads to a hypocomplementemic, immune-complex mediated glomerulonephritis, which can progress to renal sclerosis. Of patients with endocarditis, 70 to 80% have some degree of renal involvement (14). Hematuria, which is the result of microscopic infarcts of the kidney or focal or diffuse glomerulonephritis, occurs in 11 to 93% of patients, proteinuria in 35 to 88% and pyuria in 50 to 60%.

Eradicating the infection constitutes appropriate treatment in these patients. A renal biopsy, however, may be useful to exclude differential diagnoses and to obtain a prognosis. Infection control is also generally effective therapy for nephritis due to syphilis or malaria. These diseases occasionally produce heavy proteinuria associated with membranous and focal or diffuse proliferative nephropathy, respectively.

Finally, patients with persistent infections often receive long-term antibiotic therapy. In addition to direct nephrotoxicity, one is wise to consider acute interstitial nephritis among the differential possibilities (see Chapter 10). Such a diagnosis may be strongly suspected when unexplained fever, rash and eosinophilia are accompanied by significant hematuria, mild proteinuria, azotemia and urinary eosinophils. The clinical picture often varies, particularly when drugs other than the penicillins or cephalosporins are being administered. Biopsy is usually indicated to establish a firm diagnosis.

VI. Rapidly Progressive Glomerulonephritis

In the preceding sections of this chapter, real urgency in the evaluation of nephritis has been largely limited to detecting acute renal failure, when likely, and severe hypertension. Most of the categories discussed may present with an aggressive nephritic syndrome complicated not only by renal failure and hypertension, but also by the threat of sudden pulmonary hemorrhage or a central nervous system (CNS) catastrophe. Rapidly progressive glomerulonephritis (RPGN), which involves a sudden progressive deterioration in renal function, is often due to crescentic glomerulonephritis or intraglomerular extracapillary cellular proliferation (15) and demands urgent, expert nephrological evaluation. RPGN may be idiopathic or associated with membranoproliferative and membranous glomerulonephritis, IgA nephropathy, Alport's syndrome, Goodpasture's anti-GBM antibody, and systemic disorders (e.g. Henoch-Schönlein purpura, polyarteritis nodosa, SLE, postinfectious acute glomerulonephritis, Wegener's granulomatosis). The pathogenesis of this condition is not fully understood and there is no satisfactory treatment, although early plasma exchange and "pulse" therapy with methylprednisolone may sometimes be helpful.

VII. Hemolytic Uremic Syndrome

Hemolytic uremic syndrome (HUS) is a frightening disease, uncommon and unfamiliar to both patients and primary care practitioners, but recognized as potentially fulminant and life-threatening (16,17). Although 10 to 15% of the cases may follow respiratory illness, the typical antecedent is prolonged gastroenteritis, which may have begun to improve before deterioration and the appearance of pallor, lethargy, edema and decreased urine output. Anemia and renal failure are the hallmarks, but GI obstruction or perforation or CNS catastrophe may be early findings.

Physical examination should take particular note of edema, pallor, petechiae, hypertension, ileus or peritoneal signs, blood in the GI tract, and neurological status. An electrocardiogram to exclude hyperkalemic crisis and blood gas analysis may be urgently needed. General supportive measures obviously should be initiated immediately particularly since septicemia must be eliminated in the differential diagnosis.

Laboratory confirmation of HUS begins with the demonstration of anemia and microangiopathy (red blood cell fragmentation, "helmet" cells and thrombocytopenia). The presence of microangiopathic hemolytic anemia, thrombocytopenia, renal failure, hematuria and proteinuria strongly suggests HUS. The differential diagnosis includes acute renal vein thrombosis, which is rare beyond the newborn period, and infection, particularly septicemia or urosepsis associated with obstructive uropathy and renal compromise. Septicemia causing renal failure and thrombocytopenia frequently presents with hemodynamic instability, systemic coagulopathy, and a suggestive history. A renal sonogram may detect renal vein thrombosis or urinary tract anomalies.

In addition to an initial determination of renal function, electrolytes, and hematological status, effort should be directed toward identifying bacterial enteritis and ruling out concurrent urinary infection. Hypoproteinemia is common and may cause edema without gross fluid overload. Glucose intolerance occurs rarely, and dysfunction of any organ is possible, since microthrombi have been found in practically all tissues examined.

A plan of clinical and laboratory monitoring must be devised, since HUS is anything but static. During the acute, unstable period, potassium, hematocrit, and usually creatinine and platelets must be checked two to three times a day. Daily determinations of sodium, CO_2, BUN, and body weight may be needed; calcium, phosphorus, albumin, and electrolyte levels are checked less frequently. Especially important is the continuous observation of the GI and neurological status, since they may deteriorate late in the course of the disease after thrombocytopenia has substantially resolved. However, acute, spontaneous, severe hemorrhage is very rare, despite pronounced thrombocytopenia.

Overall clinical improvement generally follows closely after recovery from thrombocytopenia. Patients may be followed as outpatients when the urine output is appropriate, renal function is adequate and improving, electrolyte levels are acceptable, platelets have been over 100,000 for more than two days and hemoglobin is about 8 g/dl and reasonably stable. Very late consequences may include GI strictures, hypertension and glomerulonephritis. De novo HUS may recur or appear in subsequent renal grafts.

VIII. Diabetic Nephropathy

The new generation of diabetic nephropathy therapeutic principles are based on extremely important discoveries and hypotheses, but we remain ignorant of the basic discriminatory mechanisms separating those diabetics destined for nephropathy from those more fortunate (18,19). Nevertheless, a great deal has been learned in recent years and one can tentatively, at least, recommend a regimen of tight control, microalbuminuria monitoring, special attention to patients with early albuminuria, aggressive blood pressure normalization, and an open-minded consideration of dietary protein maneuvers and angiotensin converting enzyme inhibition. In addition, the increased incidence in diabetics of other renal conditions including various glomerulopathies, acute tubular injury, infections and hypercalciuria should keep the clinician alert for renal issues other than classic nephropathy. How often nephropathy can actually be prevented or significantly delayed in general practice remains to be established. Current data do suggest that an improvement in overall patient welfare will result from the application of the following regimen.

The initial *stabilization phase* must correct hyperglycemia, reduce the supranormal GFR and begin a crucial diabetes educational program to encourage high compliance with a regimen of strict metabolic control. The *early phase,* when clearance and resting urinary albumin excretion are normal may be followed by increased resting albumin excretion and a high risk of progression to nephropathy. This should alert the diabetologist to reexamine the patient's regimen. Many variables affect albumin excretion and attention to the details of the laboratory's sample collection procedure is extremely important. Clinical decisions should be based on data trends established by sequential samples. Determination of microalbuminuria depends on controlled protocols to ensure accuracy.

The impact of microalbuminuria monitoring and efforts to achieve "tight control" is variously thought to be "revolutionary" or "negligible." Regardless, they currently represent interesting tools in dealing with diabetic nephropathy. The use of enalapril or restriction of protein may be of benefit. Proteinuria indicates the presence of established nephropathy, but the rate of progression may be slowed in some patients.

In the *late phase* of diabetic nephropathy, aggressive treatment of hypertension may delay end-stage renal disease (ESRD) by several years. At this time, it does not appear that any available therapies can truly reverse overt diabetic nephropathy, so the clinician must accept the role of prognosticator, educator, hypertension controller, and day-to-day problem solver. The course from onset of classic proteinuria to ESRD is generally rapid (often only a few years).

Frequent renal function evaluation remains extremely important as ESRD approaches. Diabetic complications appear to be exacerbated by severe uremia, so that early institution of dialysis and transplant planning is important. Decisions as to the mode of ESRD treatment must be individualized, based on the patient's social, psychological, and medical circumstance. An illness as chronic, complex and frequently frustrating as diabetes demands such an approach.

IX. Lymphoid Malignancy

Metabolic disturbances are well known in patients with lymphoid leukemias or lymphomas of childhood and adolescence (20). Hypoglycemia, metabolic acidosis, hyperkalemia, hyponatremia and hypercalcemia are only occasionally seen, and nephrotic syndrome and renal insufficiency are similarly uncommon. However, their clinical significance in this form of systemic disease warrants some comment. Nephrotic syndrome has been reported with Hodgkins as well as non-Hodgkins lymphomas, splenic hamartoma and other conditions consistent with the current lymphokine hypotheses of altered glomerular permeability. When edema and severe proteinuria occur in lymphoid malignancy, serum and urine protein should be quantified. Renal function will generally be preserved, and a renal biopsy is likely to show minimal change disease or membranous nephropathy. With or without a histological study, appropriate antitumor therapy should be initiated and the nephrotic syndrome followed. Remission of the underlying disease will frequently be accompanied by remission of the nephrotic syndrome. Non-Hodgkins lymphomas and acute lymphocyte leukemias presenting with high white blood counts are more likely to present with compromised renal function, which is usually due to urate nephropathy, although other mechanisms certainly contribute. At serum uric acid levels above 12 mg/dl, compromised renal function is more severe and more frequent. At uric acid levels above 20 mg/

dl, compromised renal function is very common. Thus, the early workups of such patients should include serum creatinine, uric acid, electrolyte, calcium and phosphorus determinations, as well as urinalysis. If renal insufficiency is demonstrated, a renal sonogram can be used to rule out obstruction, either by tumor or stone, but it should be noted that these extrarenal mechanisms are uncommon. It should also be noted that an enlarged kidney is frequently observed and may indicate infiltration of the renal mass. Renal insufficiency at this stage demands close attention to subsequent hydration, drug dosage, and the use of prophylactic measures regarding the "tumor lysis syndrome."

Rapid tumor lysis, particularly with pre-existing renal insufficiency has been associated with such life-threatening acute metabolic disturbances as metabolic acidosis, hyperkalemia, hyperphosphatemia and hypocalcemia. These disturbances may be triggered by tissue breakdown products from a large tumor mass during chemotherapy or radiation therapy, especially in the presence of renal insufficiency. Uric acid is one these product of tumor lysis which may produce rapid acute renal failure in a patient who does not have preexisting insufficiency. Warning signs should include a very large tumor mass, indicated anatomically or as indirectly suggested by major elevations of LDH. In such patients, one must design a monitoring plan that will detect an impending crisis before basic stability is threatened. During periods of rapid change, monitoring of acid-base status, potassium, and glucose, for instance, may be required every three to four hours over a period of days.

References

1. Austin HA, Balow JE (1983) Henoch-Schönlein nephritis: prognostic features and the challenge of therapy. Am J Kid Dis 2:512–520
2. Habib R, Cameron JS (1982) Schönlein-Henoch purpura. In: Bacon PA, Hadler NM (eds) The Kidney and Rheumatic Disease. Butterworth Scientific, London, pp 178–201
3. Blau EB, Morris RF, Yunis EJ (1977) Polyarteritis nodosa in older children. Pediatrics 60:227–234
4. Hall SL, Miller LC, Duggan E, et al (1985) Wegener granulomatosis in pediatric patients. J Pediatr 106: 739–744
5. Schaller J (1982) Lupus in childhood. Clin Rheum Dis 8:219–228
6. Platt JL, Burke BA, Fish AJ, et al (1982) Systemic lupus erythematosus in the first two decades of life. Am J Kidney Dis 11 (suppl) 212–222
7. Schwartz MM (1985) The role of renal biopsy in the management of lupus nephritis. Semin Nephrol 5:255–263
8. Rush PJ, Baumal R, Shore A, et al (1986) Correlation of renal histology with outcome in children with lupus nephritis. Kidney Int 29:1066–1071
9. Bourke BE, Woodrow DF, Scott JT (1981) Proteinuria in rheumatoid arthritis—drug-induced or amyloid? Ann Rheum Dis 40: 240–244
10. Oetgen WJ, Boioe JA, Lawless OJ (1981) Mixed connective tissue disease in children and adolescents. Pediatrics 67:333–337

11. Proceedings of the First ARA Conference (1977) Rheumatic diseases in childhood. Arth Rheum 20 (Suppl): 145–636
12. Dyck RF, Katz A, Gordon DA, et al (1979) Glomerulonephritis associated with polymyocitis. J Rheum 6:336–344
13. Potter EV, Lipsohultz SA, Abidh S, et al (1982) Twelve to seventeen year follow-up of patients with poststreptococcal acute glomerulonephritis in Trinidad. Engl J Med 307:725–729
14. Barakat AY, Dakessian B (1987) The kidney in heart disease. Int J Pediatr Nephrol 7: 153–160
15. Cunningham RJ III, Gilfoil M, Cavallo T, et al (1980) Rapidly progressive glomerulonephritis in children: A report of 13 cases and a review of the literature. Pediatr Res 14:128–132
16. Kaplan BS, Proesmans W (1987) The hemolytic uremic syndrome of childhood and its variants. Semin Hematol 24:148–160
17. Karmali MA, Petric M, Lim O, et al (1985) The association between idiopathic hemolytic uremic syndrome and infection by verotoxin-producing Escherichia coli. J Infect Dis 151:775–782
18. Krolewski AS, Warram JH, Christlieb AR, et al (1985) The changing natural history of nephropathy in type I diabetes. Am J Med 78:785–794
19. Cavallo T, Pinto JA, Rajaraman S (1984) Immune complex disease complicating diabetic glomerulosclerosis. Am J Nephrol 4:347–354
20. Lynch RE (1987) Lymphoid malignancies. In: Holliday MA, Barratt TM, Vernier RL (eds) Pediatric Nephrology, 2nd edition. Williams and Wilkins, Baltimore, pp 525–527

20
Renal Transplantation

ROBERT B. ETTENGER

I. Introduction

Despite significant advances in dialysis technology, renal transplantation is the usual goal of therapy for children with end-stage renal disease (ESRD). A well-functioning kidney transplant improves a child's physical, social and psychological quality of life more than any form of dialysis.

The 1980s have witnessed a veritable explosion in transplantation technology. Numerous new immunosuppressive agents, immunological conditioning regimens and sophisticated histocompatibility typing modalities are now available (1). This has resulted in dramatic improvements in allograft outcome in adults. Results in pediatric renal transplantation have also been improving, albeit at a slower pace. Results of graft outcome in living-related donor transplantation have been equivalent to those seen in adults; cadaveric transplant success in children has been generally equivalent or somewhat inferior to what is reported in adults. Very preliminary data in 390 children from the North American

Pediatric Renal Transplant Cooperative Study (NAPRTCS) describe a six-month actuarial cadaver graft survival rate of 81%; the rate in living related transplantation is 92% (2). The current long-term graft outcome is somewhat more difficult to project since the new immunosuppressive agents have been available for only four to five years. Children on azathioprine and prednisone show a 10-year cadaveric graft survival of approximately 45% and a 10-year, non-HLA identical living-related graft survival of 50%. Patient survival rates approximate or exceed those seen in adults. Broyer and colleagues reported a three-year cumulative patient survival of 100% in pediatric recipients of living-related transplants; in cadaveric transplantation, they reported a cumulative patient survival rate of 93% at five years and 90% at ten years (3). It is likely that for children to achieve significant longevity, multiple transplants will be needed.

II. Incidence and Etiology of End-Stage Renal Disease in Children

The overall incidence of ESRD in children ranges from one to five per million total population (see Chapter 15). The etiology of ESRD in children varies by locale and, of course, by age. The causes of ESRD in children differ from those seen in adults, with an increased incidence of congenital and hereditary diseases in the pediatric age group (see Chapter 15).

III. Criteria for Acceptability for Renal Transplantation

As a general rule, almost all children with ESRD are candidates for renal transplantation. This is because transplantation permits the child (and family) a life-style that is more conducive than dialysis to optimal development and rehabilitation. There are, nevertheless, a number of issues the professional team must consider when evaluating the child with ESRD for transplantation.

A. Patient Age

Until recently, the outcome of renal transplantation in children under six years of age was suboptimal, and in children under one year of age, quite dismal (4). New developments in organ utilization and immunosuppression have improved the picture dramatically. Recent reports from the University of Minnesota have documented excellent results in nine infants under the age of one year, primarily with living-related transplantation (5). Using a sequential immunosuppressive regimen of induction therapy with anti-thymocyte globulin (ATG), prednisone and azathioprine, and maintenance with cyclosporin (CsA), prednisone and azathioprine, we have found that cadaver graft survival in children under six can exceed 90% at one year (6). We have also found that the use of kidneys from donors over the age of six years has resulted in improved graft outcome (7) and graft function (6) in these young children.

With today's improved transplantation technology, it is possible to achieve outstanding cadaveric graft outcomes in children under six years of age. Important considerations in achieving this outcome include the use of 1) optimally matched donors, 2) organs from donors over the age of six years to achieve optimal posttransplant renal function and 3) a potent immunosuppressive protocol to overcome the young child's increased immune responsiveness and propensity to mount a strong rejection response (6,7). The advent of successful peritoneal dialysis modalities for infants and young children permits us to wait until conditions for optimal transplantation can be met. We can also conclude that living-related donor transplantation yields excellent results in infants and young children.

B. Mental and Neurological Status

The infant with a significant developmental delay and the child with severe mental retardation pose difficult problems when they are evaluated for potential dialysis and transplantation. It has been our feeling that children with severe mental retardation (i.e. IQ < 40) who require custodial care should not be subjected to the rigors of dialysis and transplantation. A child with this degree of retardation cannot comprehend the need for the various procedures involved in the care and as a result reacts quite poorly to them.

It is important to recall that uremia has an adverse but often reversible effect on a child's mental functioning; it may also often cause psychological depression. Thus, it is important to detail the premorbid mental capacity of the child who presents with sudden onset ESRD and appears to be functioning at a subnormal level. If a precise premorbid determination of the child's mental functioning is unavailable, it may be necessary to initiate dialysis and alleviate the uremic symptomatology before a precise assessment of the child's mental status can be made. Initiation of dialysis often improves the picture and permits progression to transplantation in situations where it might otherwise have been predicted not to be feasible.

Infants with renal insufficiency during the first year of life frequently have concomitant neurological abnormalities, which are often profound, and include developmental delay, microcephaly, hypotonia and seizures (8). Because of these profound abnormalities, some authors have suggested preemptive renal transplantation (8), whereas others have advovocated institution of dialysis at the very earliest sign of head circumference grow-rate reduction and/or developmental fall-off (1).

C. Psychosocial Factors

Psychosocial and emotional problems in children and adolescents undergoing therapy following renal replacement frequently manifest themselves as noncompliance with the therapeutic regimen. This may occur initially when the patient is undergoing dialysis, and raises the issue of whether such a noncompliant patient should receive a renal allograft. Since noncompliance in this setting invariably leads to rejection, it is crucial to identify the potentially noncompliant patient during dialysis, if possible. Introduction of behavior modification programs or other psychological interventions may be successful in obtaining compliance. Securing family support and working with the pre-illness personality traits of the child are also keys to ensuring compliance. A child or adolescent with good self-esteem and at least one supportive family member has a high likelihood of remaining compliant with the posttransplant treatment program.

D. Pre-existing Malignancy

Wilms' tumor is the malignancy most often requiring ESRD care in childhood. Transplantation in children with Wilms' tumor should be deferred for at least one year following primary treatment of the tumor in order to detect persistence of the malignancy and to avoid the risk of overwhelming sepsis following transplantation, which may be related to chemotherapy for the tumor. Few children with primary nonrenal malignancies have been reported to have undergone renal transplantation. In the few reports available, there has been no recurrence of the primary malignancies. Thus, the presence of a primary nonrenal malignancy is not a contraindication to transplantation, although an appropriate waiting time often must be observed between tumor extirpation and transplantation.

E. Bladder Adequacy

The presence of an abnormal lower urinary tract is not a contraindication to renal transplantation. If the bladder has been defunctionalized because of a prior diversion procedure, vigorous attempts can be made to use it for transplantation. We have had excellent results utilizing a previously defunctionalized bladder for transplantation. In recipients with abnormal bladders, there is an increased incidence of posttransplant urological complications and urinary tract infections. However, graft outcome is identical to those children with normal lower urinary tracts. Bladders that have not been used for extended time periods can be hydrodilated and assessed for adequacy. If the bladder is not usable, an ileal loop or a similar diversion/augmentation can be created prior to transplantation.

If a child has a neurogenic bladder, self-catheterization can be employed successfully and safely. Problems with self-catheterization include urinary tract infection when technique is poor and noncompliance, which may lead to renal dysfunction from partial obstruction.

F. Primary Renal Disease

Primary renal disease is a most important consideration when evaluating children for renal transplantation, since, in many situations, the pathological process that caused the original renal failure can also afflict the transplanted organ. Experience with these recurrent diseases has taught us certain manipulations that can minimize their impact, e.g. deferring transplantation under certain circumstances. Thus, precise identification of the original renal disease is quite important. Recurrence of any disease as a cause of graft failure accounts for less than 2% of all graft failures; however, in children, it may account for up to 5% of graft loss (9).

The two main categories of renal disease that can potentially involve the graft are primary glomerulonephritis and inherited metabolic diseases. Specific confirmation of recurrent *glomerulonephritis* may be difficult. Often a specific histological diagnosis of the recipient's original renal disease is unavailable. In addition, all glomerulonephritic changes in the graft do not signify recurrence of an original disease. Immunological damage to the graft from the rejection process may mimic some primary glomerular diseases such as focal glomerulosclerosis (FGS) (10) and membranoproliferative glomerulonephritis (MPGN) (11). Certain types of glomerulonephritis can also occur de novo in the graft. Membranous glomerulonephritis is the most frequent de novo renal disease, occurring in as many as 9% of all pediatric renal transplants (12).

Focal glomerulosclerosis has the highest potential of all the glomerular diseases for recurrence in the allograft. The reported frequency of recurrence is approximately 25% (1). Half of the grafts in which FGS recurs will fail (1). Risk factors implicated in the development of FGS recurrence include 1) duration of original disease from onset to ESRD of three years or less, 2) presence of mesangial proliferation in addition to FGS in the native kidneys and 3) age over six years at the onset of proteinuria. Once a patient has developed FGS with graft loss, the recurrence rate in a subsequent graft approaches 80%.

Proteinuria and slow graft failure are the hallmarks of recurrent FGS. Proteinuria is often massive, occurring within hours to days after transplant; occasionally the onset of heavy proteinuria is delayed for weeks to months. Once proteinuria is established, it is usually persistent. Graft failure is not predictable; often there is a moderately long course of stable graft function punctuated by clinical problems attributable to the marked nephrotic syndrome.

Despite the morbidity attendent to recurrence of the nephrotic syndrome and the potential for graft loss, the variable incidence for recurrence and the inability to accurately predict in which child FGS will recur dictates that children with FGS not be excluded as transplant candidates. Children at high risk for recurrence should receive cadaveric rather than living-related grafts.

Histological evidence of recurrence regularly occurs in patients with MPGN Type II, and to a lesser extent in patients with MPGN type I. Clinically significant recurrence is less often the case in both of these entities. The recurrence rate in children for MPGN Type I ranges from 30 to 70% (1,4,13), with graft loss in about 30% of those with recurrence. Occasional early graft failure is associated with the presence of extracapillary crescentic glomerular changes (13). The incidence of histological recurrence of MPGN Type II approaches 100%; graft loss from recurrence ranges from 10% to 50% (1,13).

In patients with IgA nephropathy and Henoch-Schönlein purpura, histological recurrence is observed frequently. However, recurrence rarely leads to graft loss. Occasionally, however, recurrence may be severe, with crescentic glomerular disease, nephrotic syndrome and graft failure. Transplantation should be deferred in patients with Henoch-Schönlein purpura until six to twelve months after the last manifestation of purpura.

The incidence of recurrence of systemic lupus erythematosus (SLE) is less than 1%. When recurrence does occur, its clinical significance is minor.

Hebert and colleagues, using rigid criteria for diagnosing both clinical and histological recurrence, observed hemolytic uremic syndrome recurrence in 50% of patients (14). Because of the potential for recurrence, the authors suggest that the use of both cyclosporin (CsA) and antilymphocyte globulin be avoided. At UCLA, we have deferred transplantation until all clinical manifestations have completely abated. We have utilized low-dose CsA in selected patients with hemolytic uremic syndrome and their grafts are functioning well. Nevertheless, considerable caution is indicated when using CsA in patients whose original disease was hemolytic uremic syndrome. Live kidney donation must be regarded with caution in view of the report of recurrence within three weeks after living-related transplantation (14).

Inherited metabolic diseases that can involve the graft include diabetes mellitus, oxalosis, cystinosis, Fabry's disease and sickle cell anemia. Although most of the involvement of these diseases is minor, cystinosis and oxalosis are of special importance in pediatrics.

Although interstitial cystine crystals are present in the allografts of recipients with *cystinosis*, they have no adverse effect upon allograft function; there is neither recurrence of Fanconi syndrome nor deterioration of the glomerular filtration rate. In fact, cadaver donor allograft survival rates in cystinotic recipients have been reported to be superior to the rates in recipients with other primary renal diseases (3). There is no accumulation of cystine in the tubular or glomerular epithelial cells as occurs in native cystinotic kidneys; instead there is cystine deposition in the interstitium, a result of the elevated cystine content of host leukocytes that transit the transplanted organ. The major posttransplant consequences of cystinosis are extrarenal manifestations; these are not ameliorated by renal transplantation.

Until recently, patients with oxalosis (primary hyperoxaluria Type I) had been regarded as untransplantable. Recurrence of the disease, with devastating renal oxalate deposition during periods of renal insufficiency, led to an almost invariable early graft failure. However, a number of recent reports suggest that successful transplantation, both cadaveric and living-related, is possible. These reports stress the importance of vigorous preoperative lowering of serum oxalate levels with daily hemodialysis, immediate postoperative diuresis that minimizes oxalate deposition in the allograft and posttransplant management with pyridoxine, neutral phosphate, magnesium and noncalciuric diuretic therapy, as well as avoiding infection and graft dysfunction due to acute tubular necrosis or rejection.

Scheinman and colleagues reported favorable results in six children six months to eight years of age using living-related donor allografts (13). A subsequent report from the same institution documents graft loss from recurrence (15), suggesting that despite the potential for some long-term graft success in children with oxalosis, the incidence of recurrence remains significant. A potential curative alternative for children with primary oxalosis is combined hepatic and renal transplantation (16).

IV. Workup of the Potential Donor

Many centers still prefer living-related donors for the following reasons: 1) more favorable results because of a better histocompatibility match, 2) the operation can be planned, thus cutting the waiting time and 3) the supply of cadaveric organs is insufficient. The living donor should be a highly motivated blood relative, ABO compatible, and should be in excellent medical condition with normal renal function. Best results are obtained with an HLA-identical sibling; however, excellent results can also be obtained with a haploidentical relative. The potential living donor should be properly evaluated prior to kidney donation as shown in Table 20-1.

Excellent graft outcome can also be obtained utilizing a cadaveric donor (6,7). Criteria for screening potential cadaver donors are presented in Table 20-2. All donors must be ABO compatible. In addition, the HLA

TABLE 20-1. Evaluation of the Potential Living Donor

1. History, physical examination, repeated blood pressure determinations
2. ABO blood group, tissue typing, lymphocyte cross-match, mixed lymphocyte culture
3. Complete blood count, platelet count, blood urea nitrogen, creatinine, glucose, cholesterol, triglycerides, calcium, phosphorus, uric acid, prothrombin time, creatinine clearance, HIV and hepatitis-B surface antigen, CMV titer, VDRL, SGOT, SGPT, bilirubin, alkaline phosphatase, pregnancy test in females
4. Urinalysis, urine culture, 24-hour urine protein
5. Chest X-ray, electrocardiogram
6. Intravenous pyelogram, aortogram/digital subtraction angiography
7. Psychiatric evaluation

B and DR antigens should be optimally matched between donor and recipient, since this leads to fewer rejection episodes and improved long-term graft outcome. Finally, the lymphocyte cross match using donor T-lymphocytes and pretransplant recipient serum must be negative to avoid hyperacute rejection. Historical sera may be positive, but current sera must be negative.

V. Workup of the Recipient

The recipient of a kidney transplant should be thoroughly and systematically investigated (Table 20-3).

VI. Complications of Transplantation

A. Rejection

Acute rejection may appear from a few days to many months following transplantation. It may be characterized by low grade fever, malaise, graft tenderness, hypertension, weight gain, fall in renal function, reduced urine output and increased urinary protein (Table 20-4). When patients are treated with CsA, however, many of the clinical symptoms, e.g. graft tenderness and fever, will be absent. The differential diagnosis of acute rejection includes CsA toxicity, urinary obstruction or extravasation, renal artery thrombosis or stenosis, CMV and other infectious agents, recurrence of the original renal disease and drug toxicity (e.g. angiotensin converting enzyme inhibitors). Studies that are useful in differentiating rejection from other causes of renal dysfunction are shown in Table 20-4. The renal biopsy is the most certain diagnostic tool in this regard. Histologically, acute cellular rejection is characterized by interstitial edema and mononuclear cell infiltration; these inflammatory cells can often be found invading tubules and/or arterioles. The glomeruli are normal. Acute cellular rejection can often be reversed by high-dose cor-

TABLE 20-2. Criteria for Screening Potential Cadaver Donors

1. Minimum age three and preferably six years, and maximum age 65 years with no history of severe hypertension, diabetes mellitus and malignancy other than brain tumor and skin cancer
2. Absence of primary renal disease
3. Absence of generalized bacterial infection (if bacterial infection is present, donor is usable if on appropriate antimicrobial therapy for at least 24 hours) or viral infection, and negative serological studies for HIV and hepatitis B; if donor is CMV seropositive, recipient should be CMV seropositive also
4. Normal urinalysis and preterminal urine hourly output at least 0.5 ml/kg
5. Normal serum urea nitrogen and creatinine—may be elevated if donor is kept dry, i.e. prerenal azotemia is present
6. Cold ischemia time less than 48 hours, preferably less than 36 hours
7. Declaration of brain death by the patient's physician
8. ABO compatibility with recipient
9. Negative complement-dependent cytotoxicity cross-match using donor T-lymphocytes and recipient serum from the day of transplant

TABLE 20-3. Evaluation of the Renal Transplant Recipient

1. HLA typing and periodic testing for anti-HLA antibodies; antibody testing two to four weeks after every transfusion
2. Chest X-ray, electrocardiogram and echocardiogram
3. Identify and treat infection adequately (urinary tract, peritoneum, etc.)
4. Screen for HIV, hepatitis B, CMV antibody and Tb
5. Urological evaluation with cystoscopy, voiding cystourethrogram and urodynamic studies (when indicated); if massive reflux and treatment-resistant infection, consider nephrectomy, otherwise avoid
6. Control hypertension with adequate dialysis, antihypertensive agents or, as a last resort, bilateral nephrectomy
7. Diagnose and treat bone disease (hyperparathyroidism, necrosis); parathyroidectomy prior to transplant if hyperparathyroidism uncontrollable
8. Remove rejected transplanted kidneys if symptomatic
9. Control nephrotic syndrome
10. If neutropenia and/or thrombocytopenia present, control hypersplenism (partial splenectomy or embolization)
11. Establish patterns of medication compliance; psychiatric evaluation
12. Control seizures with drugs that are not hepatic p-450 enzyme inducers, if possible
13. Identify any drugs the patient is on that can interfere with prednisone, azathioprine, CsA (e.g. rifampicin, erythromycin, Tegretol, allopurinol)
14. Evaluate hepatic function; abnormalities may affect metabolism of immunosuppressive agents

ticosteroids or anti T-cell antibody preparations. Acute vascular rejection is characterized by endothelial cell swelling and proliferation, intimal proliferation and fibrinoid necrosis. Antirejection therapy here is usually ineffective.

Hyperacute rejection occurs within minutes to hours following transplantation and generally implies graft loss. This type of rejection, which

TABLE 20-4. Diagnosis of Rejection of Renal Transplant

1. Clinical picture
   Fever[a]
   Weight gain[a]
   Enlargement and tenderness of renal graft[a]
   Hypertension[a]
   Reduced urinary output[a]
   Decreased renal function
   Reduced urinary sodium excretion
   Increased proteinuria
2. Cyclosporin trough blood levels
3. Radionuclide renal studies (blood flow, excretion index, extravasation, obstruction)
4. Renal sonogram ± Doppler (kidney size, renal blood flow, corticomedullary junction, pyramid shape, obstruction)
5. Intravenous pyelogram (obstruction)
6. Renal arteriogram (major renal vessel stenosis or occlusion)
7. Computer tomography scan (perinephric masses)
8. Magnetic resonance imaging (obstruction, renal vessel stenosis or occlusion, corticomedullary junction and pyramid shape evaluation)
9. Renal biopsy ("gold standard" for rejection, CsA nephrotoxicity)
10. Immunological monitoring (e.g. circulating T-cell phenotypes, antilymphocyte antibodies, etc.)
11. Fine needle aspiration biopsy (presence in graft of inflammatory cells, tubular damage, CMV)

[a]May be absent in mild episodes.

is the result of sensitization of the recipient to HLA antigens on the donor kidney, is infrequent because of present-day, cross-matching techniques.

Chronic rejection is characterized by slowly progressive deterioration in renal function associated with proteinuria, hypertension, severe arteriolar lesions on biopsy, interstitial fibrosis and lack of response to anti-rejection treatment.

B. Other Complications

Infection is the main complication of immunosuppression and may be due to bacteria, viruses, fungi or parasites (Table 20-5). Sepsis, as well as pulmonary, urinary tract, skin, wound, central nervous system, and gastrointestinal (GI) infections may occur. Agressive workup and treatment of infection is of utmost importance for graft and patient survival. Workup of the transplant patient with suspected infection is presented in Table 20-6.

Hypertension occurs in over three quarters of posttransplant patients. In the immediate posttransplant period, it is usually related to hypervolemia, especially in the patient with acute tubular necrosis and decreased urinary output. It is also a frequent finding in acute rejection and it resolves with reversal of the rejection episode. The etiology of persistent

TABLE 20-5. Common Types of Infection
in Transplanted Patients

Bacteria
  Pneumococcus
  Staphylococcus
  Gram-negative organisms
  Legionella
  Mycobacteria
Viruses
  Cytomegalovirus
  Herpes simplex
  Varicella zoster
  Epstein-Barr
  Hepatitis B
  HIV
  Papovavirus
  Adenovirus
  Influenza A and other RNA viruses
Fungi
  Aspergillus
  Candida
  Cryptococcus
  Nocardia
Parasites
  Pneumocystis carini
  Toxoplasma
  Strongyloides

TABLE 20-6. Workup of the Transplant Patient Suspected of Having Infection

History and physical examination
Complete blood count, multiple blood cultures, serum creatinine
Urinalysis, urine cultures
Chest X-ray
Smear and cultures from:
  Sputum, transtracheal aspirate, bronchial washings, lung biopsy
    Gram, acid fast, silver and india ink stain stains
    Cultures for aerobic and anaerobic bacteria, fungi and mycobacteria
    Histology and cytology
  Any open wound
  Any subcutaneous fluid accumulation
Lumbar puncture
Acute and convalescent serum for viral and bacterial titers
Buffy coat blood culture and in situ hybridization studies for CMV
Fine needle aspiration biopsy—tubular cell staining for CMV antigens

posttransplant hypertension is due to chronic rejection (59%), renal artery stenosis (20.5%), effects of the native kidney (probably mediated by renin release) (4.5%), recurrence of primary renal disease (4.5%), nonviable kidney (1.5%) and unknown (10%) (17). Prompt diagnosis and treatment of high blood pressure is of utmost importance in these patients, since poorly controlled hypertension leads to a rapid deterioration of graft function.

Other complications of transplantation include corticosteroid toxicity (posterior subcapsular lenticular cataract, excessive weight gain), hyperlipidemia, aseptic necrosis, cardiovascular disease, GI complications (upper GI bleeding, pancreatitis, hepatitis), urological complications (obstruction, extravasation, development of calyceal-cutaneous fistula) and the development of de novo malignancy. Side effects of CsA include tremor, hypertrichosis, nephrotoxicity, hepatotoxicity, gingival hypertrophy, dysmorphic facies, hypertension and possible carbohydrate intolerence.

References

1. Ettenger RB, Marik J, Rosenthal JT, et al (1989) New modes of immunosuppression in pediatric cadaveric renal transplantation. In: Strauss J (ed) Growth, Immunosuppression and Renal Disorder in Neonates and Children. Univ of Miami Press, Coral Gables, pp 175–193
2. North American Pediatric Renal Transplant Cooperative Study (NAPRTCS) (1988) Demographics, immunotherapy and outcome of pediatric renal transplants in North America. Kidney Int 35:521 (abstract)
3. Broyer M, Gagradoux M-F, Guest G, et al (1987) Kidney transplantation in children: Results of 383 grafts performed at Enfants Malades Hospital from 1973 to 1984. In: Grunfeld J-P, Back J-F, Cromier, et al (eds) Advances in Nephrology, Vol 16. Year Book Medical Publishers, Chicago, pp 307–333
4. Fine RN, Ettenger RB (1988) Renal transplantation in children. In: Morris PJ (ed) Kidney Transplantation: Principles and Practice, 3rd edition. WB Saunders, Philadelphia, pp 635–691
5. So SKS, Nevins TE, Chang P-N, et al (1985) Preliminary results of renal transplantation in children under 1 year of age. Transplant Proc 17:182–183
6. Ettenger RB, Rosenthal JT, Marik J, et al (1989) Successful cadaveric renal transplantation in infants and young children. Transplant Proc 21:1707–1708
7. Ettenger RB, Rosenthal JT, Marik J et al (1989) Factors influencing the improvement in cadaveric renal transplant survival in pediatric recipients. Transplant Proc 21:1693–1695
8. Rotundo A, Nevins TE, Lipton M, et al (1982) Progressive encephalopathy in children with chronic renal insufficiency in infancy. Kidney Int 21:486–491
9. Mathew TH (1988) Recurrence of disease following renal transplantation. Am J Kid Dis 12:85–96
10. Ettenger RB, Hauser E, Malekzadeh MH, et al (1977) Focal glomerulosclerosis in renal allografts: association with the nephrotic syndrome and chronic rejection. Am J Dis Child 131:347–352
11. Cameron JS (1982) Glomerulonephritis in renal transplants. Transplantation 34:237–245

12. Antignac C, Hinglais N, Gubler H-C, et al (1988) De novo membranous glomerulonephritis in renal allografts in children. Clin Nephrol 30:1-7
13. Scheinman JI, Najarian JS, Mauer SM, et al (1984) Successful strategies for renal transplantation in primary oxalosis. Kidney Int 25:804–811
14. Hebert D, Sibley RK, Mauer SM (1986) Recurrence of hemolytic uremic syndrome in renal transplant recipients. Kidney Int 30:S51–S58
15. Sheldon CA, Elick B, Najarian JS, et al (1985) Improving survival in the very young renal transplant recipient. J Pediatr Surg 20:622–626
16. Watts RWE, Calne RY, Rolles K, et al (1987) Successful treatment of primary hyperoxaluria type I by combined hepatic and renal transplantation. Lancet 2:474–475
17. Broyer M, Guest G, Gagnadoux M-F, et al (1987) Hypertension following renal transplantation in children. Pediatr Nephrol 1:16–21

21
Prenatal Diagnosis of Renal and Urinary Tract Abnormalities

PHILIPPE JEANTY and MANFRED HANSMANN

I. Introduction

Prenatal diagnosis of renal and urinary tract abnormalities may be achieved by fetal ultrasonography. With improvement in techniques used to obtain and study fetal tissue, the prenatal diagnosis of conditions associated with renal disease also became possible. Sonographically diagnosed malformations occur in about 0.5% of fetuses, 50% of which are due to renal tract abnormalities (1). Of pregnancies with positive family history of renal tract anomalies, 8% were also found to have urinary tract abnormalities by ultrasound (2). In this chapter, we will review the indications and techniques of prenatal diagnosis of renal tract anomalies, present some of the commonly seen ones and touch on the management and follow-up of affected fetuses.

II. Indications for Prenatal Diagnosis of the Kidney and Urinary Tract

Incidental abnormalities of the kidney and urinary tract are often found on ultrasound examination performed routinely on pregnant women for other indications, such as assessing the gestational age, viability and growth of the fetus. Indications for prenatal study of the kidney and urinary tract may include the following: 1) family history of renal tract disease such as renal agenesis, dysplasia or hypoplasia; obstructive uropathy; congenital nephrosis and "prune-belly" syndrome; 2) presence of oligohydramnios and possibly polyhydramnios; 3) elevated maternal alpha-fetoprotein, which may suggest the presence of congenital nephrosis or obstructive uropathy; 4) "small for date" fetus and 5) presence of abnormalities of other systems or chromosomal aberrations in the fetus or family members.

III. Methods Used in the Prenatal Diagnosis of Renal Tract Disease

A. Ultrasound

Widely used since the mid seventies, ultrasonography is a noninvasive technique that utilizes non-ionizing acoustical energy. With the advances in fetal ultrasonography, prenatal diagnosis of renal tract abnormalities has become rather accurate (3–5). The fetal bladder is usually visible by 13 to 14 weeks gestation, and the kidneys a few weeks later. Intrarenal anatomy becomes distinguishable and the cortex, medulla and collecting system can be differentiated after 20 weeks gestation. Later on, even the arcuate arteries are visible.

The amniotic fluid is essentially produced by fetal urination around nine weeks gestation. Oligohydramnios, which suggests the presence of a urinary tract abnormality, can be identified as early as 14 to 15 weeks gestation. Oligohydramnios may be due to increased removal of fluid from the amniotic cavity (premature rupture of the membrane) or decreased production of urine by the fetus. Decreased urine production can be due to mechanisms that affect the urinary system at three levels: 1) prerenal due to low perfusion states (placental insufficiency or growth retardation), 2) renal (agenesis or dysplasia) and 3) postrenal (obstructive disease such as ureteropelvic junction stenosis and posterior urethral valves).

The size and volume of the fetal kidney may also be measured. The renal volume is changed, for example, in cystic renal disease, renal agenesis and renal tumors. Measurement of growth of the fetal kidney is also possible, and charts of renal volume as a function of fetal age have been devised (6). Renal functions may also be assessed by measurement of amniotic fluid and urine volume. Ultrasonography may also detect hourly fetal urine production with or without maternal furosemide administration. However, failure to visualize the urinary bladder following maternal furosemide does not necessarily indicate absent fetal kidneys, since this may occur in the growth-retarded fetus with decreased renal perfusion

(7). The use of fetal ultrasound in the diagnosis of renal tract abnormalities is presented in Figure 21-1.

B. Other Methods

Elevated levels of alpha-fetoprotein in the maternal serum or amniotic fluid may suggest the presence of congenital nephrosis, renal agenesis or obstructive uropathy. Determination of enzyme activity, demonstration of storage products of fetal tissues and analysis of amniotic fluid and fetal blood components are the methods used in the prenatal diagnosis of metabolic and hereditary disorders associated with renal disease (8). Fetal cells may be obtained by amniocentesis, chorionic villus sampling (CVS) and percutaneous umbilical blood sampling (PUBS). Amniocentesis, which is considered a safe and accurate procedure, is performed under ultrasound guidance at around 16 to 18 weeks gestation. Chorionic villus sampling yields about 10 to 15 mg of fetal material, sufficient for enzyme assays and chromosome and DNA analysis. This procedure, which can be performed at 8 to 12 weeks gestation, may be complicated by fetal loss in 1 to 2% and maternal infection in 0.3% of cases. One to five milliliters of pure fetal blood can be obtained by PUBS at around 15 to 38 weeks gestation, with a risk of fetal loss of 1/500.

Recently, the mutation for autosomal dominant (adult) polycystic kidney disease (APKD) has been localized to the short arm of chromosome

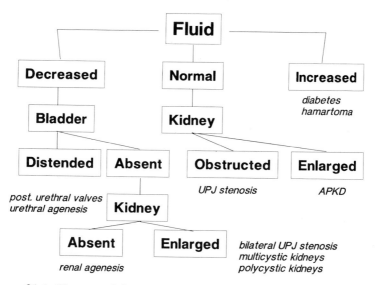

FIGURE 21-1. The use of fetal ultrasonography in the diagnosis of renal tract abnormalities (UPJ: ureteropelvic junction; APKD: autosomal dominant adult polycystic kidney disease).

16 by demonstrating a genetic linkage with the alpha chain of hemoglobin (9). These techniques have been also used successfully in the prenatal diagnosis of this condition (10). DNA studies may be performed on fetal material obtained by CVS or fetal blood obtained by PUBS. DNA linkage has also been used to identify Lowe's oculocerebrorenal syndrome and Wilms' tumor-aniridia complex (11). Marker loci have also been identified in the middle of the long arm of the X chromosome of patients with Alport's syndrome (12,13).

IV. Renal and Urinary Tract Abnormalities Diagnosed Prenatally

The renal and urinary tract abnormalities that can be diagnosed prenatally, the ultrasonographic findings (Figures 21-2 to 21-5) and other methods used in the diagnosis are presented in Table 21-1.

These abnormalities are frequently associated with anomalies of other organ systems and chromosomal aberrations. About one-half of the cases with cystic kidneys and subvesical obstruction may have a structural

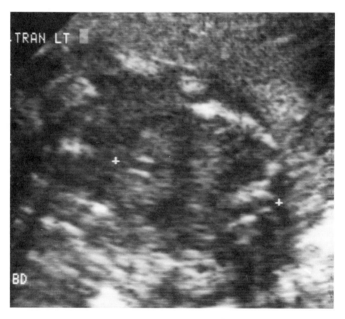

FIGURE 21-2. Bilateral renal agenesis. The fetus is difficult to distinguish from the placenta because of the absence of amniotic fluid. The film, which is obtained at the level of the renal fossa, reveals no evidence of renal tissue.

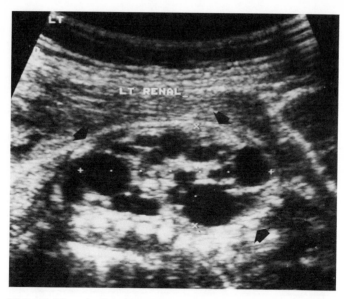

FIGURE 21-3. Multicystic dysplastic kidney (between arrows) showing disorganized cysts varying from a few millimeters to 2 cm in diameter, which distinguish this condition from hydronephrosis.

anomaly of other organ systems (2), and around one-fourth of fetuses with obstructive uropathy have a chromosomal aberration (14). The workup of every fetus with congenital abnormality of the kidney or urinary tract should therefore include a sonogram of other organs and chromosomal karyotyping.

V. Conditions and Syndromes Associated with Renal Disease That Can Be Diagnosed Prenatally

Various conditions that are associated with renal disease can be diagnosed prenatally. With the possible exception of the "prune-belly" and Meckel syndromes, in which renal involvement may be severe and require a decision concerning the outcome of the fetus, renal involvement in the other conditions (see Appendix IV) is usually not so severe, and the disease is managed taking into consideration the basic pathophysiological abnormality and outcome of that particular disease. Conditions with renal involvement that can be diagnosed prenatally are presented in Table 21-2.

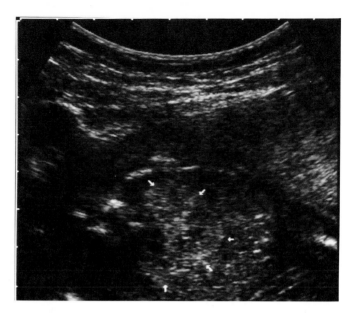

FIGURE 21-4. Autosomal recessive (infantile) polycystic kidney disease. A transverse film through the renal area reveals a large echogenic mass representing large kidneys (between arrows). The increased echogenicity is due to numerous small cysts that are too small to be visible as cysts. Also note the absence of amniotic fluid.

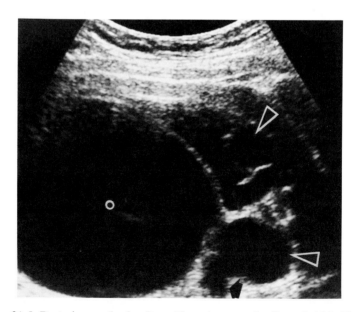

FIGURE 21-5. Posterior urethral valves. Note the severely distended bladder (circle), distended tortuous ureters (arrows) and the hydronephrotic kidneys (triangles).

TABLE 21-1. Renal and Urinary Tract Abnormalities Diagnosed Prenatally

Abnormality	Ultrasound findings	Other tests
Renal agenesis, bilateral (Figure 21-2)	Severe oligohydramnios, absence of kidneys and bladder	Elevated alpha-fetoprotein in maternal serum and amniotic fluid
Renal multicystic dysplasia (Figure 21-3)	Oligohydramnios, multiple cysts of variable size, usually unilateral	
Renal hypoplasia	Oligohydramnios, small kidneys	
ARPKD[a] (Figure 21-4)	Large bilateral echogenic kidneys, severe oligohydramnios	
ADPKD[b]	Oligohydramnios, cysts of various sizes	DNA markers on chromosome 16
Congenital nephrosis		Elevated alpha-fetoprotein in maternal serum and amniotic fluid
Renal tumors	Increased renal volume, solid mass	
Hydronephrosis	Oligohydramnios, pelvicalyceal distension	
Obstructive uropathy	Oligohydramnios, hydronephrosis, possibly large bladder	Elevated alpha-fetoprotein in amniotic fluid
Ureteropelvic junction obstruction	Dilated collecting system, normal bladder	
Posterior urethral valves (Figure 21-5)	Severe oligohydramnios, severely distended bladder	

[a]Autosomal recessive (infantile) polycystic kidney disease.
[b]Autosomal dominant (adult) polycystic kidney disease.

VI. Management of Renal Tract Anomalies in the Fetus

Prenatal diagnosis of renal tract anomalies allows early treatment to decrease renal damage and the occurrence of end-stage renal disease. When such an anomaly is discovered in the fetus, the degree of renal damage and renal function should be assessed and abnormalities of other organ systems and chromosomal aberrations should be looked for. The strategy of management and the prognosis of the fetus should be discussed by a committee that includes a perinatologist, ultrasonographer, urologist, pediatric nephrologist, neonatologist, social worker, psychologist and specialists in ethical and legal matters. The subject should be also discussed with the family before reaching a decision on the final management plan.

TABLE 21-2. Conditions with Renal Involvement That Can Be Diagnosed Prenatally

"Prune-belly" syndrome	Meckel's syndrome
Robert's syndrome	Osteogenesis imperfecta
Ehlers-Danlos syndrome	Sickle-cell disease
Thanatophoric dwarfism	Glycogen storage disease, Type I
Fabry's disease	Gangliosidosis
Gaucher's disease	Mucolipidosis, Type II
Hurler's syndrome	Metachromatic leukodystrophy
Niemann-Pick disease	Cystinosis
Aminoacidurias	Oxalosis
Lesch-Nyhan syndrome	Zellweger syndrome
Tyrosinemia, Type I	Chromosomal aberrations

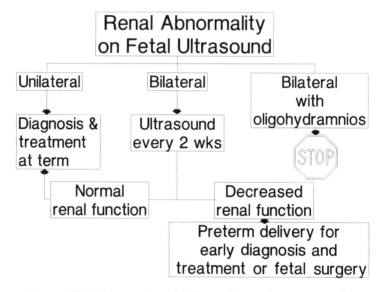

FIGURE 21-6. Approach to the fetus with renal tract anomalies.

Generally, fetuses with unilateral renal involvement or bilateral involvement with persistently normal renal function on follow-up can be diagnosed and treated following a term delivery. Fetuses with severe bilateral renal involvement and severe oligohydramnios have a grave prognosis and the parents may choose to terminate the pregnancy. Fetuses with bilateral renal involvement, who on follow-up show impaired renal function, may have preterm delivery for early diagnosis and treatment if they are viable. Our plan of approach to a fetus with renal tract anomalies is similar to that of Helin and Persson (2) and is presented in Figure 21-6.

When preterm delivery is not possible because of immature lungs or other reasons, these fetuses may benefit from fetal surgery. At present, this consists of decompression of distal obstruction, particularly posterior urethral valves, by a shunt placed between the fetal bladder and amniotic fluid cavity (15,16). The main complication of the procedure is spontaneous abortion or precipitation of premature labor. Figures from the Report of the International Fetal Surgery Registry, however, reveal a procedure-related fetal death rate of 4.6% (17). Pulmonary hypoplasia continues to be the primary cause of death in both treated and untreated patients. The enthusiasm for fetal surgery has dwindeled somewhat. The concept of "fetus-as-patient," however, creates an ethical issue related to the accuracy of diagnosis, acceptability of abortion, expected benefit and risks of treatment and medicolegal problems (18). The need for more defined criteria for premature delivery and fetal surgery is clearly evident.

References

1. Helin I, Persson P-H (1986) Prenatal diagnosis of urinary tract abnormalities by ultrasound. Pediatrics 78: 879–883
2. Reuss A, Wladimiroff JW, Niiermeijer MF (1987) Antenatal diagnosis of renal tract anomalies by ultrasound. Pediatr Nephrol 1: 546–552
3. Hansmann M, Hackelöer B-J, Staudach A (1986) Ultrasound Diagnosis in Obstetrics and Gynecology. Springer-Verlag, Berlin, pp 223–237
4. Romero R, Pilu GL, Jeanty P, et al (1987) Prenatal Diagnosis of Congenital Anomalies. Appleton and Lange, Norwalk, pp 301–311
5. Barakat AY, Awazu M, Fleischer AC (1989) Antenatal diagnosis of renal abnormalities: a review of the state of the art. South Med J 82: 229–234
6. Jeanty P, Dramaix-Wilmet M, Elkhazen N, et al (1982) Measurement of fetal kidney growth on ultrasound. Radiology 144: 159–162
7. Raghavendra BN, Young BK, Greco MA, et al (1987) Use of furosemide in pregnancies complicated by oligohydramnios. Radiology 165: 455–458
8. Harms E (1987) Prenatal diagnosis of inborn errors of metabolism with renal manifestations. Pediatr Nephrol 1: 540–545
9. Reeders ST, Breuning MH, Davies KE, et al (1985) A highly polymorphic DNA marker linked to adult polycystic kidney disease on chromosome 16. Nature 317: 542–544
10. Reeders ST, Gal A, Propping P, et al (1986) Prenatal diagnosis of autosomal dominant polycystic kidney disease with DNA probe. Lancet 2: 6–8
11. Ostrer H, Hejtmancik JF (1988) Prenatal diagnosis and carrier detection of genetic diseases by analysis of deoxyribonucleic acid. J Pediatr 112: 679–687
12. Menlove L, Kirschner N, Nguyen K, et al (1985) Linkage between Alport syndrome-like hereditary nephritis and X-linked PFLPs. Cytogenet Cell Genet 40: 697–698
13. Flinter FA, Bobrow M, Chantler C (1987) Alport's syndrome or hereditary abnormalities of other systems nephritis? Pediatr Nephrol 1: 438–440
14. Nicolaides KH, Rodeck CH, Gosden CM (1986) Rapid karyotyping in non-lethal fetal malformations. Lancet 1: 283–287

15. Harrison MR, Golbus MS, Filly RA, et al (1982) Fetal surgery for congenital hydronephrosis. N Engl J Med 306: 591–593
16. Golbus MS, Harrison MR, Filly RA, et al (1982) In utero treatment of urinary tract obstruction. Am J Obstet Gynecol 142: 383–388
17. Report of the International Fetal Surgery Registry (1986) Catheter shunts for fetal hydronephrosis and hydrocephalus. N Engl J Med 315: 336–340
18. Arant BS, Jr (1987) Prevention of hereditary nephropathies by antenatal interventions. Ethical considerations. Pediatr Nephrol 1: 553–560

22
The Role of Early Diagnosis and Intervention in the Prevention of Kidney Disease

Amin Y. Barakat

I. Introduction

Renal disease is a major cause of morbidity and mortality. It may be overt or asymptomatic, escaping medical attention. Equal attention should be paid to children with asymptomatic renal disease, as well as symptomatic and sick children. Kidney disease should be suspected in children with a family history of certain renal conditions (Alport's syndrome, polycystic kidney disease and vesicoureteral reflux) and in those with congenital abnormalities of other organ systems (cardiovascular, gastrointestinal, central nervous system, genital), chromosomal aberrations, urinary tract infections and various genetic and systemic diseases (see Chapter 1 and Appendix IV).

Urinary tract infection (UTI) is a major cause of end-stage renal disease (ESRD) in children. Often bacteriuria is asymptomatic, and children may present with subtle symptoms not related to the urinary tract such as failure to thrive, unexplained fevers and gastrointestinal symptoms and sometimes normal urinalysis, which makes the recognition of UTI more difficult. Between 5 to 10% of children with symptomatic UTI develop renal scars, which, in some cases, lead to hypertension and uremia (1).

The overall incidence of kidney and urinary tract abnormalities is approximately 5%, and reaches about 10% in males under the age of 18 years (2). Urinary tract abnormalities represent 50% of the total ultrasonographically diagnosed malformations, which occur in 0.25% of fetuses (3). These abnormalities, along with hereditary diseases of the kidney and UTI, account for 50 to 90% of children with ESRD (4,5). Early diagnosis and treatment of many of these conditions will decrease the occurrence of renal damage and ESRD.

The best available treatment for ESRD at the present time is renal transplantation, and as a temporary measure, chronic peritoneal dialysis or hemodialysis. Renal transplantation yields excellent results, but it is expensive and can be complicated by rejection and, sometimes, recurrence of the disease in the transplanted kidney. Additionally, the available facilities and number of renal grafts are not adequate to cover all patients requiring this treatment. Chronic dialysis is not the ideal treatment and is also expensive. Furthermore, technical problems are encountered in obtaining arterial access in children, thus making chronic hemodialysis difficult to maintain in the pediatric age group. Peritoneal dialysis may be complicated by metabolic derangements and infection, which often interfere with adequate peritoneal exchange.

The ideal "treatment" of ESRD in children, therefore, is prevention. In this chapter, I will briefly discuss the role of early diagnosis and intervention in the prevention of kidney disease, or the favorable alteration of its natural course.

II. Early Diagnosis

A. Prenatal Diagnosis

Various renal and urinary tract abnormalities, particularly obstructive uropathy, may be diagnosed prenatally by ultrasonography. Although obstruction before 15 weeks gestation may result in renal dysplasia, late obstruction of the urinary tract may produce hydronephrosis and cystic changes, with functionally normal kidneys at birth (6). Some of these conditions are amenable to intervention; others are not.

Different conditions and syndromes associated with renal tract abnormalities can be diagnosed by chromosomal karyotyping, enzyme determination in amniocytes and alpha-feto protein determination in maternal blood and amniotic fluid. Recently, the mutation for adult polycystic kidney disease (APKD), which is one of the most common autosomal dominant diseases of man (one to three per thousand) has been localized, to the short arm of chromosome 16 (7). This has made possible the prenatal and early detection of asymptomatic patients and opened the way for the use of genetic markers in the early detection of other genetic diseases of the kidney.

Although prenatal diagnosis of various renal tract abnormalities contributes significantly to early intervention to decrease renal damage, this modality has its limitations and it raises complex ethical questions, such as the accuracy of diagnosis, termination of pregnancy in conditions that are compatable with life and the adequacy of fetal surgery (8). The indications and methods used in the prenatal diagnosis of renal disease are discussed in detail in Chapter 21.

B. Postnatal Diagnosis

1. History

A high index of suspicion for renal disease and urinary tract abnormalities should be kept at all times, and an accurate patient and family history of renal and urinary tract disease should be obtained (Chapter 2). Subtle signs and symptoms, which may often appear unrelated to the urinary tract, such as unexplained fevers, failure to thrive, anemia, acidosis and gastrointestinal symptoms should be looked for. Family history of early deafness, renal failure, hypertension, diabetes or urological surgery are also important. Vesicoureteral reflux, a major cause of renal scarring, may be familial in up to 45% of cases (9). Over 300 genetic conditions may be associated with renal and urogenital abnormalities (10–12) (see Appendix IV).

2. Blood Pressure

Hypertension in children is defined as average systolic and/or diastolic blood pressure (BP) equal or greater than the 95th percentile for age and sex on at least three occasions. Renal parenchymal and renovascular lesions are the commonest causes of hypertension in children. Occurring in 1 to 3% of children, hypertension may be a sign of renal disease and is a major risk factor in heart disease. There is definite evidence that primary hypertension in adults may be preceded by high BP in childhood (13). If inadequately treated, elevated BP may be complicated by arteriosclerosis, nephrosclerosis and cerebral hemorrhage; therefore, early diagnosis and control of hypertension are very important in preventing morbidity from this disease.

Although mass screening programs for hypertension in children do not seem to be cost-effective, it should be realized that there is general lack of awareness that hypertension occurs in the pediatric age group and that many children do not have their BP determined because they are not under continuous medical care. If such programs are instituted, they should include trained personnel and resources for counseling, referral and follow-up (13). The workup of the child with hypertension is discussed in Chapter 16.

3. Urinalysis and Urine Culture

A urinalysis should be performed routinely once a year,and urine culture during the first year of life, and when indicated thereafter (Chapter 9). An abnormal urinalysis may be the first sign of renal disease. The presence of hematuria, proteinuria and casts suggests glomerular disease. Pyuria is usually a sign of UTI, but it may be present with inflammation, renal calculi or a urinary tract abnormality. A preschool child with UTI, however, may have no pyuria and a urine culture is necessary to make this diagnosis. A defect in the concentrating ability of the urine can occur in diabetes mellitus or diabetes insipidus, renal failure and sickle cell disease.

4. Imaging of the Urinary Tract

About one-third of children in their first attack of pyelonephritis are found to have a developmental anomaly of the urinary tract (14). Vesicoureteral reflux occurs in about 35% (50% in the first year of life), and obstructive uropathy in 10% of children with symptomatic or asymptomatic UTI (15). Children who develop UTI should be studied by a voiding cystogram and renal ultrasound or intravenous pyelography (IVP). Imaging of the urinary tract is also indicated in the presence of abnormalities of other systems such as congenital heart disease, gastrointestinal and central nervous system abnormalities, supernumerary nipples, chromosomal aberrations and other syndromes associated with renal disease (Chapter 6). Individuals with a family history of certain renal and urinary tract abnormalities such as renal agenesis, polycystic kidney disease and vesicoureteral reflux should be also studied.

5. Genetic Screening

The use of DNA markers in the early and prenatal diagnosis of APKD has opened the way for the use of these markers in other genetic diseases of the kidney. This will allow genetic counseling, as well as early treatment to reduce the risk of developing ESRD. It will also help to avoid transplanting an affected kidney from an asymptomatic donor. DNA linkage has been also used to identify Lowe's oculocerebrorenal syndrome and Wilms' tumor-aniredia complex (16). Significant linkage was also found between the gene of Alport's syndrome and marker loci in the middle of the long arm of the X chromosome (17).

III. Mass Screening

The morbidity rate of chronic glomerular disease is about 40 to 50 per one hundred thousand hospitalized children (18), and two to four times more when asymptomatic cases are picked up by mass screening for hematuria and proteinuria in school children (19). In the Japanese Nephritis Study, positive urinary findings were found in 0.17% of primary and 0.29% of junior high school children following the second urine screen (20). In this study, children with asymptomatic hematuria without proteinuria tended to have minor histological changes with focal segmental lesions. Diffuse proliferative lesions were seen more in those with hematuria and proteinuria, severe lesions being more common in children with heavy proteinuria and hematuria. Over 70% of IgA nephropathy and 65 to 80% of membranoproliferative glomerulonephritis were detected by mass school urine screening (21).

Asymptomatic bacteriuria occurs in 1.2% of school girls and 2% of young women (Chapter 9). The cumulative incidence of UTI in school girls followed over a 10-year span was found to be 5% (22).

Although it is debatable whether mass urine screening programs are cost-effective, they can definitely contribute to the diagnosis of many asymptomatic children who do not have routine medical care. These programs may be conducted on school children to detect the presence of hematuria, pyuria or proteinuria, which may suggest UTI, and congenital abnormalities of the kidney and urinary tract or glomerular disease, allowing early treatment, adequate follow-up and, when indicated, investigation of other members of the family to detect asymptomatic renal disease.

Screening programs should be accurate, practical and economical. They should be performed by individuals capable of interpreting the results and following up children with positive results, and backed up by an institution to assure continuity. Efforts should be made to obtain the support and cooperation of the Departments of Health and Education as well as the School Board, students, their families and the community as a whole. The procedure should be clearly explained to parents, students and teachers, detailing clearly the exact aim of the screening and the benefits obtained from it. Public education to explain the signs and symptoms of renal disease and the benefits obtained from these screening programs through the use of the news media is also very effective.

Mid-voided urine should be collected in school under supervision, and examined by the simple dipstick method (such as Multistix® 8 SG, Ames Division, Miles Laboratories, Inc., Elkhart, IN 46515). The use of an automated urine chemistry analyzer gives faster and more objective results (we have used Clinitek 200, Ames Division, Miles Laboratories, Inc., Elkhart, IN 46515). From there on, steps are followed according to the algorithm shown in Figure 22.1.

Children with positive findings may be studied according to the specific abnormality, as described elsewhere in this book. A quick screen to exclude the presence of renal disease includes:

1. History and physical examination including blood pressure determination
2. Urinalysis
3. Urine culture, colony count and antibiogram
4. Serum urea nitrogen, creatinine, electrolytes, calcium, phosphorus, and C_3 complement
5. A 24-hour urine (creatinine, protein and calcium). Urine protein/creatinine and calcium/creatinine ratios correlate with the timed collections

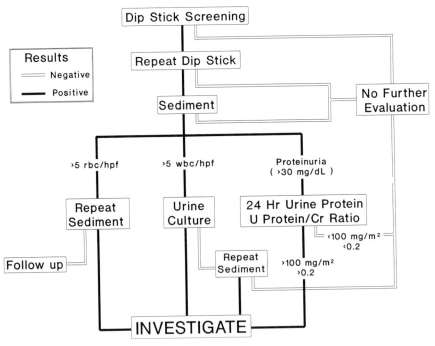

FIGURE 22-1. Algorithm showing the suggested steps in mass urine screening of children.

6. Creatinine clearance
7. Renal ultrasound and voiding cystourethrogram ± intravenous pyelogram (IVP) and renal scan
8. Other studies as necessary

IV. Kidney Disease Prevention Programs

Early diagnosis and treatment of renal disease may be achieved by establishing regional kidney disease prevention programs, which, in collaboration with a pediatric nephrology service, should promote 1) public education, 2) school screening, 3) genetic screening and family counseling and 4) prenatal diagnosis of obstructive uropathy and genetic diseases of the kidney.

V. Intervention

Early diagnosis of kidney and urinary tract disease allows early intervention to prevent renal damage. Although the discussion of treatment does not fall within the scope of this book, early intervention is an integral part in the prevention of ESRD, and will be outlined briefly.

A. Congenital Abnormalities

When a congenital urinary tract abnormality is discovered in a fetus, anomalies of other organs and chromosomal aberrations should be excluded, and the degree of renal function assessed. With unilateral renal malformation, investigation and treatment may be started following term delivery. Fetuses with bilateral hydronephrosis should be followed up weekly or biweekly with sonograms. Those with no evidence of impairment will be investigated at term, and those with decreased renal function will undergo preterm delivery to institute early diagnosis and treatment; if this is not possible, fetal surgery may be attempted (23).

Fetal surgery, which mainly consists of decompression of obstructive lesions of the urinary tract, is controversial. In addition to the ethical dilemma involved and the risk of mortality to the fetus, it is still doubtful whether fetal surgery offers much advantage over early neonatal surgery.

Fetuses with oligohydramnios and bilateral renal agenesis or cystic malformations carry a very poor prognosis for life, and parents may choose to terminate the pregnancy.

Affected newborns should be managed as early as possible. Various factors affect the severity of renal failure in obstructive uropathy, including volume status, diet and the timing of obstruction (24). Relief of obstruction under the age of six months may be associated with improvement in renal function (25). It should be kept in mind that a diseased kidney is more vulnerable to infection, obstruction, hemorrhage, stone formation and, consequently, morbidity and further deterioration in renal function. Early treatment of these complications will help also to prevent additional renal damage.

B. Urinary Tract Infection

Delay in the treatment of UTI is an important determinant of renal scarring and damage (26). Successful treatment of UTI in children consists of suspecting the condition, prompt and accurate diagnosis, adequate therapy, radiological investigation of the urinary tract, correction of any urological abnormality present, and close follow-up with urine cultures. Prolonged suppressive antibiotic therapy also plays a role in preventing recurrence.

C. Hypertension

The optimal treatment of hypertension in children consists of the least amount of intervention required to reduce BP successfully, while maintaining a high degree of compliance, which is a major problem in children (13). Management of hypertension consists of pharmacological and non-pharmacological therapy; the latter consists of weight reduction, dietary modification and physical conditioning. Dietary salt restriction appears to be beneficial in the prevention and treatment of hypertension in infants and children. Children with renal disease require effective antihypertensive therapy to preserve renal function (13). Public education should promote routine BP determination, weight control and low salt intake.

D. Glomerular Disease

It is not well known whether treatment of most glomerular diseases can prevent progression of the disease to renal failure. Evaluation of treatment in these conditions is generally confusing since they are heterogeneous, may represent similar end-organ responses to different pathological processes and may undergo a spontaneous recovery. There is some evidence, however, that treatment of some of these conditions, such as membranoproliferative, anti-GBM and rapidly progressive glomerulonephritis (RPGN) may prevent or delay the development of renal failure (27). Pulse therapy with methylprednisolone and plasma exchange, for example, were found to be effective in RPGN. A low protein diet with or without essential amino acid or ketoacid supplements may have some beneficial effect in slowing the rate of progression of renal failure, although an effect on renal histology has not been confirmed (28). Phosphate and sodium restriction, antihypertensive treatment and the use of oral adsorbants may also help to delay progression of renal failure (28). Patients at risk to develop diabetic nephropathy (diabetics with elevated microalbuminuria and elevated glomerular filtration rate) should be given optimal therapy and aggressively controlled (29).

VI. Responsibility of the Practicing Physician

The practicing physician should keep a high index of suspicion for UTI and congenital and hereditary diseases of the kidney. The following suggestions contribute to the early diagnosis of these conditions:

1. Obtain accurate patient and family history of renal disease, urinary tract malformations and abnormalities of other organ systems that may be associated with renal involvement.
2. Determine blood pressure on every child as a part of the physical examination.
3. Perform a urinalysis on every child once a year, and more frequently if indicated.
4. Perform a urine culture at least once within the first year of life, and when indicated thereafter. It is important to keep in mind that a normal urinalysis in preschool children does not exclude a UTI.
5. Perform a voiding cystourethrogram, and renal ultrasound or IVP on every child, whether boy or girl, with a well-documented UTI.
6. Investigate the renal tract in children with congenital abnormalities of other organ systems and systemic diseases known to be associated with renal abnormalities.
7. When indicated, investigate family members of affected children for evidence of renal disease (Alport's syndrome, polycystic kidney disease, familial hematuria, vesicoureteral reflux, etc.).
8. Recommend prenatal diagnosis on high-risk pregnant women and those with a family history of hereditary renal disease (congenital nephrotic syndrome, obstructive uropathy, Meckel's syndrome, possibly polycystic kidney disease etc.)
9. Coordinate and consult with a pediatric nephrologist.

If there is any indication of renal tract involvement, a more thorough screening should be performed, as outlined in section III, and a pediatric nephrologist consulted.

VII. Conclusion

More effort should be directed toward preventing renal and urinary tract diseases. This may be achieved by early diagnosis and treatment of these diseases by making physicians more aware of the occurrence and presentation of renal disease, mass screening by urinalysis and blood pressure determination, public education and establishing regional kidney disease prevention programs. Although these programs will have a considerable impact on reducing morbidity and mortality from renal disease, certain limitations still exist and further research in the fields of pathogenesis and treatment of various renal diseases is needed before more effective prevention is possible.

References

1. Winberg J (1978) Urinary tract infections in infants and children. In: Edelmann CM, Jr (ed) Pediatric Kidney Disease. Little, Brown and Co, pp 1123–1144
2. Barakat AY, Drougas JG (1989) Occurrence of congenital abnormalities of the kidney and urinary tract in 13,775 autopsies. Urology, in press.
3. Helin I, Persson P-H (1986) Prenatal diagnosis of urinary tract abnormalities by ultrasound. Pediatrics 78: 879–883
4. Fine RN (1982) Renal transplantation in children. In: Chaterjee SN (ed) Organ Transplantation. John Wright, Boston, p 243
5. Habib R, Broyer M, Benmaiz H (1973) Chronic renal failure in children. Causes, rate of deterioration and survival data. Nephron 11: 209–220
6. Temple JK, Shapira E (1981) Genetic determinants of renal disease in neonates. Clin Perinatol 8: 361–373
7. Reeders ST, Breuning MH, Davies KE, et al (1985) A highly polymorphic DNA marker linked to adult polycystic kidney disease on chromosome 16. Nature 317: 542–544
8. Arant BS (1987) Prevention of hereditary nephropathies by antenatal interventions—ethical considerations. Pediatr Nephrol 1: 553–560
9. Van den Abbeele AD, Treves ST, Lebowitz RL, et al (1987) Vesicoureteral reflux in asymptomatic siblings of patients with known reflux: radionuclide cystography. Pediatrics 79: 147–153
10. Barakat AY, Der Kaloustian VM, Mufarrij AA, et al (1986) The Kidney in Genetic Disease. Churchill Livingstone, Edinburgh
11. Barakat AY, Seikaly MG, DerKaloustian VM (1986) Urogenital abnormalities in genetic disease. J Urol 136: 778–785
12. Barakat AY, Butler MG (1987) Renal and urinary tract abnormalities associated with chromosome aberrations. Intern J Pediatr Nephrol 8: 215–226
13. Task Force on Blood Pressure Control in Children (1987) Report of the second Task Force on Blood Pressure Control in Children—1987. Pediatrics 79: 1–25
14. Hutchison JH, Cockburn F (1986) Pyelonephritis. In: Hutchison JH (ed) Practical Pediatric Problems, 6th edition. Lloyd-Luke, London, p 400
15. Gauthier B, Edelmann CM, Jr, Barnett HL (1982) Urinary tract infection. In: Gauthier B, Edelmann CM, Jr, Barnett HL (eds) Nephrology and Urology for the Pediatrician. Little, Brown and Co, Boston, pp 73–85
16. Ostrer H, Hejtmancik JF (1988) Prenatal diagnosis and carrier detection of genetic diseases by analysis of deoxyribonucleic acid. J Pediatr 112: 679–687

17. Flinter FA, Bobrow M, Chantler C (1987) Alport's syndrome or hereditary nephritis? Pediatr Nephrol 1: 438–440
18. Koide K (1976) Epidemiology of chronic glomerulonephritis and nephritic syndrome. Gendai Iryo 8: 503
19. Kitagawa T (1985) Screening for asymptomatic hematuria and proteinuria in school children. Relationship between clinical laboratory findings and glomerular pathology or prognosis. Acta Paediatr Jpn 27: 366–373
20. Sakai T (1987) Epidemiology—Japan. In: Holliday MA, Barratt TM, Vernier RL (eds) Pediatric Nephrology. Williams and Wilkins, Baltimore, pp 358–359
21. Kitagawa T (1988) Lessons learned from the Japanese nephritis screening study. Pediatr Nephrol 2: 256–263
22. Kunin CM (1970) A ten-year study of bacteriuria in school girls: Final report of bacteriologic, urologic and epidemiologic findings. J Infect Dis 122: 382–393
23. Barakat AY, Awazu M, Fleischer AC (1989) Antenatal diagnosis of renal abnormalities: A review of the state of the art. Southern Med J 82: 229–234
24. Awazu M, Barakat AY, Chevalier RL, et al (1989) The cause of uremia in obstructed kidneys. J Pediatr 114: 179–186.
25. McCrory WW, Shubaya M, Leumann E, et al (1971) Studies of renal function in children with chronic hydronephrosis. Pediatr Clin North Am 18:445–465
26. Winberg J (1987) Clinical aspects of urinary tract infection. In: Holliday MA, Barratt TM, Vernier RL (eds) Pediatric Nephrology, 2nd ed. Williams and Wilkins, Baltimore, pp 626–646
27. Haycock GB (1988) The treatment of glomerulonephritis in children. Pediatr Nephrol 2: 247–255
28. Klahr S, Schreiner G, Ichikawa I (1988) The progression of renal disease. N Engl J Med 318: 1657–1666
29. Mogensen CE, Christensen CK, Christiansen JS, et al (1986) On predicting and preventing diabetic nephropathy. In: Friedman EA, L'Esperance FA Jr (eds) Diabetic Renal Retinal Syndrome, vol 3. Grune & Stratton, Orlando, pp 81–109

23
The Use of Computers in Clinical Nephrology

MARSHALL SUMMAR and RAYMOND M. HAKIM

One of the real challenges to today's clinician and researcher is the evolving, and often confusing role of computers in medicine. This confusion has been caused, in part, by the explosion of technology that has made a multitude of both hardware and software available. Changes occur so quickly that systems, particularly software, often become obsolete by the time they are installed. In this chapter, we will present briefly some of the current uses of this technology in clinical medicine and, particularly, in nephrology. This chapter is meant to be an introduction to the subject and is not exhaustive by any means.

The traditional role of computers was designed around the structure of the machine. The early models were large, bulky, difficult to program and prohibitively expensive for small group purchase or use. Early studies involved using large sets of patients and cumbersome, somewhat inflexible data entry formats. This led to a certain static nature in these studies, since modification in midstream was virtually impossible. Data were usually concentrated in regional centers and encoded and processed in large batches. Results were often delayed by months and the individual researchers would often obtain their results when the original question had ceased to be relevant. This system tended to discourage small independent studies that would require the rigorous mathematical handling of a computer.

The development of the mass-produced silicon chip has changed this framework. Now there are small, cost-effective machines that are in some respects much more powerful than their larger predecessors. Microcomputers with megabyte working systems are now commonplace, and the delays and frustrations of time-sharing are gone. However, what has happened as a result of this newer aspect of computer technology is not quite as impressive, and a large untapped potential remains.

Unlike our colleagues in business and engineering for whom spreadsheet analysis and CAD (computer-aided design) drawings have revolutionized the operation of their business, one often finds the physician's computer acting as little more than a glorified typewriter or billing system.

Physicians and medical researchers have little time to learn a completely new technology, especially one with so many available options. What often happens is that software specialists are brought in to custom design a system for a particular use; this works very well until some unforeseen problem arises or some change is desired. This can quickly become cost-prohibitive at the salary rates of most programmers. Fortunately, there are now some alternatives available and affordable with respect to both time and money.

Probably one of the best developments has been in the field of database management (note, this is one field in which science and business uses overlap heavily). The third and upcoming fourth generation of database programs have incorporated performance with flexibility and ease of use. These programs are designed to run on small desktop systems with only a minimun of preparation. Programmers have also developed and included in these systems subprograms that will actually guide the user through the design applications for the database, ensuring the proper syntax and wording of the commands. Data types can now be modified easily even after large amounts of data have been entered. Help keys have been added to guide the user through difficult commands. This has made available an easy, yet powerful tool for following patients with large volumes of data. Patients with metabolic diseases can be followed graphically and trends can be easily plotted. Patients with renal disease benefit from having all their data at hand in a form that can be easily manipulated mathematically and graphically. Comments about the patient's course can be stored beside the patient's laboratory data. In more extensive databases, patient billing, medical records, laboratory values and scheduling can all be managed from one database. Clinic schedules can be generated and quarterly reviews become a matter of searching the database electronically. This allows better control of the physician's time in being able to better spot trends and clusters and anticipate these for clinic scheduling. From a research standpoint, the database allows identification of subgroups of patients without lengthy record reviews. Statistical analysis becomes much easier, since most database programs allow output of files compatible with statistical packages such as BMDP(1), SPSS (2) and others. The role of the computer in patient care is presented in Figure 23-1.

In our genetics laboratory, for example, we have designed a system for handling our DNA samples. Using this system, we can determine where a sample is, how much of it remains and what restriction enzyme and probe combinations have been used on it. This ties in with a pedigree file that places the data in perspective and will directly output preformatted files to linkage analysis programs. The benefits from this are that repeat digests are often avoided, digests can be designed quickly with the amount of reagents precalculated and the system keeps track of how much DNA remains on a patient. We use this system for autosomal dominant

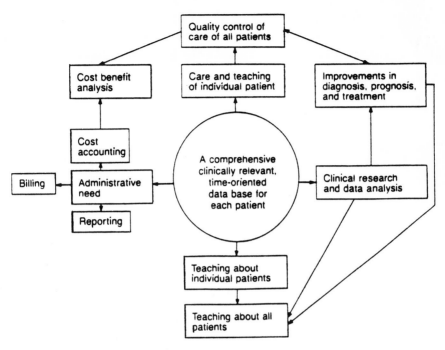

FIGURE 23-1. Diagrammatic representation of the role of the computer in patient care. Reproduced with permission from Pollak VE (1985) The computer in medicine: Its application to medical practice, quality control and cost containment. JAMA 253:62–68. Copyright 1985, American Medical Association.

polycystic kidney disease patients and others. This system is cross referenced to our database, and our cytogenetics laboratory, so that patient data are rapidly available to all users.

For ease of entry, these programs allow on-line formatting of screen forms for prompt entry of information, thus allowing data entry by almost anyone, including nonmedical personnel. The programs will accept a wide range of text values, thus eliminating the need for bulky and cumbersome coding systems while preserving the ability to identify selected groups. Preformatted letters can be used for appointment reminders and letters about laboratory results. By using a local system network, the physician, technician, office manager and researcher can all access the same data from their individual machines. Built into these systems are numerous safeguards for patient confidentiality. Passwords and scrambling of data make it possible to limit access to authorized individuals only. Access can be layered as well, with only certain personnel able to access data of a certain type.

The benefits for the patient are also quite numerous. Obviously, quick ready access to a patient's records will make treatment more effective and rapid. Patients with complicated treatment programs can benefit from the use of preset treatment regimens, which are automatically modified by selected parameters. This is especially useful for patients with chronic diseases. One example is the ARTEMIS system used in France, in which over 20,000 hypertensive patients are currently followed (3). In this system, information is entered interactively by nurses, physicians and secretaries. Used for personalized recall letters and summary reports, this system has replaced the written record. An expert system that checks patient records for trends, abnormal values, missed appointments and medication doses has been added to this system. It also makes recommendations for further studies, dose changes or follow-up based on predefined parameters. This system also gives physicians the differential diagnosis of hypertension. For patients with complicated medical courses and multiple medication schedules, the computer can be used to print up day-by-day dosing schedules, which are especially useful when tapering medications. Use of monitoring programs can remind the physician when to update medications for changing biophysical parameters, and as new regimens become available, the database can be used to identify those patients who need to be changed and arrange contact. Emergency treatment programs can be printed out, based on weight, surface area or any other parameters and these can be given to patients, especially those living out of town or who are traveling, which can greatly aid other physicians seeing a patient for the first time.

Using the newer programs, the physician now has active control over the structure and form of the data collected, but, more importantly, significant trends can be developed and spotted much earlier. Programs, such as BMDP, with multiple linear regression, cluster analysis, survival tables and a host of probability tests can now all be run on the average microcomputer. An example of this would be the chronic renal failure database developed at Cincinnati (4), which is used to monitor the dialysis of each patient as well as his or her long-term course. This system benefits the patient by providing more accurate control of the dialysis process and provides physicians with organized information so that future modifications in the treatment program can be made. The use of microcomputers would allow widespread use of such a system in smaller centers without the benefits of a large central computer system. This can greatly improve the quality of dialysis care, and the benefit of having a central collection system would allow more of data to be analyzed. A spin-off of this could be the development of on-line consultation for problem patients. The flexibility of today's commercial databases would allow one to collect both the study data as well as information that might only be pertinent locally.

Morgan and Will (5) describe the use of sequential data display (creatinine, reciprocal creatinine, log creatinine) in following patients with renal failure (Figure 23-2). The point is made that certain trends could

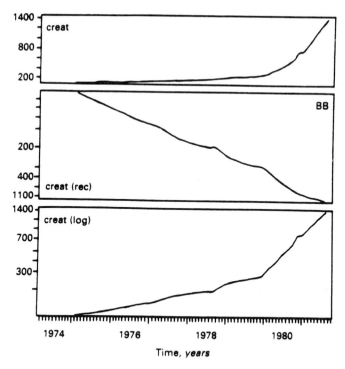

FIGURE 23-2. The changes of serum creatinine with time in a patient with polycystic renal disease and progressive renal impairment. When plotted as a reciprocal (middle panel), a rectilinear decline in glomerular filtration rate is
apparent, but logarithmically (lower panel), the plot is curvilinear. The change
in slope occurring in December 1980 might indicate an intercurrent cause of
accelerated decline in renal function. In fact, no change in management was made
at this time, and the clinical status of the patient was stable. From Morgan DB,
Will EJ (1983) Selection, presentation and interpretation of biochemical data in
renal failure. Reprinted from Kidney Int 24:438–445 with permission

only be spotted using graphic display and sequential collection. The use
of database structures for this could shorten the lag in detecting these.
There are currently available a wide range of commercial data display
programs that can quickly and attractively arrange and graph data. This
becomes useful clinically both for evaluation of the treatment course and
for use as a teaching tool for the patient. It is well documented that patient
compliance increases when some visible result is perceived. In the treatment of renal patients, these trends are very often difficult for the patient
to spot until they are visualized graphically, and with the often long
clinical course involved, the use of graphics can help the patient understand his or her disease and the effects of treatment better.

Looking ahead to the future (and in some places, the present) the computer holds great potential as an on-line consultation service. The use of flowcharts in diagnosis is ideally suited to electronic manipulation and, although computers will never replace clinical experience or knowledge, the availability of applicable differential diagnoses with suggested confirmatory testing may be a welcome addition to the physician's armamentarium. In rural areas where consultants are hard to come by, this may be especially welcome, bringing up-to- date information on the diagnosis and treatment process.

The picture painted above seems quite rosy and sensible; however, there are a few problems. With the widespread use of individual databases, standardization for analysis of large groups will become more and more difficult. There is a degree of compatibility in architecture between the various systems but this requires some time and effort. This will eventually become the responsibility of the subspecialists who will impose their own standardization while maintaining a level of creativity. Patient confidentiality also becomes an issue, but with the passwords and safety features included in database programs, this need not be a problem. Finally, what of the busy clinician who has never had the time to learn the use of computers or the rudiments of programming. It is hoped that the benefits of computer use will become attractive, and that the desire to remain competitve in today's increasingly more competitive market will remain strong. If this is not enough, the developers of software continue to make the programs more and more "user friendly," so that eventually one may not need to know any more than where the power switch is.

References

1. University of California: BMDP Statistical Software. 1964 Westwood Blvd, Suite 202. Los Angeles, CA 90025
2. SPSS, Inc: Statistical Package for the Social Sciences. Suite 3300, 444 North Michigan Avenue. Chicago, IL 60611
3. Devries C, Deqoulet P, Jeunemaitre X, et al (1987) Integrating management and expertise in a computerized system for hypertensive patients. Nephrol Dial Transplant 2:327–331
4. Pollak VE, Peterson DW, Flynn J (1986) The computer in quality control of hemodialysis patient care. Q Rev Biophys 12:202–210
5. Morgan DB, Will EJ (1983) Selection, presentation, and interpretation of biochemical data in renal failure. Kidney Int 24:438–445

Appendix I: Reference Intervals

AMIN Y. BARAKAT

The following reference intervals are guidelines usually needed in the diagnosis and management of renal disease. Values may vary according to the methodology used. Laboratory values are given in conventional and international units. A few references have been used in the formulation of this table (1–5); values from other sources have been referenced separately. The prefixes for units are the standard ones approved by the Conférence Générale des Poids et Mesures, 1964, the International Union of Pure and Applied Chemistry and the International Federation of Clinical Chemistry. Few other abbreviations are used:

B, blood; Ca, calcium; d, day; EDTA, ethylenediaminetetraacetate, edetic acid; f, female; hr, hour; m, male; min, minute; mo, month; RBC, red blood cell; P, plasma; S, serum; U, urine; wk, week; yr, year.

Test	Specimen		Conventional units	International units
			g/dl	g/L
Albumin	S	Premature	3.0–4.2	30–42
		NB	3.6–5.4	36–54
		Infant	4.0–5.0	40–50
		Thereafter	3.5–5.0	35–50
	U	*Look under* urine protein		
			ng/dl	nmol/L
Aldosterone	P (heparin, EDTA)	Newborn:	5–60	0.14–1.7
	S	1 wk–1 yr:	1–160	0.03–4.4
		1–3 yr:	5–60	0.14–1.7
		3–5 yr:	<5–80	<0.14–2.2
		5–7 yr:	<5–50	<0.14–1.4
		7–11 yr:	5–70	0.14–1.9
		11–15 yr:	<5–50	<0.14–1.4

Test	Specimen		Conventional units	International units
			ng/dl	nmol/L
		Adult:		
		Average sodium diet		
		Supine:	3–10	0.08–0.3
		Upright F:	5–30	0.14–0.8
		M:	6–22	0.17–0.61
		2–3 × higher during pregnancy		
		Adrenal vein: 200–800 ng/dl		5.5–22
		Low sodium diet: increases 2–5 fold		
		Florinef suppression: <4 ng/dl		<0.11
		ACTH or angiotensin stimulation,		
		1 hr: 2–5 fold		

			ng/dl	
or (6,7)	P	Premature	110–250	
		Full-term	110–200	
		3–12 mo	49–71	
		Adult	13.38–14.84	

U, 24 hr	Total U Na mmol/d	Plasma renin activity ng angiotensin I/ml/hr	U Aldosterone mg/d	U Aldosterone nmol/d
	< 20	5–24	35–80	<97–220
	50	2–7	13–33	36–91
	100	1–5	5–24	14–66
	150	0.5–4	3–19	8–53
	200		1–16	3–44
	250		1–13	3–36

(assuming normal serum Na, K and extracellular volume)

			μg/d	
or (7)		Premature	2.5– 4.1	
		Newborn	6.4– 9.2	
		Adult	9.8–12.0	

Test	Specimen			U/L	
Alkaline phosphatase	S	Infant:		150–400	Same
		Child,	2–10 yr	100–300	
			11–18 yr,	50–375	
			M:	30–300	
			F:	30–100	
		Adult:			
Angiotensin I	P (EDTA)	Peripheral vein		11–88 pg/ml	11–88 ng/L
Angiotensin II	P (EDTA)	Arterial:		1.2–3.6 ng/dl	12–36 ng/L
		Venous:		50–75% of arterial conc.	Fraction of arterial conc. 0.50–0.75
Anion gap [Na−(Cl+CO₂)]	P (heparin)			7–16 mmol/L	Same

Test	Specimen		Conventional units	International units
Antidiuretic hormone (ADH, vasopressin)	P (EDTA)	Plasma mOsm/kg	Plasma ADH pg/ml	Plasma ADH, ng/L
		270–280:	<1.5	Same
		280–285:	<2.5	
		285–290:	1–5	
		290–295:	2–7	
		395–300:	4–12	
Anti-nDNA antibody		<1:20		
Anti-nuclear antibody titer (ANA)		<1:20		
Anti-streptolysin (ASO) titer	S	≤ 166 Todd units (170–330 in school-aged children)		
			mmol/L	
Base excess	B (heparin)	Newborn:	−10 to −2	Same
		Infant:	−7 to −1	
		Child:	−4 to +2	
		Thereafter:	−2 to +3	
			mEq/L	mmol/L
Bicarbonate (HCO₃⁻)	S	Premature	18–26	Same
		Infant	20–26	
		1–2 yr	20–25	
		>2 yr	22–26	
Blood volume	B (heparin)	M: 52–83 ml/kg		M: 0.052–0.083 L/kg
		F: 50–75 ml/kg		F: 0.050–0.075 L/kg
			pg/mL	ng/L
Calcitonin	S, P (heparin, EDTA)	Newborn term:		
		cord	30–240	Same
		48 h:	91–580	
		7 d:	77–293	
		Premature, cord:	30–265	
		48 hr:	108–670	
		7 d:	79–570	
		Adult, M:	<100	
		F:	4× lower (increases in pregnancy)	
		Concentrations decrease with age		
			mg/dl	mmol/L
Calcium, ionized	S, P, B			
		Newborn		
		3–24 hr:	4.3–5.1	1.07–1.27
		24–48 hr:	4.0–4.7	1.00–1.17
		Thereafter:	4.48–4.92 or	1.12–1.23
			2.24–2.46 mEq/L	1.12–1.23
			mg/dl	mmol/L
Calcium, total	S	Cord:	9.0–11.5	2.25–2.88

Test	Specimen		Conventional units	International units
			mg/dl	mmol/L
		Newborn		
		Premature:	6.1–11.6	1.52–2.90
		3–24 hr:	9.0–10.6	2.3 –2.65
		24–48 hr:	7.0–12.0	1.75–3.0
		4–7 d:	9.0–10.9	2.25–2.73
		Child:	8.8–10.8	2.2 –2.70
		Thereafter:	8.4–10.2	2.1 –2.55
	U	*Look under* urine calcium		
			mm Hg	kP$_a$
Carbon dioxide, partial pressure (pCO₂)	B (heparin)	Newborn:	27–40	3.6–5.3
		Infant:	27–41	3.6–5.5
		Thereafter M:	35–48	4.7–6.4
		F:	32–45	4.3–6.0
			mmol/L	
Carbon dioxide, total (tCO₂)	S, P (heparin)	Cord:	14–22	Same
		Premature:	14–27	
		Newborn:	13–22	
		Infant:	20–28	
		Child:	20–28	
		Thereafter:	23–30	
			pg/ml	pmol/L
Catecholamines, fractionated	P (EDTA)	Norepinephrine		
		Supine	100–400	591–2364
		Standing	300–900	1773–5320
		Epinephrine		
		Supine	< 70	<382
		Standing	<100	<546
		Dopamine (no postural change)	< 30	<196
	U, 24 hr	Norepinephrine	μg/d	mmol/d
		0–1 yr:	0–10	0–59
		1–2 yr:	0–17	0–100
		2–4 yr:	4–29	24–171
		4–7 yr:	8–45	47–266
		7–10 yr:	13–65	77–384
		Thereafter:	15–80	87–473
		Epinephrine		
		0–1 yr:	0–2.5	0–13.6
		1–2 yr:	0–3.5	0–19.1
		2–4 yr:	0–6.0	0–32.7
		4–7 yr:	0.2–10	1.1–55
		7–10 yr:	0.5–14	2.7–76
		Dopamine		
		0–1 yr:	0–85	0–555
		1–2 yr:	10–140	65–914
		2–4 yr:	40–260	261–1697
		Thereafter:	65–400	424–2611

Test	Specimen		Conventional units	International units
			μg/d	
Catecholamines, total free	U, 24 hr	0–1 yr:	10–15	Same
		1–5 yr:	15–40	
		6–15 yr:	20–80	
		Thereafter:	30–100	
			mg/dl	μmol/L
Ceruloplasmin	S	Newborn:	1–30	0.06–1.99
		6–12 mo:	15–50	0.99–3.31
		1–12 yr:	30–65	1.99–4.30
		Thereafter:	14–40	0.93–2.65
			mmol/L	
Chloride	S, P (heparin)	Cord:	96–104	Same
		Premature:	100–117	
		Newborn:	97–110	
		Thereafter:	98–106	
	U	*Look under* urine chloride		
			mmol/L	
	Sweat	Normal	0–35	Same
		Marginal	30–60	
		Cystic fibrosis	60–200	
		Increases by 10 mmol/L during lifetime		
			mg/dl	mmol/L
Cholesterol, total	S, P (EDTA or heparin)	Cord:	45–100	1.17–2.59
		Newborn:	53–135	1.37–3.50
		Infant:	70–175	1.81–4.53
		Child:	120–200	3.11–5.18
		Adolescent:	120–210	3.11–5.44
		Adult:	140–250	3.63–6.48
Complement, total hemolytic	P (EDTA)		75–160 U/ml or <33% of plasma CH_{50}	Same
classic pathway components			mg/dl	mg/L
Clq	S	Cord:	1.0–14.9	10–149
		1 mo:	2.2– 6.2	22– 62
		6 mo:	1.2– 7.6	12– 76
		Adult:	5.1– 7.9	51– 79
C3			mg/dl	mg/L
RID	S	Cord:	65–112	0.65–1.12
		1 mo:	61–130	0.61–1.30
		Adult:	111–171	1.11–1.71
		Maternal:	161–175	1.61–1.75
		At birth, conc. is 50–75% of adult values		
Nephelom- etry	S	Newborn:	58–120	0.58–1.20
C4				
RID	S	Newborn:	16–39	160–390 mg/L
		Adult:	15–45	150–450

Test	Specimen		Conventional units	International units
			mg/dl	mg/L
Nephelom- etry	S	Newborn: Adult:	10–26 13–37	100–260 130–370
			mg/dl	mg/L
Properdin	S	Cord: 1 mo: 6 mo: Adult:	1.3–1.7 0.6–2.2 1.3–2.5 2.0–3.6	13–17 6–22 13–25 20–36
			μg/dl	μmol/L
Copper	S	Birth–6 mo: 6 yr: 12 yr: Adult, M: F:	20–70 90–190 80–160 70–140 80–155	3.14–10.99 14.13–29.83 12.56–25.12 10.99–21.98 12.56–24.34
	U, 24 hr		0–30 μg/d	0–0.47 μmol/d
			μg/dl	nmol/L
Cortisol	S, P (heparin)	Newborn: Adults: 08:00 hr 16:00 hr 20:00 hr	1–24 5–23 3–15 ≤50% of 08:00 h	28–662 138–635 82–413 Fraction of 08:00 hr ≤0.50
			μg/d	nmol/d
Cortisol, free	U, 24 hr	Child: Adolescent: Adult:	2–27 5–55 10–100	5.5–74 14–152 27–276
			mg/dl	μmol/L
Creatinine *Jaffe, kinetic or* *enzymatic*	S, P	Cord: Newborn: Infant: Child: Adolescent: Adult M: F:	0.6–1.2 0.3–1.0 0.2–0.4 0.3–0.7 0.5–1.0 0.6–1.2 0.5–1.1	53–106 27–88 18–35 27–62 44–88 53–106 44–97
Jaffe, manual	S, P		0.8–1.5 mg/dl	70–133
	U, 24 hr		mg/kg/d	μmol/kg/d
		Premature: Full-term: Infant: Child: Adolescent: Adult, M: F:	8–20 10–16 8–20 8–22 8–30 14–26 11–20	71–180 90–144 71–180 71–195 71–265 124–230 97–177
			mg/d	mmol/d
		or M: F:	800–1800 600–1600	7 –15.9 5.2–14.1

Test	Specimen		Conventional units	International units
Cyclic AMP	P (EDTA)		ng/ml	nmol/L
		M:	5.6–10.9	17–33
		F:	3.6–8.9	11–27
	U, 24 hr		<3.3 mg/d or <1.64 mg/g creatinine	1000–11,500 nmol/d, <6000 nmol cAMP/g creatinine
Erythropoietin	S		mU/ml	U/L
RIA			<5–20	Same
Hemagglutination			25–125	
Bioassay			5–18	
α-Fetoprotein (8)	S		Fetal peak of 200–400 mg/dl in first trimester	
			ng/ml	
		Premature	134,734 ±41,444	
		Newborn	48,406 ±34,718	
		2–4 wk	2,654 ± 3,080	
		2 mo	323 ± 278	
		3 mo	88 ± 87	
		4 mo	74 ± 56	
		5 mo	46.5± 19	
		6 mo	12.5± 9.8	
		7 mo	9.7± 7.1	
		8 mo	8.5± 5.5	
		1 yr	<30	
		Adult	<40	
		weeks:	mg/dl	mg/L
	Amniotic fluid	10–12	0.5–3.3	5–33
		13–14	0.3–3.7	3–37
		15–16	0.4–2.7	4–27
		17–18	0.1–2.6	1–26
		19–20	<0.1–1.14	<1–14
		21–22	<0.1–1.1	<1–11
		23–24	<0.1–0.7	<1–7
Fibrin degradation products	B (thrombin and proteolytic inhibitor in tube)		<10 μg/mL	<10 mg/L
Agglutination (Thrombo-Wellco test®)	U: 2 ml in similar tube		<0.25 μg/ml	<0.25 mg/L
Fibrinogen	B (sodium citrate)	Newborn:	125–300 mg/dl	1.25–3.00 g/L
		Adult:	200–400	2.00–4.00
Folate	S	Newborn:	7.0–32 ng/ml	15.9–72.4 nmol/L
		Thereafter:	1.8–9	4.1–20.4
	RBC (EDTA)	150–140 ng/ml cells		340–1020 nmol/L cells

Functions, renal (9)

	GFR[a] ml/min/1.73m²	PAH Clearance[b] ml/min/1.73m²	Tm PAH[c] mg/min/1.73m²	Concentrating capacity m Osm/kg water		
				Basal	Dehydration	Pitressin
Preterm				190–300	370–680	
27 wk	2–10					
32	4–12					
34	5–15					
36	6–40					
37	12–26					
Term NB	8–42	33–162	6–26	180–400	210–650	
4– 7 d	20–53	38–162				
8–12 d	40–60	120–188				
15–30 d	30–90	103–260	3.7–22	776	780–1100	
2 mo	42–90	203–321	13.3–93		870–1200	400–960
3	46–125	154–345	41–58			450–1030
4	56–120	204–327			950–1260	500–1060
6	89–144	392–601	57–68			550–1120
8	58–160	262–781	46			600–1160
12	63–150	332–557	21–88		1000–1310	640–1220
18	105–235	503–724	52		1020–1330	700–1280
2 yr	105–172	503–724	77–84		1040–1390	
3	101–179	624–754				820–1340
4	100–184	632–723	84		1060–1410	
5	120–184					
6	79–170	497–872	65			
7	110–156		31–100			
8	90–148	680–711	75		1100–1420	820–1340
9	88–166	490–744	88			
10	95–162	566–704	95			
11	110–146	562–784	82			
12	110–136	551–747	95		1110–1430	820–1340
13–19	110–136	482–662			1130–1460	
Adult						
M	110–152	561–833	80 ± 12	800–1400	1200–1500	
F	101–133	92–696	77 ± 11	800–1400	1200–1500	

[a] GFR (glomerular filtration rate): >age 40 yr, decreases ~6.5 ml/min/1.73 m²/decade
[b] PAH clearance (paraaminohippurate; renal plasma flow), >age 40 yr, decreases ~75 ml/min/1.73 m²/decade
[c] Tm PAH (maximum tubular excretory capacity)
[a,b] In malnourished children, 45% of normal (10)

Test	Specimen		Conventional units	International units
			mg/dl	mmol/L
Glucose	S, Fasting	Cord:	45–96	2.5–5.33
		Premature:	20–60	1.1–3.3
		Neonate:	30–60	1.7–3.3
		1 d:	40–60	2.2–3.3
		>1 d:	50–80	2.8–5.0
		Child:	60–100	3.3–5.5
		Adult:	70–105	3.9–5.8
	U	*Look under* urine glucose		

Test	Specimen		Conventional units	International units
Glucose, 2 hr postprandial	S		<120 mg/dl	<6.7 mmol/L
		6–12 yr:	35–45%	
		Adult M:	41–53%	
		F:	36–46%	
			g/dl	mmol/L
Hemoglobin (Hb)	B (EDTA)	Cord:	14.5–22.5	2.25–3.49
		1–3 d (capillary):	14.5–22.5	2.25–3.49
		2 mo:	9.0–14.0	1.40–2.17
		6–12 yr:	11.5–15.5	1.78–2.09
		12–18 yr M:	13.0–16.0	2.02–2.48
		F:	12.0–16.0	1.86–2.48
		18–49 yr M:	13.5–17.5	2.09–2.71
		F:	12.0–16.0	1.86–2.48
			mg/dl	mg/L
Immunoglobulins A (IgA)	S	Cord:	0–5	0–50
		Newborn:	0–2.2	0–22
		1/2–6 mo:	3–82	30–820
		6 mo–2 yr:	14–108	140–1080
		2–6 yr:	23–190	230–1900
		6–12 yr:	29–270	290–2700
		12–16 yr:	81–232	810–2320
		Thereafter:	60–380	600–3800
D (IgD)		Newborn:	None detected	None detected
		Thereafter:	0–8 mg/dl	0–0.44 μmol/L
E (IgE)		M:	0–230 IU/ml	0–230 kIU/L
		F:	0–170	0–170
			mg/dl	g/L
G (IgG)		Cord:	760–1700	7.6–17
		Newborn:	700–1480	7–14.8
		1/2–6 mo:	300–1000	3–10
		6 mo–2 yr:	500–1200	5–12
		2–6 yr:	500–1300	5–13
		6–12 yr:	700–1650	7–16.5
		12–16 yr:	700–1550	7–15.5
		Adults: (higher in blacks)	600–1600	6–16
Ketone bodies	S		0.5–3 mg/dl	5–30 mg/L
			mg/dl	mmol/L
Lactate	B (heparin)	Capillary, newborn:	≤ 30	≤ 3.0
		child:	5–20	0.56–2.25
		Venous	5–18	0.5 –2
		Arterial	3–7	0.3 –0.8
Lactate/pyruvate	B (heparin)		10	
Lysozyme (11)	P	Neonate:	0.9–2.3 mg/dl	
		Adult:	1.1–1.7	

Test	Specimen		Conventional units	International units
			mEq/L	mmol/L
Magnesium	S	Newborn:	1.5–2.3	0.75–1.15
		Adult:	1.4–2.0	0.7 –1
Nitrogen (NPN)	S		<35 mg/dl	<25.0 mmol/L
			mOsm/kg H$_2$O	
Osmolality	S, Child, Adult:		275–295	
	U		*Look under* urine osmolality	
Osmolality ratio	U/S		1.0–3.0	
			> 3.0 after 12-hr fluid restriction	
			mm Hg	kP$_a$
Oxygen, partial pressure (pO$_2$)	B, arterial (heparin)	Birth:	8–24	1.1–3.2
		5–10 min:	33–75	4.4–10.0
		30 min:	31–85	4.1–11.3
		>1 hr:	55–80	7.3–10.6
		1 d:	54–95	7.2–12.6
		Thereafter:	83–108	11–14.4
		(decreases with age)		
Oxygen saturation	B, arterial (heparin)			Fraction saturated:
		Newborn:	40–90%	0.40–0.90
		Thereafter:	95–99%	0.95–0.99
Parathyroid hormone (PTH)	S	Varies with laboratory:		
		Mayo Clinic Bioscience:		
		N-terminal	230–630 pg/ml	230–630 ng/L
		C-terminal	410–1760 pg/ml	410–1760 ng/L
		Nichols Institute:		
		C-terminal	40–100 μlEq/ml	40–100 mEq/L
Peritoneal surface area (12)		Infant:	383 cm^2/kg	
		Adult:	177 cm^2/kg	
				H$^+$ concentration
pH	B (arterial heparin)	Premature (48 hr)	7.35–7.50	31–44 nmol/L
		Newborn: full-term	7.11–7.36	43–77
		5–10 min:	7.09–7.30	50–81
		30 min:	7.32–7.38	41–61
		>1 hr:	7.26–7.49	32–54
		1 d:	7.29–7.45	35–51
		Thereafter:	7.35–7.45	35–44
		Must be corrected to body temperature		
	U	*Look under* urine pH		
			mg/dl	mmol/L
Phosphorus, inorganic	S	Cord:	3.7–8.1	1.2–2.6
		Premature (1 wk):	5.4–10.9	1.7–3.5
		Newborn:	4.3–9.3	1.4–3.0
		Child:	4.5–6.5	1.45–2.1
		Thereafter:	3.0–4.5	0.97–1.45
			On nonrestricted diet:	
			0.4–1.3 g/d	12.9–42.10 mmol/d
Plasma volume	P (heparin)	M:	25–43 ml/kg	0.025–0.043 L/kg
		F:	28–45	0.028–0.045

Test	Specimen		Conventional units	International units
			mmol/L	
Potassium	S	Premature:	4.6–6.7	Same
		Full-term newborn:	3.9–5.9	
		Infant:	4.1–5.3	
		Child:	3.4–4.7	
		Thereafter:	3.5–5.1	
	P (heparin)		3.5–4.5	
	U	*Look under* urine potassium		
			ng/hr/1.73 m^2	
Prostaglandin E2		Premature:	16.4–21.4	
(13,14)		Newborn:	20.6–41.2	
		3–12 mo:	31.1–43.9	
		Adult:	227–295	
Protein selectivity index (Cl ratio of IgG/albumin) (15,16)			<10%: highly selective	
			>20%: poorly selective	
			g/dl	g/L
Protein, serum	S	Premature:	4.3–7.6	43–76
total		Newborn:	4.6–7.4	46–74
		Child:	6.2–8.0	62–80
		Adult:		
		Recumbent:	6.0–7.8	60–78
		Ambulatory:	∼0.5 g higher	∼5 g higher
			g/dl	g/L
Electrophoresis		Albumin		
		Premature:	3.0–4.2	30–42
		Newborn:	3.6–5.4	36–54
		Infant:	4.0–5.0	40–50
		Thereafter:	3.5–5.0	35–50
		α_1-Globulin		
		Premature:	0.1–0.5	1–5
		Newborn:	0.1–0.3	1–3
		Infant:	0.2–0.4	2–4
		Thereafter:	0.2–0.3	2–3
		α_2-Globulin		
		Premature:	0.3–0.7	3–7
		Newborn:	0.3–0.5	3–5
		Infant:	0.5–0.8	5–8
		Thereafter:	0.4–1.0	4–10
		β-Globulin		
		Premature:	0.3–1.2	3–12
		Newborn:	0.2–0.6	2–6
		Thereafter:	0.5–1.1	5–11
		γ-Globulin		
		Premature:	0.3–1.4	3–14
		Newborn:	0.2–1.0	2–10
		Infant:	0.3–1.2	3–12
		Thereafter:	0.7–1.2	7–12
		(higher in blacks		
Protein, urine	U, 24 hr	*Look under* urine protein		
Total				

Test	Specimen		Conventional units	International units
		Average % of total protein		Fraction of total
Electrophoresis		Albumin	37.9	0.379
		Globulin α_1	27.3	0.273
		α_2	19.5	0.195
		β	8.8	0.088
		γ	3.3	0.033
			ng/ml/hr	µg/L/hr
Renin activity;	P (EDTA)	Premature (17)	18.2 ± 5.1	Same
(PRA)		0–3 yr:	<16.6	
		3–6 yr:	< 6.7	
		6–9 yr:	< 4.4	
		9–12 yr:	< 5.9	
		12–15 yr:	< 4.2	
		15–18 yr:	< 4.3	
		Normal sodium diet		
		Supine:	0.2–2.5	
		Upright:	0.3–4.3	
		Low sodium diet		
		Upright:	2.9–24	
			ng/ml/hr	
or (6,7,18)		Premature, 1–3 d:	61.3–67.30	
		Full-term, 1–3 d:	9.95–13.45	
		3–12 mo:	5.02–7.48	
		Adult, supine:	0.15–1.65	
		upright:	0.66–8.10	

Size, kidney (9)

Age	Kidney weight (g)	Kidney length (cm)
Preterm		
27 wk	10.5	
28	11	
32	16	
34	19	
36	22	
Term newborn	24	4.8
15–30 d	26	5
2 mo	29	
4		5.3
6	40	
8	60	5.9
12	72	6
2 yr	85	7
4	100	8

Age	Kidney weight (g)	Kidney length (cm)
5	106	8.5
6	112	8.9
7	120	9.3
8	128	9.7
9	138	10.1
10	150	10.44
11	164	10.81
12	178	11.19
13–19	196–282	11.19
Adult, M:	290	13.4
F:	248	13.4

Test	Specimen		Conventional units	International units
			mmol/L	
Sodium	S, P (heparin)	Newborn,		
		premature, full-term:	134–146	Same
		Infant:	139–146	
		Child:	138–145	
		Thereafter:	136–146	
	U	Look under urine sodium		
	Sweat	Normal	10–40	
		Cystic fibrosis	>70	
			mg/dl	mmol urea/L
Urea nitrogen	S, P	Cord:	21–40	7.5–14.3
		Premature (1 wk):	3–25	1.1–9
		Newborn:	3–12	1.1–4.3
		Infant/child:	5–18	1.8–6.4
		Thereafter:	7–18	2.5–6.4
Urea nitrogen/ creatinine	S		10–15	
			mg/dl	μmol/L
Uric acid Phosphotungstate	S	Newborn:	2.0–6.2	119–369
		Adult M:	4.5–8.2	268–488
		F:	3.0–6.5	178–387
Uricase		Child:	2.0–5.5	119–327
		Adult M:	3.5–7.2	208–428
		F:	2.6–6.0	155–357

Urine
Acidifying capacity (9)

Age	pH Control	pH After NH$_4$Cl or CaCl$_2$	H$^+$ Excretion (μEq/min/1.73 m^2) Control	H$^+$ Excretion After NH$_4$Cl or CaCl$_2$
Term newborn	4.9–6.8			
4–7 d	5.7–7.4			
2 mos	4.9–6.3	5.02–5.4	54–168	67–230
3	5.4–6.6	4.6–6.4	30–113	
4	5.2–7.3	4.7–6.4	8–68	83–172
5	5.0–5.4	5.0–5.1	86–125	165–197
6	6.5–7.2	4.9–5.0		
8	5.5–6.8	4.6–5.0	43–73	109–113
2–5 yr	5.3–6.7	4.7–5.6	9–48	62.1–164
6–11	5.67–6.83	4.7–5.04	23–58	108.7–150.8
12–16	5.23–5.90	4.80–5.0	59–111	89–148
Adult (M and F)	5.4–7.02	4.5–7.0	10–50	60–130

Acidity, titratable
  Premature: 0–12 μM/min/m^2
  Full term: 0–11
  Child: 20–50 mEq/d

Addis count (12-hr specimen)
  Red cells: < 1 million
  White cells: < 2 million
  Casts: 10,000
  Protein: <55 mg

Ammonia
  2–12 mo: 4–20 μEq/min/m^2
  1–16 yr: 6–16 μEq/min/m^2

Amount
  Preterm: 1–3 ml/kg/d
  Term newborn (1–2 d):   15–60 mL
  Neonate,   4–12 d: 100–300
                 15–60 d: 250–450
  Infant,   6–12 mo: 400–600
  Child,   2–4 yr: 500–750
                 6–7 yr: 650–1000
                 8–19 yr: 700–1500
  Adult: 1000–1600

Varies with intake and other factors: Extreme dehydration, 0.2–0.3 ml/min; extreme hydration, 16 ml/min

Bladder capacity (19)
  32 × age in yr + 73 (ml)
  2 + age yr (oz)

Calcium
                  Usually < 4 mg/kg/d, or
  1st wk: < 2 mg/d
  Child: 10–25 md/d
  Adult: 50–400 mg/d
  Fractional excretion: < 2%

Calcium/creatinine (20,21)
Preterm newborn	0.3–2.3
Term newborn	0.05–1.2
Infant and child	< 0.21

Chloride
Infants:	1.7–8.5 mmol/24 hr
Children:	17–34
Adults:	140–240
	Varies with chloride intake

Citrate (22)	439 ± 49 mg/g creatinine
Copper	*Look under* copper
Cortisol	*Look under* cortisol
Creatinine	*Look under* creatinine
Cyclic AMP	*Look under* cyclic AMP
Cystine (23)	<75 mg/g creatinine

Frequency
3–6 mo	20 times/d
6–12	16
1–2 yr	12
2–4	9
12	4–6

Glucose
Qualitative	Negative
	Dipstick detects 75–125 mg/dl
Quantitative	
Newborn, full term	12–32 mg/dl
preterm	60–130 mg/dl
Adult	<15 mg/dl or 30–300 mg/1.73 m^2/d

Glucose, maximal tubular
reabsorption of (TmG) (24)
	$mg/min/1.73\ m^2$
Infant	142–284
Child	266–458
Adult	289–361

Glucose, renal threshold (24)
	mg/ml
Premature	2.21–2.84
Infant	2.20–3.68
Child	2.36–3.30
Adult	1.98–2.78

Hemoglobin	Negative
Hypoxanthine (23)	5.9–13.2 mg/d
Ketone bodies	2 mg/dl
	20 mg/d

Lysozyme/creatinine (tubular
proteinuria) (11)
	$\mu g/mg$
Neonate	1.2–19
1 yr	0.1–23
2–12 yr	0.1–5
Adult	0.1–14

Magnesium (25)	180 ± 10 mg/1.73 m^2/d

| *Magnesium/calcium* (26) | 1.56 |

Osmolality — mOsm/L

Infant	50–600
Child	50–1400
12-hr restriction	> 850
24-hr urine	~300–900
Malnourished children (10)	201–275

| *Oxalate* (23) | <50 mg/1.73 m^2/d |

pH

Newborn/neonate:	5–7	0.1–10 mmol/L
Thereafter:	4.5–8	0.01–32
Average	~ 6	~ 1.0
F	7.0–7.5	31–100

| *Phosphorus* | *Look under* phosophorus |
| *Phosphorus, tubular reabsorption* | 78–97% |

Porphyrins

Qualitative	Negative
Coproporphyrins	< 160 µg/d
Uroporphyrins	< 30 µg/d

Potassium (7)
26–123 mmol/L
0.4–5.2 mEq/kg/d
varies with diet

Fractional excretion (7)	< 30% (Normal renal function and regular diet)
Newborn	18.5–32.9
1–12 mo	7.5–25.7
2–20 yr	7.0–23.8

Protein

qualitative	< 20 mg/dl
quantitative	<100 mg/m^2/d
Proteins, Bence-Jones	Negative

| *Protein/creatinine ratio* (27) | <0.2 (>3.5 in nephrotic syndrome) |

Sediment
Casts

Hyaline:	occasional (0–1) casts/hpf
RBC:	not seen
WBC:	not seen
Tubular epithelial:	not seen
Transitional and squamous epithelial:	not seen
RBC:	0–2/hpf
WBC:	
M	0–3/hpf
F and children	0–5/hpf
Bacteria, unspun:	no organisms/oil immersion field
spun:	<20 organisms/hpf

Sodium

Infants:	0.3–3.5 mmol/d
	(6–10 mmol/m^2)
Children and adults:	5.6–17 mmol/d
	(varies with intake
	and other factors)

Sodium/potassium (7)

Prematures and newborns	1.4–7.9
Infants 1–12 mo	1.1 ± 1.5
Children	0.5–2.5
Infants on milk	0.7
Generally (28)	> 1

Specific gravity, random

Newborn:	1.006–1.008
Adult:	1.002–1.030
After 12 hr of fluid restriction:	>1.025
After 24 hr:	1.015–1.025

Uric acid (29)

		5–12 mg/kg/d
	Child	$520– \pm 147$ mg/d
	Adult	250–750 mg/d

Urobilinogen   1–4 mg/d

Vanillylmandelic acid (VMA)	U, 24 hr	md/d	μmol/d
	Newborn:	<1.0	<5.0
	Infant:	<2.0	<10.1
	Child:	1–3	5–15
	Adolescent:	1–5	5–25
	Thereafter:	2–7	10–35
	or:	1.5–7 μg/mg creatinine	0.86–4 mmol/mol creatinine

Xanthine (23)   4.1–8.6 mg/d

Vasopressin (14,30)	P	pg/ml	
		Full-term, 1–3 d	5.0
		Adult, supine	0.8–3.2
		upright	1.9–10.5
	U, 24 hr,	ng/24 hr	
		Newborn	1.0–1.4
		3–12 mo	4.8–6.0
		Adult	32.5–39.5

Vitamin D	S		
		25(OH) D	30 ± 5 ng/ml
		1,25(OH) 2 D	20–80 pg/ml
		24,25(OH) 2 D	1–5 ng/ml

References

1. Tietz NW, Logan NM (1987) Reference ranges. In: Tietz NW (ed) Fundamentals of Clinical Chemistry, 3rd edn. WB Saunders, Philadelphia, pp 928–975
2. Mabry CC (1987) Reference ranges for laboratory tests. In: Behrman RE, Vaughn VC III (eds) Nelson Textbook of Pediatrics, 13th edn. WB Saunders, Philadelphia, pp 1535–1558
3. Silver HK, Kempe CH, Bruyn HB, Fulginiti VA (1987) Handbook of Pediatrics, 15th edn. Appleton & Lange, Norwalk, pp 834–854
4. Rowe PC (ed) (1987) The Harriet Lane Handbook, 11th edn. Year Book Medical Publishers, Chicago
5. Scully RE, McNeely BU, Mark EJ (eds) (1986) Normal reference laboratory values. N Engl J Med 314: 39–49
6. Siegler RL, Crouch RH, Hackett TN, Jr, Wilker M, Jubiz W (1977) Potassium-renin-aldosterone relationships during the first year of life. J Pediatr 91: 52–55
7. Sulyok E, Nemeth M, Tenyi I, Csaba IF, Varga F, Gyory E, Thurzo V (1979) Relationship between maturity, electrolyte balanceand the function of the renin-angiotensin-aldosterone system in newborn infants. Biol Neonate 35: 60–65
8. Wu JT, Book L, Sudar K (1981) Serum alpha-fetoprotein (AFP) levels in normal infants. Pediatr Res 15: 50–52
9. Papadopoulou ZL, Tina LU, Sandler P, Jose PA, Calcagno PL (1978) Size and function of the kidneys. In: Johnson TR, Moore WM, Jeffries JE (eds) Children are Different: Developmental Physiology, 2nd edn. Ross Laboratories, Columbus, pp 97–102
10. Alleyne GAO (1987) Renal function in malnourished children. In: Holliday MA, Barratt TM, Vernier RL (eds) Pediatric Nephrology, 2nd edn. Williams and Wilkins, Baltimore, pp 170–172
11. Barratt TM, Crawford R (1970) Lysosome excretion as a measure of renal tubular dysfunction in children. Clin Sci 39: 457–465
12. Esperanca MJ, Collins DL (1966) Peritoneal dialysis efficacy in relation to body weight. J Pediatr Surg 1: 162–169
13. Joppich R, Scherer B, Weber PC (1979) Renal prostaglandins: Relationship to the development of blood pressure and concentrating capacity in pre- and full-term healthy infants. Eur J Pediatr 132: 253–259
14. Godard C, Vallotton MB, Favre L (1982) Urinary prostaglandins, vasopressin and kallikrein excretion in healthy children from birth to adolescence. J Pediatr 100: 898–902
15. Soothill JF (1962) The estimation of eight serum proteins by gel diffusion precipitation technique. J Lab Clin Med 59: 859–870
16. Cameron JS, Blandford G (1966) The simple assessment of selectivity in heavy proteinuria. Lancet 2: 242–247
17. Sulyok E, Seri I, Tulassay T, et al (1985) The effect of dopamine administration on the activity of the renin-angiotensin-aldosterone system in sick preterm infants. Eur J Pediatr 143: 191–193
18. Richer C, Hornych H, Amiel-Tison C, et al (1977) Plasma renin activity and its postnatal development in pre-term infants. Biol Neonate 31: 301–304

19. Berger RM, Maizels M, Moran GC, et al (1983) Bladder capacity (ounces) equals age (years) plus 2 predicts normal bladder capacity and aids in diagnosis of abnormal voiding patterns. J Urol 129: 347–349

20. Karlen J, Aperia A, Zetterstrom R (1985) Renal excretion of calcium and phosphate in preterm and term infants. J Pediatr 106: 814–819

21. Stapelton FB, Noe HN, Jerkins G, et al (1982) Urinary excretion of calcium following an oral calcium loading test in healthy children. Pediatrics 69: 594–597

22. Miller LA, Stapleton FB (1985) Urinary citrate excretion in children with hypercalciuria. J Pediatr 107: 263–266

23. Stanbury JB, Wyngaarden JB, Fredrickson DS, et al (eds) (1983) The Metabolic Basis of Inherited Disease, 5th edn. McGraw-Hill, New York

24. Brodehl J, Oemar BS, Hoyer PF (1987) Renal glucosuria. Pediatr Nephrol 1: 502–508

25. Rudman D, Dedonis JL, Fountain MT, et al (1980) Hypocitraturia in patients with gastrointestinal malabsorption. New Engl J Med 303: 657–661

26. De Sants NG, Di Ioris B, Capodicasa G, et al (1987) Renal excretion of calcium, oxalate and magnesium between 3 and 16 years: the value of overnight urine. Contrib Nephrol 58: 8–15

27. Ginsberg JM, Chang BS, Matarese RA, et al (1983) Use of single voided urine samples to estimate quantitative proteinuria. New Engl J Med 309: 1543–1546

28. Schwartz GJ, Feld LG (1987) Potassium. In: Holliday MA, Barratt TM, Vernier RL (eds) Pediatric Nephrology, 2nd ed. Williams and Wilkins, Baltimore, pp 114–127

29. Stapleton FB, Linshaw MA, Hassanein K, et al (1978) Uric acid excretion in normal children. J Pediatr 92: 911–914

30. Pohjavuori M, Fyhrquist F (1980) Hemodynamic significance of vasopressin in the newborn infant. J Pediatr 97: 462–465

Appendix II: Formulas

AMIN Y. BARAKAT

The following conversions and formulas are commonly used in nephrology to assist in the clinical workup of a patient. The clinician should keep in mind that these are estimates, and the results should be interpreted in the context of the clinical picture (1-4).

A. Conversions

$$mEq/l = \frac{mg/dl}{MW} \times 10 \times valence \text{ or } \frac{mg/dl \times 10}{Eq\ W}$$ (MW: molecular weight; Eq W: equivalent weight)

$$mg/dl = \frac{mEq/L}{10} \times Eq\ W$$

$$Eq\ W = \frac{Atomic\ weight}{valence}$$

Temperature: $C = \frac{5\ (F-32)}{9}$ $F = \frac{(C \times 9)}{5} + 32$ (C: centigrade; F: Fahrenheit)

1 in = 2.54 cm; 1 cm = 0.3973 in
1 lb = 0.454 kg = 16 oz; 1 kg = 2.204 lb
1 oz = 28.350 g
1 L = 1.06 qt = 33.81 oz
1 dl = 100 ml
mm Hg $\times$ 1.36 = cm water; cm water $\times$ 0.735 = mm Hg

Compound	mEq/g salt	mg salt/mEq
NaCl	17	58
$NaHCO_3$	12	84
KCl	13	75
$CaCO_3$	20	50
$CaCl_2 \cdot 2\,H_2O$	14	73
Ca gluconate $\cdot$ 1 H_2O	4	224
Ca lactate $\cdot$ 5 H_2O	6	154
$MgSO_4 \cdot 7\,H_2O$	8	123
NH_4Cl	19	54

B. Measurements

Ideal Body Mass (5)

< 5 ft (males and females): $\text{Height}^2 \dfrac{\text{(cm)} \times 1.65}{1000}$

> 5 ft: Males: Kg = 39 + 2.27 (Height, in. − 60)
                Lb = 86 + 5   (Height, in. − 60)

      Females: Kg = 42.2 + 2.27 (Height, in. − 60)
                Lb = 93   + 5   (Height, in. − 60)

Body Surface Area (m^2), Approximation to Weight (kg)

1–5 kg	0.05 $\times$ Weight + 0.05
6–10 kg	0.04 $\times$ Weight + 0.10
11–20 kg	0.03 $\times$ Weight + 0.20
21–70 kg	0.02 $\times$ Weight + 0.40
10 kg	0.5 m^2
30 kg	1.0 m^2

Kidney Size in Normal Children   (6)

Length (cm) (5–13 yr) = 0.379 $\times$ Age (yr) + 6.65 $\pm$ 1.45

Sectional area (cm^2) = 1.0126 $\times$ Height (in.) − 9.272 $\pm$ 10.24
          or   7.23 $\times$ Kidney length (cm) − 29.37 $\pm$ 9.8
          or   28.47 $\times$ Body surface (m^2) + 12 $\pm$ 9.94

Urinary Bladder Capacity (Values level off after age 9 yr)   (7)

(ml) = 32 × Age (yr) + 73
(oz) =   2 + Age (yr)

C. Clearance (C)

$$C_k = \frac{U_k V}{S_k}$$ (k is any substance; U: urine; S: serum; V: volume)

$CH_2O = V(1 - U/S \text{ Osm})$

GFR

Full-term infants: (ml/min/1.73 m²) = 1.1 × Body length (cm)   (8)

Children:

$$(\text{ml/min/1.73 m}^2) = \frac{K \times \text{Body length (cm)}}{S_{Cr} \text{ (mg/dl)}}$$ (Cr: creatinine)   (9)

    K in low birth weight infants <1 yr = 0.33 (0.2–0.5)
        term infants <1 yr   = 0.45 (0.3–0.7)
        children (2–12 yr)   = 0.55 (0.4–0.7)
        females (13–21 yr)   = 0.55 (0.4–0.7)
        males (13–21 yr)   = 0.70 (0.5–0.9)

Adolescent boys = 1.5 × Age (yr) + $\dfrac{0.5 \times \text{Length (cm)}}{S_{Cr} \text{ (mg/dl)}}$ (10)

Adults (18–92 yr): Males (ml/min) = $\dfrac{140 - \text{Age in years}) \times \text{Weight (kg)}}{72 \times S_{Cr} \text{ (mg/dl)}}$ (11)

Females: 85% of males

D. Fluids and Electrolytes

Total body water	60% body weight
Intracellular fluid	40%
Extracellular fluid	20%
Interstitial fluid volume	15%
Plasma volume	~50ml/kg
Blood volume	~75 ml/kg

Potassium

Total body potassium   55 mEq/kg
    Falls ~ 370 mEq for each 1 mEq/L fall in measured serum potassium
    Serum K concentration increases by 0.6 mEq/L for every 0.1 decrease
    in serum pH

Chloride

Decrease in 1 mEq/L of serum chloride = decrease of 1% of total body chloride

Correction of Electrolyte Abnormality

mEq needed = (Desired level − Actual level) × Distribution factor × Baseline weight in kg

Distribution factor: HCO_3 0.4–0.5
 Cl   0.2–0.3
 Na   0.6–0.7

Correction of Serum Na

Hyperlipidemia: Reduction of Na (mEq/L) = plasma lipids (mg/dl) × 0.002

Hyperproteinemia: Reduction of Na (mEq/L) = amount of protein >8 (g/dl) × 0.25

Hyperglycemia: Expected Na (mEq/L) = measured Na + 0.028 (glucose − 100)

Hyperglycemia with insulin treatment: Expected Na (mEq/L) = measured Na + 0.16 (glucose − 100)

Total CO_2 Exhaled

$$= 3.2 \text{ ml/kg/min; } 7\% \text{ increase } °C \text{ of fever}$$

$$pH = \log \frac{1}{H^+}$$

$$pH = 6.1 + \log \frac{(HCO_3^-)}{0.03 \ pCO_2}$$

$$H^+ = 24 \frac{(P_aCO_2)}{HCO_3^-}$$

Metabolic Acidosis

pCO_2 decreases 1–1.5 mm Hg for each mEq/L decrease in HCO_3^-

pCO_2 = last 2 digits of pH
pCO_2 = 1.5 HCO_3^- + 8
HCO_3^- + 15 = last 2 digits of pH

Metabolic Alkalosis

pCO_2 increases 0.5–1 mm Hg for each mEq/L increase in HCO_3^-

pCO_2 = last 2 digits of pH

Respiratory Acidosis

HCO_3^- increases 0.35 mEq/L for each mm Hg increase in pCO_2

Respiratory Alkalosis

HCO_3^- decreases 0.5 mEq/L for each mm Hg decrease in pCO_2

Prediction of Compensatory Response in Simple Acid-Base Disturbances (12)

Metabolic acidosis $P_aCO_2 = (1.5 \times HCO_3^-) + 8 \pm 2$

Metabolic alkalosis $P_aCO_2 = (0.9 \times HCO_3^-) + 9 \pm 2$

Respiratory alkalosis $\Delta HCO_3^- = \dfrac{\Delta P_aCO_2}{10} \times 4$

Respiratory acidosis $\Delta HCO_3^- = \dfrac{\Delta P_aCO_2}{10} \times 2.5$

Osmolality

Estimated serum osmolality (mOsm/kg water) = 2 Na (mEq/L) +

$\dfrac{Glucose}{18} + \dfrac{BUN}{2.8} + \dfrac{(Mannitol}{18} + \dfrac{Ethyl\ alcohol)}{4.6}$ (all in mg/dl)

(Normal ~ 290)

Osmolar gap (mOsm/kg water) = Measured osmolality − Calculated osmolality

(Normal < 10)

E. Tubular

$FE_K = U_K/S_K \times S_{Cr}/U_{Cr} \times 100$ (FE: fractional excretion; K: HCO_3^-, PO_4, Na, etc.)

Tubular reabsorption of phosphate (TRP%) = $(1 - FE_{PO_4}) \times 100$

$Tm_{PO_4} = P_{PO_4}$ (threshold) $\times$ GFR   (13)

TP/GFR   (13):
  Newborn   : 6.9 ± 1.2
  1 mo–12 yr : 4.4 ± 0.6
  12–16 yr   : 4.0 ± 0.6
  > 16 yr   : 3.2 ± 0.4

% Na (or water) delivery = $\dfrac{V}{GFR} \times 100$

% distal Na reabsorption = $\dfrac{C_{H_2O}}{C_{H_2O} + C_{Na}} \times 100$

F. Renal Failure Indices

$$FE_{Na} (\%) = U_{Na}/S_{Na} \times S_{Cr}/U_{Cr} \times 100 \quad (14)$$

Acute tubular necrosis: > 3 (adults)
Prerenal and others: < 1 (adults); < 2 (neonates)
(In small prematures, may normally reach as high as 5%)

$$\frac{U \text{ urea (mg/dl)}}{S \text{ urea (mg/dl)}} \quad \begin{array}{ll} \text{Acute tubular necrosis} & : \quad < 14 \\ \text{Prerenal failure} & : \quad > 14 \end{array} \quad (15)$$

$$\text{Renal failure index (RFI)} = \frac{U_{Na} \text{ (mEq/L)} \times P_{Cr} \text{ (mg/dl)}}{U_{Cr} \text{ (mg/dl)}} \quad (16, 17)$$

Acute tubular necrosis: Adults : > 1.98
                        Infants : > 3
                        Neonates: > 2
Prerenal < 1.5

G. Others

Creatinine, Serum

(age 1–20 yr) (mg/dl) =
  Males : $0.35 + (0.025 \times \text{Age, yr})$ (18)
  Females: $0.37 + (0.018 \times \text{Age, yr})$

Creatinine, Urine

Children (mg/kg/24 hr) = $15 + (0.5 \times \text{Age, yr}) \pm 3$ (19)
Adults   (mg/kg/24 hr) = $28 - (0.2 \times \text{Age, yr})$ (11)

Protein Selectivity Index (PSI) =

(U IgG $\times$ P IgG / U albumin $\times$ S albumin) $\times$ 100 (20)
  $< 10\%$: Selective
  $> 20\%$: Nonselective

Calcium

Corrected serum calcium in hypoalbuminemia:
  Serum calcium (mg/dl) $-$ serum albumin (g/dl) $+ 4$ or
  Each g/dl of albumin binds ~ 0.8 mg/dl calcium or
  % calcium bound = 8 (albumin) + 2 (globulin) + 3

Uric Acid

Acute uric acid nephropathy suspected if spot urine $\dfrac{\text{Uric acid}}{\text{Creatinine}} > 1$

References

1. Behrman RE, Vaughn VC III (eds) (1987) Nelson Textbook of Pediatrics, 13th edition. WB Saunders, Philadelphia
2. Holliday MA, Barratt TM, Vernier RL (1987) Pediatric Nephrology, 2nd edition. Williams and Wilkins, Baltimore
3. Rollings RC (1984) Facts and formulas. Rollings and Rollings, Nashville
4. Rowe PC (ed) (1987) The Harriet Lane Handbook, 11th edition. Year Book Medical Publishers, Chicago
5. DuBose TD (1983) Clinical approach to patients with acid-base disorders. Med Clin North Am 67: 799–813
6. Stark H, Eisenstein B, Tieder M (1983) TP/GFR as a measure of normal PO4 handling in children. Europ J Pediatr 140: 181 (abstract)
7. Soothill JF (1962) The estimation of eight serum proteins by gel diffusion precipitation technique. J Lab Clin Med 59: 859–870
8. Traub SL, Johnson CE (1980) Comparison of methods of estimating creatinine clearance in children. Am J Hosp Pharm 37: 195–201
9. Hodson CJ, Drewf JA, Karn MN, et al (1962) Renal size in normal children. A radiographic study during life. Arch Dis Child 37: 616–622
10. Berger RM, Maizels M, Moran GC, et al (1983) Bladder capacity (ounces) equals age (years) plus 2 predicts normal bladder capacity and aids in diagnosis of abnormal voiding patterns. J Urol 129: 347–349
11. Schwartz GJ, Feld LG, Langford DJ (1984) A simple estimate of glomerular filtration rate in full-term infants during the first year of life. J Pediatr 104: 849–854
12. Espinel CH (1976) The FENa test. Use in the differential diagnosis of acute renal failure. JAMA 236: 579–581
13. Luke RG, Linton AL, Briggs JD, et al (1965) Mannitol therapy in acute renal failure. Lancet 1: 980–982
14. Mathew OP, Jones AS, James E, et al (1980) Neonatal renal failure: usefulness of diagnostic indices. Pediatrics 65: 57–60
15. Handa SP, Morrin PAF (1967) Diagnostic indices in acute renal failure. Canad Med Ass J 96: 78–82
16. Schwartz GJ, Haycock GB, Chir B, Spitzer A (1976) Plasma creatinine and urea concentration in children: Normal values for age and sex. J Pediatr 88: 828–830
17. Ghazali S, Barratt TM (1974) Urinary excretion of calcium and magnesium in children. Arch Dis Child 49: 97–101
18. Schwartz GJ, Ganthier B (1985) A simple estimate of glomerular filtration rate in adolescent boys. J Pediatr 106: 522–526
19. Schwartz GJ, Brion LP, Spitzer A (1987) The use of plasma creatinine concentration for estimating GFR in infants, children and adolescents. Pediatr Clin North Am 34: 571–590
20. Cockcroft DW, Gault MH (1976) Prediction of creatinine clearance from serumn creatinine. Nephron 16: 31–41

Appendix III: Curves

AMIN Y. BARAKAT

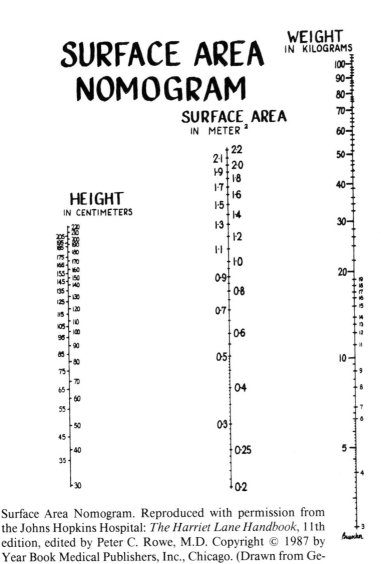

Surface Area Nomogram. Reproduced with permission from the Johns Hopkins Hospital: *The Harriet Lane Handbook*, 11th edition, edited by Peter C. Rowe, M.D. Copyright © 1987 by Year Book Medical Publishers, Inc., Chicago. (Drawn from Gehan and George, Cancer Chemotherapy Reports 54: 225, 1970.)

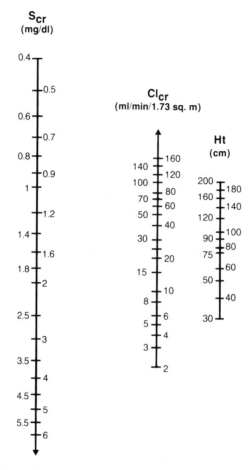

Nomogram used to estimate creatinine clearance in patients 1 to 18 years of age. A straight line connecting the child's serum creatinine value (S_{Cr}) and height (Ht) will intersect the center line at a value approximating creatinine clearance (Cl_{Cr}). Originally published in Traub SL, Johnson CE (1980) Comparison of methods of estimating creatinine clearance in children. Am J Hosp Pharm 37: 195–201. Copyright © 1980 American Society of Hospital Pharmacists, Inc. All rights reserved. Reprinted with permission.

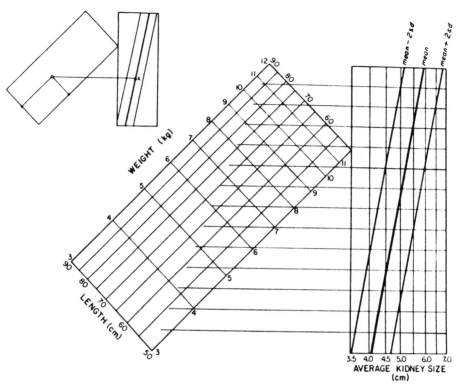

Nomogram to determine normal infant kidney length. The infant's weight and length determine two oblique lines on the left of the plot. The intersection should then be extended parallel to the horizontal rulings to its intersection with the heavy (mean) line on the right graph. The predicted kidney length is indicated on the abscissa. From Blane CE, Bookstein FL, DiPietro MA, Kelsch RC (1985) Sonographic standards for normal infant kidney length. AJR 145: 1289–1291, with permission, © by American Roentgen Ray Society.

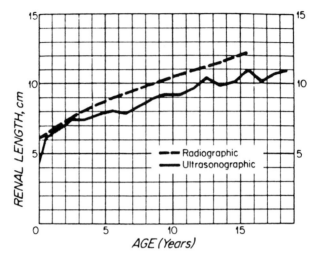

Sonographic and radiographic renal length as function of age. From Rosenbaum DM, Korngold E, Teele RL (1983) Sonographic assessment of renal length in normal children. AJR 142: 467–469, with permission, © by American Roentgen Ray Society.

GIRLS: BIRTH TO 36 MONTHS
PHYSICAL GROWTH
NCHS PERCENTILES*

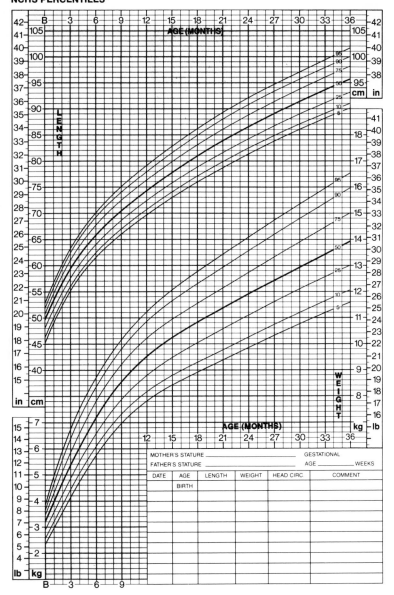

Growth Charts. Adapted from Hamill PVV, Drizd TA, Johnson CL, Reed RB, Roche AF, Moore WM (1979) Physical growth: National Center for Health Statistics percentiles. Am J Clin Nutr 32: 607–629. Copyright Ross Laboratories, 1982. Reproduced by permission of Pediatrics 41:106, Copyright 1968.

GIRLS: 2 TO 18 YEARS
PHYSICAL GROWTH
NCHS PERCENTILES*

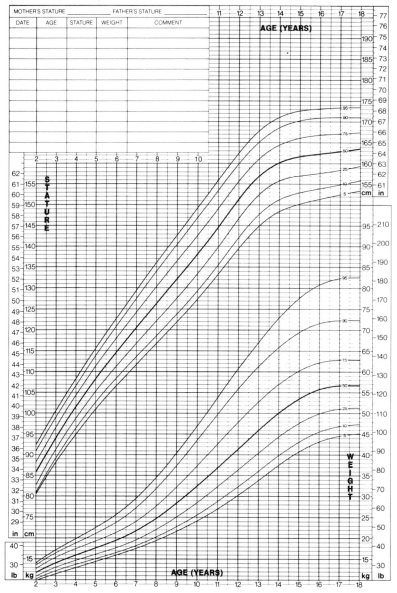

BOYS: BIRTH TO 36 MONTHS
PHYSICAL GROWTH
NCHS PERCENTILES*

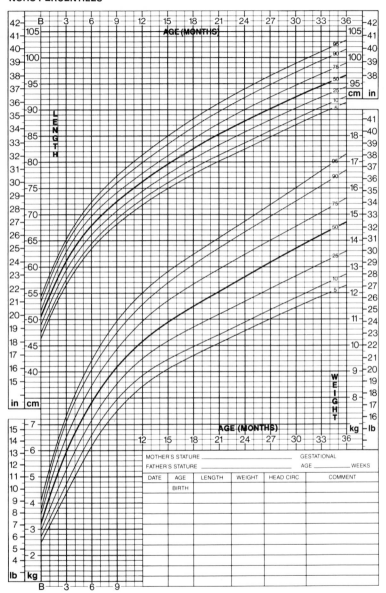

BOYS: 2 TO 18 YEARS
PHYSICAL GROWTH
NCHS PERCENTILES*

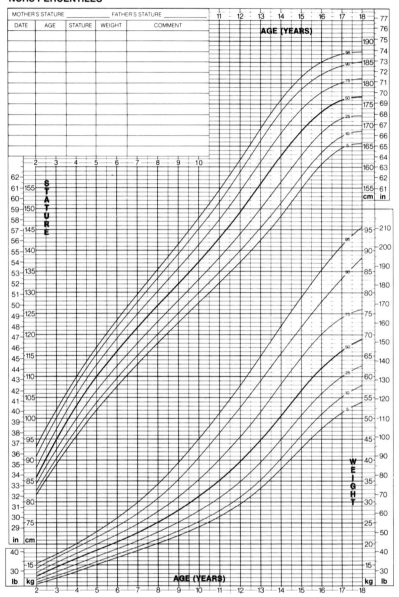

GIRLS: BIRTH TO 36 MONTHS
PHYSICAL GROWTH
NCHS PERCENTILES*

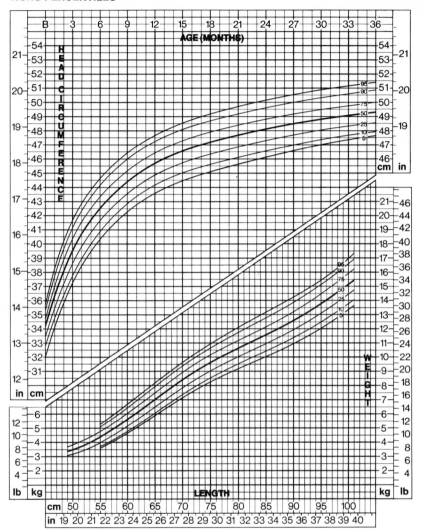

BOYS: BIRTH TO 36 MONTHS
PHYSICAL GROWTH
NCHS PERCENTILES*

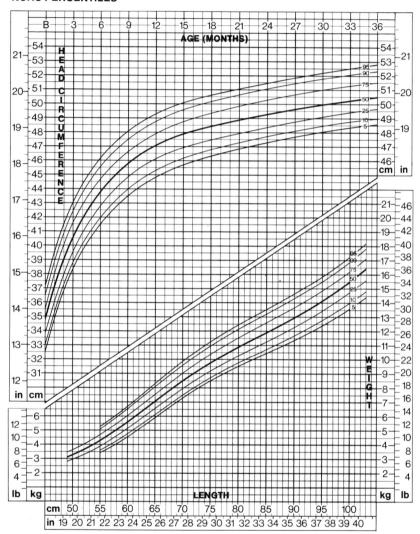

GIRLS: PREPUBESCENT
PHYSICAL GROWTH
NCHS PERCENTILES*

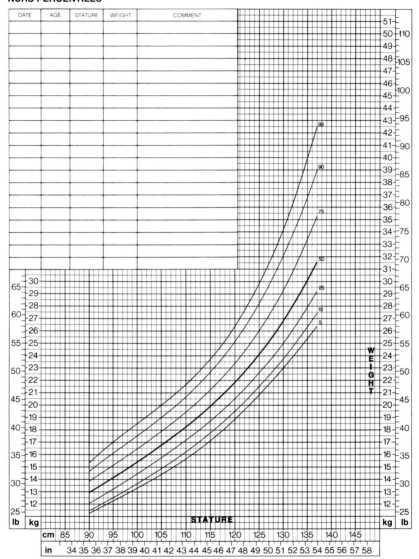

**BOYS: PREPUBESCENT
PHYSICAL GROWTH
NCHS PERCENTILES***

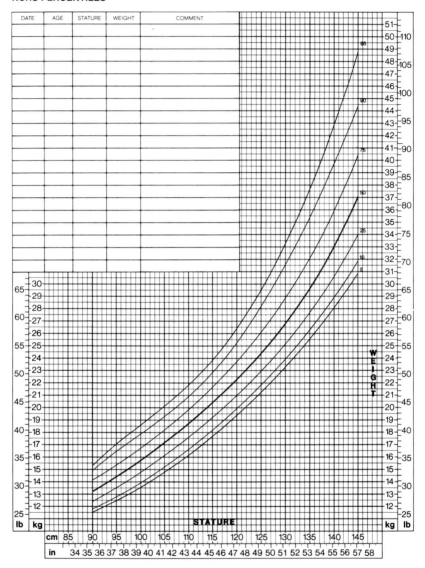

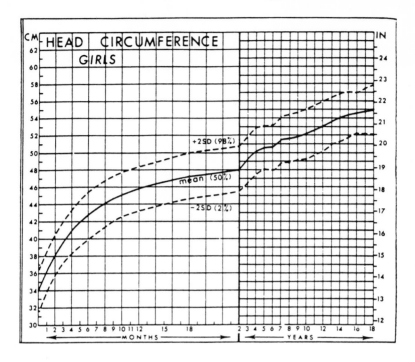

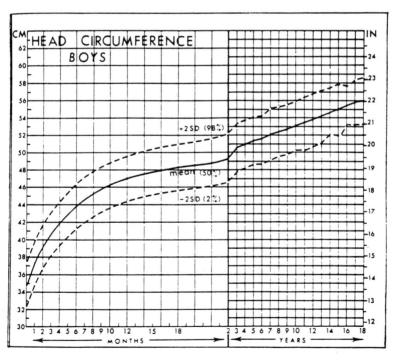

Appendix IV: Conditions and Syndromes Associated with Renal Abnormalities

Amin Y. Barakat

Syndrome, Disease, Condition	Main Features	Renal and Urinary Tract Abnormalities	Inheritance
Abruzzo-Erickson syndrome	Cleft palate, coloboma, hypospadias, deafness, short stature, radial synostosis	Horseshoe kidney, hypospadias	?AD; ?XL
Achondrogenesis	Micromelic dwarfism, short trunk, fetal hydrops	Hydronephrosis, hydroureter, double collecting system	AR
Acrocephalopolydactylous dysplasia, Elejalde	Acrocephaly, hexadactyly of hands, gigantism, thick skin, visceromegaly, connective tissue hyperplasia	Cystic renal dysplasia	?AR
Acrocephalosyndactyly Type I (Apert; ACS I)	Irregular craniosynstosis, midfacial hypoplasia, syndactyly, broad distal phalanx of thumb and big toe	Polycystic kidneys, hydronephrosis	AD
Acrocephalopolysyndactyly Type II (Carpenter, ACPS II)	Acrocephaly, peculiar facies, brachysyndactyly of hands, mental retardation	Hydronephrosis, hydroureter	AR
Acrorenal syndrome	Acral anomalies of hands and feet, urinary tract abnormalities	Ectopic, aplastic, and hypoplastic kidneys; bladder neck obstruction	Sporadic
Adams-Oliver syndrome	Growth deficiency, absence defects of limbs, scalp and skull	Double collecting system	
Adenine phosphoribosyltransferase (APRT) deficiency	Signs and symptoms associated with renal stones	Urolithiasis, renal failure	AD
Adrenal hyperplasia III (21-OH-ase deficiency)	Virilization, adrenal insufficiency	Unilateral renal agenesis, UP junction obstruction, double collecting system	AR

Syndrome, Disease, Condition	Main Features	Renal and Urinary Tract Abnormalities	Inheritance
Adrenal insufficiency and renal disease	Same	Renal microangiopathy, renal failure	Sporadic
Aglossia-adactylia (Hanhart) syndrome	Aglossia, micrognathia, hypoadactyly, cranial nerve palsy	Unilateral renal agenesis	Sporadic
AIDS	Abnormality in cellular immunity, infections, Kaposi sarcoma	Proteinuria, focal glomerular sclerosis, diffuse mesangial proliferation, minimal glomerular changes, acute and chronic renal failure, Type IV renal tubular acidosis, interstitial nephritis, nephrocalcinosis, membranoproliferative glomerulonephritis, Type I	—
Alcohol embryopathy	Prenatal and postnatal growth retardation, microcephaly, short palpebral fissues, joint contractures, mental retardation	Unilateral renal agenesis and hypoplasia, hydronephrosis, duplication of urinary tract, other	—
Aldosteronism, primary	Hyperaldosteronism, low renin secretion, systemic hypertension	Proteinuria, impairment of urinary concentrating ability, hypertension	Sporadic
Aldrich (Wiskott-Aldrich)	Congenital thrombocytopenia, bloody diarrhea, eczema, recurrent infections, elevated serum IgA	Hematuria, proteinuria, nephrotic syndrome, renal failure	XL
Alkaptonuria	Dark urine, pigmentation of sclerae, chronic arthropathy	Nephrocalcinosis	AR
α1-antitrypsin deficiency, emphysema, necrotizing angitisitis and glomerulonephritis	Same	Glomerulonephritis	Sporadic
Alstrom syndrome	Retinitis pigmentosa, nerve deafness, obesity, diabetes mellitus	Proteinuria, renal failure	AR
Amelogenesis imperfecta and nephrocalcinosis (enamel-renal; ERS)	Amelogenesis imperfecta, nephrocalcinosis, impaired renal concentration and possible abnormality of calcium metabolism	Nephrocalcinosis, impaired renal concentration	?AR

Syndrome, Disease, Condition	Main Features	Renal and Urinary Tract Abnormalities	Inheritance
Amyloidosis	Macroglossia, peripheral polyneuropathy, hepatosplenomegaly	Glomerular amyloid deposition, proteinuria, hypertension, nephrosis, positive renal biopsy in 87% of cases	
Angiokeratoma, diffuse (Fabry disease, alpha-galactosidase A deficiency	Pain; skin lesions; cerebral, ocular, cardiac and renal manifestations	Abnormal lipid deposition in epithelial and endothelial cells	XL
Aniridia, partial, unilateral renal agenesis, psychomotor retardation	Same	Unilateral renal agenesis	?AR
Antley-Bixler (trapezoidocephaly synostoses)	Cranio- and humeroradial synostosis, midface hypoplasia, abnormal ears, narrow chest and pelvis, digital abnormalities	Ectopia, duplication of kidney and ureter, renal hypertension	?AR
Anus, imperforate with hand, foot and ear anomalies (Townes-Brocks)	Anal stenosis, dysgenetic ears; digital, renal and cardiac abnormalities	Renal hypoplasia, aplasia, dysplasia; proteinuria; VU reflux; posterior urethral valves; meatal stenosis	AD
Arteriohepatic dysplasia (Alagille)	Unusual facies, vertebral and eye anomalies, chronic cholestasis, peripheral pulmonary stenosis	Unilateral renal agenesis, proteinuria, tubular acidosis, renal insufficiency, mesangial lipidosis with foam cells	AD
Arthro-dento-osteodysplasia (Hajdu-Cheney)	Acroosteolysis, generalized osteoporosis, joint laxity, small stature, persistent cranial sutures, early loss of teeth	Polycystic kidneys	AD
Arthrogryposis multiplex congenita with renal and hepatic abnormality	Same	Renal tubular cell degeneration, nephrocalcinosis	?XLR
Asphyxiating thoracic dystrophy of the newborn (Jeune)	Hypoplastic thorax, respiratory difficulty, protruding abdomen, polydactyly, tapetoretinal degeneration	Proteinuria, hypertension, renal failure, Fanconi-like syndrome, cystic dysplasia, nephronophthisis, VU junction stenosis	AR
Asplenia (Ivemark)	Congenital asplenia; cardiac, GI, GU and skeletal abnormalities	Agenetic, hypoplastic, dysplastic, horseshoe, ptotic and cystic kidneys; ureteral and urethral valves; hydronephrosis; double collecting system	Sporadic ?AR

Syndrome, Disease, Condition	Main Features	Renal and Urinary Tract Abnormalities	Inheritance
Asymmetric crying facies	Asymmetric crying facies, cardiovascular and other anomalies	Unilateral agenetic, ectopic, cystic and dysplastic kidney; fetal lobulation	?
Bacterial endocarditis	Evidence of heart disease, fever, renal involvement	60–80% of patients are affected; hematuria (90%), proteinuria (35–88%), renal infacts (57%), focal or diffuse GN, renal failure	—
Barakat syndrome	Familial nephrosis, nerve deafness, hypoparathyroidism	Proteinuria, steroid-resistant nephrosis, renal failure	AR? XL?
Bartter syndrome (hypokalemic alkalosis)	Hypokalemic alkalosis, hyperaldosteronism, normal BP, hyperplasia	Hyperplasia of juxta glomerular apparatus	AR
Beeturia (Beta-cyaninuria)	Asymptomatic except for red urine following oral ingestion of beets	Red urine	?
Behcet syndrome	Recurrent inflammatory lesions of mouth, genitalia and eyes	Proteinuria, hematuria, nephrotic syndrome, renal failure, glomerulonephritis, anyloidosis, rapidly progressive glomerulonephritis	?
Biliary atresia, extrahepatic	Biliary atresia, renal and cardiac malformations	Renal aplasia or hypoplasia, nephrosis, polycystic kidneys, megaloureter, atresia of ureter	?AR
Biliary malformation with renal tubular insufficiency	Proximal renal tubular insufficiency, cholestatic jaundice, failure to thrive, predisposition to infection, other congenital anomalies	Proximal renal tubular disease, renal tubular acidosis, proteinuria	?XLR ?AR
Bird-headed dwarf (Seckel type dwarfism)	Severe short stature, microcephaly, narrow face, beak-like nose	Renal ectopy and hypoplasia, nephritis	AR
Bloom syndrome	Growth failure, facial telangiectasia, defective immunity	Wilms' tumor	AR
Blue diaper syndrome	Bluish discoloration of diapers, failure to thrive, hypercalcemia, infections	Azotemia, nephrocalcinosis, interstitial nephritis	?AR, ?XL

Syndrome, Disease, Condition	Main Features	Renal and Urinary Tract Abnormalities	Inheritance
Blue rubber bleb nevus (BEAN)	Rubbery, bluish to black cutaneous nevi, nocturnal pain, regional hyperhydrosis	Hypernephroma	AD
Bowen-Hutterite syndrome (Bowen-Conradi)	Microcephaly, prominent nose, micrognathia, joint deformities	Horseshoe kidney, double collecting system	AR
Brachio-oto-renal dysplasia (BOR)	Preauricular pits, cervical fistulae, hearing loss, renal abnormalities	Ectopic, aplastic, hypoplastic, dysplastic and polycystic kidneys; chronic interstitial nephropathy with renal failure; glomerular segmental and focal hyalinization	AD
Brachymesomelia-renal syndrome	Brachymesomelia of upper limbs, craniofacial dysmorphism, corneal opacities, renal anomalies	Glomerulocystic dysplasia	?
C (Opitz trigonocephaly) syndrome	Trigonocephaly, polysyndactyly, abnormal ears, joint dislocations	Unilateral renal agenesis, hypospadias	AR
Camptobrachydactyly	Brachydactyly of hands and feet, polydactyly, flexion contractures of fingers, septate vagina	Urinary incontinence	AD
Campomelic dwarfism (dysplasia)	Congenital bowing of long bones, abnormal facies, dwarfism, other defects	Hydronephrosis, hydroureter, hypoplastic and cystic kidneys	AR
Cardio-vertebro-renal syndrome	Severe obstructive left heart abnormalities, verteral and renal anomalies	Calyceal and ureteral ectasia, bifid pelvis, papillary necrosis	?AR
Carnitine deficiency, myopathic	Lethargy, nonketotic hypoglycemia, hepatomegaly and cardiomegaly	Renal tubular defect in carnitine transport	AR
Caroli disease	Segmental cystic dilation of intrahepatic bile ducts, cholelithiasis, hepatic fibrosis, congenital anomalies, failure to thrive	Medullary sponge, infantile polycystic kidneys	Sporadic
Caudal regression, sironemelia sequence	All degrees of severity, from imperforate anus to sironomelia	Agenetic, dysplastic, and horsehoe kidney; duplication of urinary tract	Sporadic
Cerebral gigantism (Sotos)	Acceleration of growth, acromegalic appearance, characteristic facies, variable mental retardation	Urethral stricture, Wilms' tumor	AD

Syndrome, Disease, Condition	Main Features	Renal and Urinary Tract Abnormalities	Inheritance
Cerebro-costo-mandibular syndrome	Cerebral maldevelopment, micrognathia, severe costovertebral abnormalities	Renal ectopia, medullary cysts	?AR; ?AD
Cerebro-hepato-renal (Passarge) syndrome	Hypotonia, abnormal ears, hepatomegaly, renal cysts, failure to thrive	Cortical cysts, proteinuria, renal failure, hypospadias	?AR
Cerebro-hepato-renal (Zellweger) syndrome	Failure to thrive, cerebral, renal and skeletal abnormalities; severe hypotonia, liver disease, distinctive facies, death in early infancy	Renal cysts and dysplasia	AR
Cerebro-oculo-facio-skeletal (COFS) syndrome	Microcephaly, ocular, facial and skeletal abnormalities	Horseshoe kidney, bilateral renal agenesis, double collecting system	AR
Charcot-Marie-Tooth (CMT) disease	Slowly progressive weakness and muscle atrophy, ocular abnormalities, cardiopathy	Hyalinization and hypercellularity of glomeruli; focal segmental sclerosis with IgM and C3 deposits	AD XL
CHILD syndrome (ichthyosiform erythroderma and limb defects)	Congenital hemidysplasia, unilateral ichthyosiform erythroderma, ipsilateral limb defects	Ipsilateral renal agenesis	?XL; ?AR
Chloride diarrhea, familial	Defective intestinal transport of chloride; diarrhea, salt and water wasting	Juxtaglomerular hyperplasia, nephrocalcinosis	AR
Chondrodysplasia punctata, rhizomelic form	Flat face, microcephaly, cataract, short femur and humerus, stippled epiphysea	Micromulticystic kidneys	AR
Chromosome aberrations	See p. 483		
Central nervous system dysgenesis, microcephaly, mental retardation	Microencephaly with dysmyelination, spastic cerebral palsy, seizures, severe mental retardation, biliary duct hypoplasia	Hydronephrosis, hydroureter	AR
Cockayne syndrome	Cachectic dwarfism, precocious senile appearance, microcephaly, deafness, mental retardation, skin hypersensitivity to sun	Nephrosclerosis, thickened glomerular basement membrane, tubulointerstitial disease	AR
Cohen syndrome	Hypotonia, obesity, prominent incisors	UP junction obstruction	AR

Syndrome, Disease, Condition	Main Features	Renal and Urinary Tract Abnormalities	Inheritance
Cold hypersensitivity (familial cold urticaria)	Cold urticaria, pain and swelling of joints, fever	Renal failure, amyloid nephropathy	AD
Coloboma of macula with Type B brachydactyly	Pigmented macular coloboma, Type B brachydactyly	Unilateral renal agenesis	?AD
Complement component Clq deficiency	Lupus-like illness	Glomerulonephritis	?
Complement component C3 deficiency	Life-threatening infections, lupus-like picture with fever, arthralgias and cutaneous vasculitis	Proteinuria, hematuria, membranoproliferative glomerulonephritis	AD
Connective tissue disease, mixed	Arthritis, sclerobactyly, Raynaud's phenomenon, lymphadenopathy, anemia	Proteinuria, membranous and proliferative glomerulonephritis, renal failure	—
Coloboma, cardiac defect, other anomalies	Same	Unilateral renal agenesis, ectopia, double collecting system, posterior urethral valves, UP junction obstruction, hypospadias	?
Coloboma, cataracts, iris anomalies, myopia, hypertelorism, deafness, umbilical hernia, mental retardation	Same	Proteinuria, generalized aminoaciduria, VU reflux, hydroureter	?AR
Cornelia de Lange syndrome	Pre- and postnatal growth deficiency, dysmorphic facies, hirsutism, mental retardation	Renal cystic dysplasia and hypoplasia, hydronephrosis, hypospadias	Sporadic
Cranio-carpo-tarsal dystrophy (Freeman-Sheldon)	Mask-like "whistling" face, ulnar deviation of hands, talipes equinovarus	Renal hypoplasia with contralateral hydronephrosis	AD
Craniosynostosis with radial defects (Baller-Gerold)	Craniosynostosis, radial hypoplasia or aplasia, other skeletal abnormalities	Crossed renal ectopia	AR
Crome syndrome	Brain malformations, epilepsy, cataracts, renal damage	Sclerotic glomeruli, necrotic tubules	AR
Cryoglobulinemia, familial mixed (Meltzer syndrome)	Vasculitis of skin with recurrent purpura, arthralgias, hepatic disease, infection	50% of cases affected; hypertension, proteinuria, nephrosis, renal tubular acidosis, papillary necrosis, glomerulonephritis	AD

Syndrome, Disease, Condition	Main Features	Renal and Urinary Tract Abnormalities	Inheritance
Cryptophthalmos with other malformations (Fraser)	Unilateral or bilateral absence of palpebral fissures with other abnormalities	25% of cases have renal and ureteral aplasia, hypospadias or urethral meatal stenosis	AR
Cystathioninuria	Variable mental retardation, thrombocytopenia	Urolithiasis	AR
Cystic fibrosis	Failure to thrive, respiratory and gastrointestinal involvement, lethal	Microscopic nephrocalcinosis, hypercalciuria	AR
Cushing's disease	Obesity, osteoporosis, growth retardation, hypertension	Urolithiasis, renal dysplasia	Sporadic
Cytochrome C oxidase deficiency	Myopathy, lactic acidosis, failure to thrive, weakness, death from respiratory failure in early infancy	Fanconi-like syndrome	AR
Dalmatian (renal) hypouricemia	Hypouricemia, uric acid urolithiasis	Increased renal clearance of uric acid	AR
Denys-Drash (Drash) syndrome	Pseudohermaphroditism, nephropathy, and Wilms' tumor in various combinations	Wilms' tumor, nephrotic syndrome, glomerulonephritis, diffuse mesangial sclerosis	Sporadic
Deafness, progressive; cataracts, myopia, marfanoid habitus, renal disease	Same	Proteinuria, renal failure	AD?
Dermatomyositis	Myositis with muscle weakness, cutaneous lesions, edema, low-grade fever	Proteinuria, arteriolar fibrosis, vasculitis, nephrotic syndrome, various glomerular lesions, renal insufficiency	—
Dermatomyositis	Myositis with muscle weakness, cutaneous lesions, edema, low-grade fever	Proteinuria, arteriolar fibrosis, vasculitis, nephrotic syndrome, various glomerular lesions, renal insufficiency	—
Diabetes mellitus	Hyperglycemia, polyuria, polydipsia, diabetic ketoacidosis	Proteinuria, hypertension, clinical diabetic nephropathy develops 10–20 years after diagnosis; 7% of cases are affected	Multifactorial AD, AR?
Diabetic embryopathy	Infants of diabetic mothers, skeletal, cardiac, GI and other malformations	Hydronephrosis, renal agenesis, double ureter	—

Syndrome, Disease, Condition	Main Features	Renal and Urinary Tract Abnormalities	Inheritance
Diaphragmatic hernia, familial, congenital	Congenital diaphragmatic hernia, respiratory distress at birth	Aplastic, polycystic, horseshoe, double and ectopic kidney; hydronephrosis, hydroureter	Multifactorial
Diethylstilbesterol, exposure in utero	Abnormalities and neoplasm of genital tract	Urethral stenosis, hypospadias	—
DiGeorge syndrome	Absence of thymus and parathyroid glands, immunodeficiency, congenital heart defect, characteristic facies	Hydronephrosis, malrotation	Sporadic
Disaccharide (sucrose) intolerance	Diarrhea	Urolithiasis	AR
Diverticula, multiple calyceal, sensorineural deafness	Same	Calyceal diverticula, attenuation of the pelvicalyceal system	AD
Dubowitz syndrome	Short stature, microcephaly, peculiar facies, eczema	Hypospadias	AR
Dysautonomia, familial (Riley-Day)	Reduced or absent tear production, postural hypotension, excessive perspiration, relative indifference to pain, emotional lability	Glomerulosclerosis secondary to renal vascular denervation	AR
Dyschondrosteosis	Mesomelic dwarfism with hereditary nephritis	Nephritis	AD?
Dyssegmental dwarfism	Short trunk and limbs, narrow chest, vertebral defects, reduced joint mobility, death in neonatal period	Hydronephrosis, hydroureter	AR?
Ectrodactyly-ectodermal dysplasia-clefting (EEC, Rapp-Hodgkin)	Ectrodactyly, ectodermal dysplasia, cleft lip/palate	Unilateral renal agenesis, hypospadias	AD
Ehlers-Danlos syndrome	Hyperelasticity and fragility of skin and blood vessels, hypermobility of joints	UP junction abnormality, dissected or hypoplastic renal artery, polycystic or medullary sponge kidney, renal tubular acidosis, bladder neck obstruction	AD AR XL Sporadic
Elliptocytosis	Mild anemia, if any	Renal tubular acidosis	AD
Ellis-van Creveld syndrome (Chondroectodermal dysplasia)	Acromelic dwarfism, polydactyly, hypoplasia and dystrophy of nails and teeth, cardiac malformation	Nephrocalcinosis, glomerulosclerosis, unilateral renal agenesis, megaureter	AR

Syndrome, Disease, Condition	Main Features	Renal and Urinary Tract Abnormalities	Inheritance
Epidermal nevus	Midfacial nevus, seizures, mental deficiency	Renal hamartoma, nephroblastoma, renal artery stenosis	Sporadic
Epidermolysis bullosa dystrophica	Subepidermal blisters, ulceration of mucosae, flexion contractures of fingers, osteoporosis	Hydronephrosis, hydroureter, renal amyloidosis	AD
Exomphalos-macroglossia-gigantism (EMG, Beckwith-Wiedemann)	Omphalocele, macroglossia, nephromegaly, increased birth weight, facial flame nevus, characteristic ear helix anomaly, hypoglycema	Renal medullary dysplasia, Wilms' tumor, hydronephrosis, hydroureter, ectopic and double kidney, renocortical cysts	AD
Facio-cardio-renal syndrome	Characteristic facies, severe mental retardation, cardiac defects, horseshoe kidney	Horseshoe kidney, hydroureter	AR?
Facio-oculo-acoustico-renal (FOAR) syndrome	Ocular and craniofacial anomalies, deafness	Proetinuria, aminoaciduria, VU reflux	AR?
Familial thrombocytopenia	Bleeding tendency	Hydronephrosis	AD
Fanconi-Bickel syndrome	Defect in renal tubular transport and glycogenosis; failure to thrive, hepatomegaly	Glycosuria, calciuria, proteinuria, organic aciduria, glycogen accumulation in proximal tubular cells	AR
Fanconi pancytopenia	Pancytopenia, hyperpigmentation, skeletal deformities, absent or hypoplastic thumb	33% of patients affected; aplastic, ectopic, and horsehoe kidney, duplication of urinary tract, hydronephrosis, renal cysts	AR
Fatty metamorphosis of the viscera (visceral steatosis)	Hypoglycemia, hypotonia, death in neonatal period	Vacuolization of renal proximal tubular epithelium	AR
Femoral-facial syndrome	Femoral hypoplasia, unusual facies, cleft palate	Hemangioma of urinary tract	Sporadic
FG syndrome	Congenital hypotonia, macrocephaly, mental retardation, imperforate anus, partial agenesis of corpus callosum	Dilation of urinary tract, urolithiasis	XL
Focal dermal hypoplasia (Goltz)	Atrophy and linear pigmentation of skin, dysplastic nails, anomalies of hands and vertebrae	Horseshoe kidney	XLD

Syndrome, Disease, Condition	Main Features	Renal and Urinary Tract Abnormalities	Inheritance
Frontometaphyseal dysplasia	Prominent supraorbital ridges, metaphyseal dysplasia, joint limitations, conductive deafness	Double collecting system, UV obstruction, pyelonephritis	XL
Frontonasal dysplasia	Median cleft face, ocular hypertelorism	Unilateral renal agenesis	?sporadic ?AR
Fryns syndrome	Characteristic facies, corneal opacities, cleft lip/palate, pulmonary hypoplasia, distal digital hypoplasia, urogenital abnormalities	Cystic dysplasia, duplication of urinary tract	AR
Fructose intolerance, hereditary	Hypoglycemia, liver cirrhosis	Renal tubular acidosis, proteinuria, aminoaciduria	AR
Fundus flavimaculatus, cystic kidneys	Same	Polycystic kidneys	?
Galactosemia	Cataracts, hepatosplenomegaly, failure to thrive, variable mental retardation	Proteinuria, aminoaciduria	AR
Galloway syndrome	Microcephaly, hiatus hernia, nephrosis	Nephrosis, microcystic dysplasia, focal glomerulosclerosis, focal basement membrane thickening,	AR
Gangliosidoses	Severe cerebral degeneration, skeletal deformities, accumulation of ganglioside in different organs	cytoplasmic ballooning and accumulation of ganglioside in renal glomerular epitheliam cells	AR
Gaucher's disease (β-glucosidase deficiency)	Hepatosplenomegaly, Gaucher cells in bone marrow	Gaucher cells in glomeruli and interstitium	AR
Glycinuria	Renal colic	Oxalate urolithiasis	?AD
Glycogen storage disease I (Von Gierke)	Short stature, hepatomegaly, hypoglycemia, hyperuricemia	Enlarged kidneys, Fanconi-like syndrome, vacuolated renal tubular cells	AR
Glycogen storage disease (McArdle)	Crampy muscle pain on exertion, myoglobinuria	Acute renal failure	AR
Goldston syndrome	Dandy-Walker malformation, celebellar malformations, dysplastic kidneys	Cystic renal dysplasia	AR

Syndrome, Disease, Condition	Main Features	Renal and Urinary Tract Abnormalities	Inheritance
Gout	Hyperuricemia, arthritis, tophi	Uric acid urolithiasis, nephropathy with acute renal failure, chronic urate nephropathy with nephrosclerosis and hypertension	?
Granulomatous disease, chronic	Neutrophil dysfunction, recurrent bacterial infections	Cystitis	XL
Hall-Pallister syndrome	Hypothalamic hamartoblastoma, hypopituitarism, imperforate anus, polydactyly	Agenesis, dysplasia, horseshoe and cross ectopia of kidney	Sporadic
Heart, congenital malformations	Cardiac murmur and other findings depending on nature of malformation	Renal agenesis, dysgenesis, ectopia and hypoplasia; 25% of ventricular septal defect have renal abnormalities, particularly hypoplasia	?
Heart disease, congenital, cyanotic	Cyanosis and hypoxia secondary to cardiac malformation	Glomerular enlargement, proteinuria, decreased renal plasma flow, proximal renal tubular acidosis, glomerular sclerosis, others	?
Heart failure, congestive	Tachypnea, tachycardia, hepatomegaly, edema, poor perfusion	Proteinuria (85%), hematuria, pyuria, infarcts, arteriolar sclerosis, inability to concentrate urine (27–77%), prerenal azotemia, glomerulonephritis	—
Hemihypertrophy	Total or partial asymmetry, hemihyperesthesia, hemiareflexia, scoliosis	Wilms' tumor, enlarged kidneys, nephrocalcinosis medullary sponge kidneys, hypospadias	?AR
Hemolytic-uremic syndrome (HUS)	Coombs' negative hemolytic anemia, thrombocytopenia, acute renal failure	Renal microangiopathy, acute renal failure	?
Hemophilia A and B	Factor VIII or Factor IX deficiency, bleeding episodes	Filling defects, calculi, papillary necrosis, hydronephrosis	XL
Henoch-Schönlein purpura	Purpuric skin rash, arthralgia, abdominal pain, nephritis	Hematuria, proteinuria; nephritis of variable severity and histology in 20–30% of cases	—

Syndrome, Disease, Condition	Main Features	Renal and Urinary Tract Abnormalities	Inheritance
Hepatic fibrosis, congenital	Hepatic fibrosis, congenital heart disease	Cystic, dysplastic kidneys	?AR
Hepatic fibrosis, polycystic kidney, coloboma, encephalopathy	Same, other dysmorphic features	Polycystic kidneys	?AR
Hepatitis, viral	Jaundice, abnormal liver functions, positive hepatitis antigens	Proteinuria, hematuria, cylindruria, decreased GFR, immune complex glomerular disease with HB$_s$Ag	—
Hypermethioninemia	Hepatic cirrhosis, pancreatic cell hyperplasia	Enlarged kidneys, aminoaciduria	AR
Hyperoxaluria	Renal colic	Hematuria, nephrocalcinosis, oxalate urolithiasis	AR
Hyperparathyroidism, familial primary	Hypercalcemia and related symptoms, osteitis fibrosa	Nephrocalcinosis, urolithiasis, salt wastage, medullary sponge kidney	AD
Hyperparathyroidism, neonatal	Respiratory distress, hypotonia, seizures, polyuria, failure to thrive	Nephrocalcinosis	?AR
Hyperprolinemia, Type I (proline oxidase deficiency)	Elevated plasma levels of L-proline, nephropathy, photogenic epilepsy	Familial nephropathy, hematuria, renal hypoplasia, pyelonephritis	AR
Hypertelorism, microtia facial clefting (HMC)	Hypertelorism, microtia, clefting, psychomotor retardation, atretic auditory canals	Ectopic kidneys	AR
Hypertelorism with esophageal abnormality and hypospadias (G; Opitz-Frias)	Ocular hypertelorism, dysphagia, hoarse cry, hypospadias	Unilateral duplication of renal pelvis and ureters, VU reflux, hypospadias	?XLD
Hypertension, essential	Asymptomatic elevation in blood pressure, atherosclerotic damage to other organs	Proteinuria, nephrosclerosis	?
Hypertension with adrenal, genital and renal defects; deafness	Same, abnormal steroidogenesis, hyporeninemia	Focal nephritis, malignant nephrosclerosis, renal failure	?AR
Hyperuricemia, ataxia, deafness	Same	Hereditary nephropathy, renal failure	?XLD
Hypoaldosteronism	Hypoaldosteronism, hyporeninemia, hyperkalemia	Distal tubular acidosis, renal insufficiency	Sporadic

Syndrome, Disease, Condition	Main Features	Renal and Urinary Tract Abnormalities	Inheritance
Hypophosphatasia, infantile	Low alkaline phosphatase, hypercalcemia, rickets	Nephrocalcinosis	AR
Hypospadias; mental retardation	Also microcephaly, craniofacial dysmorphysm, joint laxity, beaked nails	Hypospadias	?AR ?XLR
Hypouricemia, hypercalciuria and decreased bone density	Hypouricemia, hypercalciuria, decreased bone density, decreased renal clearance of uric acid	Defect in renal tubular reabsorption of uric acid	?AR
Ichthyosis, familial, dwarfism, mental retardation, renal disease	Same, hypogonadism, spasticity	Chronic pyelonephritis, glomerulosclerosis, double kidney and ureter, vacuolization of proximal tubular cells, renal insufficiency	?AR
Ichthyosis, split hairs and aminoaciduria syndrome	Same	Aminoaciduria	?AR
Intestinal pseudoobstruction, familial	Intermittent episodes of abdominal pain or distension, megaduodenum, smooth muscle degeneration	Hydronephrosis, VU reflux, megacystis	AD
Intrahepatic cholestasis, renal disease	Same	Tubulointerstitial nephropathy	?AR
Radial ray defects, hearing impairment, internal ophthalmoplegia, thrombocytopenia (IVIC syndrome)	Radial ray hypoplasia, hearing impairment, internal ophthalmoplegia, thrombocytopenia	Renal ectopia	AD
Johanson-Blizzard syndrome	Hypoplastic alae nasi, hypothyroidism, congenital deafness, pancreatic achylia	Hydronephrosis	AR
Kallmann syndrome	Anosmia, color blindness, hypogonadism	Unilateral renal agenesis	AD
Kartagener syndrome	Dextrocardia, bronchiectasis, sinusitis, immotile cilia syndrome	Mesangiocapillary glomerulonephritis	AR
Kaufman oculo-cerebrofacial syndrome	Growth and mental retardation, microcephaly, hypotonia, hypertelorism, other eye abnormalities	Caleictasis, ureterectasia, bifurcation of renal pelvis	AR
Kaufman-McKusick syndrome	Hydrometrocolpos, polydactyly, congenital heart malformation	Polycystic kidneys, hydronephrosis, bladder neck obstruction	AR

Syndrome, Disease, Condition	Main Features	Renal and Urinary Tract Abnormalities	Inheritance
Kawasaki disease (mucocutaneous lymph node)	Fever, desquamation of skin, rash, lymphoadenopathy, arthritis, urethritis	Urethritis, renal artery involvement in 50% of cases	—
Keratoconus, cleft lip/palate, genitourinary abnormalities, short stature, mental retardation	Same	Double ureters, splitting of renal pelvis	?AR
Klippel-Feil deformity, conductive deafness and absent vagina	Short stature, absent vagina, conductive deafness, Klippel-Feil deformity of cervical spine	Renal agenesis and ectopia	?
Klippel-Trenaunay-Weber syndrome	Asymmetric limb hypertrophy, hemangiomas	Diffuse bilateral nephroblastoma, hemangioma of urinary tract	Sporadic
Lacrimo-auriculo-dento-digital syndrome	Nasolacrimal duct obstruction, cup-shaped pinnas, enamel dysplasia, digital malformations	Unilateral renal agenesis	AD
Larsen syndrome	Flat facies, multiple joint dislocations	Hydronephrosis, unilateral agenesis	AD AR
Laurence-Moon syndrome	Retinitis pigmentosa, mental retardation, obesity, short stature, hypogonadism, polydactyly	Pyelonephritis; glomerulonephritis; cystic, dysplastic, hypoplastic and hydronephrotic kidneys; VU reflux; nephrosclerosis	AR
Lecithin: cholesterol acyltransferase (LCAT) deficiency	Diffuse corneal opacities, anemia, proteinuria, renal insufficiency	Proteinuria, hematuria, renal failure, hypertension, glomerular foam cells, deposits in intima of renal arterioles	AR
Leprechaunism	Failure to thrive, peculiar facies, emaciation, hirsutism, endocrine disorders	Tubular ectasia, medullary calcification	AR
Leprosy	Chronic infection affecting skin, neural tissue and mucous membranes, typical acid-fast mycobacteria in scrapings	Interstitial nephritis, chronic pyelonephritis, renal amyloidosis, proliferative glomerulonephritis, glomerulosclerosis, uremia	—
Leptospirosis	Headache, fever, chills, myalgias, jaundice, rash	Occur in 80% of patients; proteinuria and pyuria (65%), hematuria and cylindruria (5–10%), tubulointerstitial nephritis, acute renal failure	—

Syndrome, Disease, Condition	Main Features	Renal and Urinary Tract Abnormalities	Inheritance
Lesch-Nyhan syndrome	Self-mutilation, extrapyramidal signs, delayed motor development, excessive uric acid production	Uric acid urolithiasis and nephropathy, shrunken kidneys	XLR
Leukonychia totalis	White nails, sebaceous cysts, renal calculi	Renal calculi	AD
Limb deficiency, distal and oral defects	Distal limb deficiency, oral defects, micrognathia	Oligomeganephronia	Sporadic
Lipodystrophy, acquired total (Lawrence)	Progressive, generalized loss of adipose tissue, liver cirrhosis, hyperlipemia, insulin-resistant nonketotic diabetes	Nephromegaly, glomerular sclerosis, renal insufficiency	Sporadic
Lipodystrophy, concenital total (Seip)	Generalized loss of fat, hypertrichosis, increased pigmentation, hepatosplenomegaly, acceleration of somatic growth, enlarged genitalia, insulin-resistant nonketotic diabetes	Nephromegaly, hydronephrosis, hydroureter, urolithiasis, nephrosis, renal insufficiency	AR
Lipodystrophy partial (Barraquer-Simmonds)	Loss of adipose tissue from face and upper body, hypertriglyceridemia, hypocomplementemia	Mesangiocapillary glomerulonephritis	Sporadic
Lissencephaly (Miller-Dieker)	Microcephaly, incomplete brain development, vertical ridge in forehead, mental deficiency	Unilateral renal agenesis, cystic renal dysplasia	AR
Liver cirrhosis, congenital and renal tubular defects	Same	Fanconi-like syndrome	?
Liver disease, subepidermal immunoprotein, and membranoproliferative glomerulonephritis	Small liver with hepatocellular damage, hypersplenism, papulosquamous dermatitis, IgC in skin	Proteinuria, membranoproliferative glomerulonephritis	?AR
Lowe oculo-cerebro-renal syndrome	Growth and mental retardation, hypotonia, metabolic acidosis, generalized aminoaciduria, proteinuria, rickets, eye changes	Aminoaciduria, proteinuria, hematuria, pyuria, decreased tubular absorption of phosphate, renal failure	XL
Lupus erythematosis, systemic (SLE)	Collagen disease with multisystem involvement, arthritis, fever, malar rash, autoantibody abnormality	Proteinuria, abnormal urine sediment, lupus nephritis, nephrotic syndrome, hypertension, renal failure	?

Syndrome, Disease, Condition	Main Features	Renal and Urinary Tract Abnormalities	Inheritance
Lymphangiectasia, intestinal	Protein-losing enteropathy	Nephrotic syndrome	AD
Lymphedema, hypoparathyroidism	Congenital lymphdema, hypoparathyroidism, nephropathy, mitral valve prolapse, brachytelephalangy	Proteinuria, hypoplastic kidneys, renal failure	?AR ?XLR
Lymphogenic hypergammaglobulinemia, antibody deficiency, autoimmune hemolytic anemia, glomerulonephritis	Same	Glomerulonephritis	AR
Lymphopenic immune defect	Lymphopenia, T-cell deficiency, recurrent infections, photophobia, short stature	Glycosuria, focal glomerular sclerosis	XL
Macrothrombocytopathia, nephritis, deafness	Same	Nephritis similar to acute or hereditary glomerulonephritis, hypertension, progressive renal failure	AD
Magnesium, defect of renal tubular transport of	Hypomagnesemia with secondary hypocalcemia, convulsions, tetany	Nephrocalcinosis, renal interstitial fibrosis	AR
Malaria	Paroxysmal fevers, anemia, splenomegaly	Nephrotic syndrome, membranous and rarely proliferative, immune complex glomerulonephritis	—
Malignancy, disease	Depends on the type and site of disease	Acute renal failure secondary to renal parenchymal involvement, obstruction or urate nephropathy, immune complex glomerulopathy	?
Malignancy, therapy	Tumor lysis syndrome	Increased serum urate and creatinine, drug nephrotoxicity	—
Mammorenal syndrome	Lateral displacement of nipples, bilateral renal hypoplasia or duplication	Bilateral renal hypoplasia or duplication	Sporadic
Marden-Walker syndrome	Blepharophimosis, microphthalmia, cleft palate, congenital joint contractures, failure to thrive	Microcystic renal disease, dilated collecting system	AR

Syndrome, Disease, Condition	Main Features	Renal and Urinary Tract Abnormalities	Inheritance
Marfan syndrome	Musculoskeletal abnormalities, hypotonia, excessive length of limbs, cardiovascular abnormalities, ectopia lentis and other eye changes	Hydronephrosis and hydroureter; polycystic, extopic and medullary sponge kidney; unilateral renal agenesis; nephrolithiasis, ureteral stenosis, duplication of urinary tract	AD
Marshall-Smith syndrome	Failure to thrive, accelerated skeletal maturation, craniofacial dysmorphism, psychomotor retardation	Hydronephrosis, hydroureter	?
Meckel-Gruber syndrome	Occipital encephalocele, microcephaly, abnormal facies, cleft lip/palate, polydactyly	Dysplastic, polycystic, hypoplastic, horseshoe, hydronephrotic and medullary sponge kidney; dilated ureters; renal vascular abnormalities	AR
Mediterranean fever, familial (FMF)	Fever, pleuritis, peritonitis, arthritis	Anyloid nephropathy	AR
Megacolon, aganglionic (Hirschsprung)	Congenital megacolon	Obstructive uropathy	Multifactorial
Megaduodenum and/or megacystis	Megacystis, dilated small bowel, malrotation, intestinal hypoperistalsis	Megacystis, hydronephrosis, hydroureter	AD
Metachromatic leukodystrophy (sulfatide lipidosis)	Weakness, hypotonia, macular changes, mental deterioration	Metachromatic granules in tubular cells, sulfatide in lysosomes	AR
Metatropic dwarfism (dysplasia)	Short-limbed dwarfism, narrow thorax with short ribs, progressive kyphoscoliosis	Bilateral hydroureter	AR
Microphthalmia with associated anomalies (Lenz dysplasia)	Micro- or anophthalmia, renal dysgenesis, cryptorchidism, abnormality of limbs, clavicles and teeth	Renal failure, dysgenesis or aplasia; hydroureter, hypospadias	XL
Miranda syndrome	Brain malformations, renal and liver dysplasia	Cystic renal dysplasia	AR
Mitochondrial cytopathy, with ragged red fibers	Ataxia, seizures, retinitis pigmentosa, ophthalmoplegia, failure to thrive, abnormal mitochondria on muscle biopsy	Glomerulosclerosis, tubular atrophy, renal failure, Fanconi syndrome	AR

Syndrome, Disease, Condition	Main Features	Renal and Urinary Tract Abnormalities	Inheritance
Mucopolysaccharidosis Type I (MPS I, Hurler syndrome; α-L iduronidase deficiency)	Coarse facies, stiff joints, mental deficiency, cloudy cornea	Metachromatic granules in glomerular epithelium	AR
Mulibrey nanism	Progressive growth failure, hydrocephaloid head, ocular abnormalities, hypotonia, hepatomegaly	Wilms' tumor	AR
MURCS association	Short stature, Müllerian duct aplasia, renal anomalies, cervical defects	Renal agenesis and/or ectopia	Sporadic
Myotonic dystrophy	Myotonia, muscle wasting, cataract, hypogonadism	Polycystic kidneys	AD
N syndrome	Mental retardation, visual impairment, deafness, spasticity	Hypospadias	AR?
Nail patella syndrome (hereditary osteo-onycho-dysplasia)	Dystrophic nails, hypoplastic/absent patella, dysplastic elbows, iliac horns	Nephropathy in 30–55% of patients, proteinuria, renal insufficiency	AD
Nephropathy, familial, retinitis pigmentosa, cerebellar ataxia, skeletal abnormalities	Tapetoretinal degeneration, ataxia, peripheral dysostosis,, renal anomalies	Nephronophthisis	AR
Nephrosis with deafness; urinary tract and digital malformations	Same, bifid uvula	Nephrosis, ureteral constriction, double collecting system, UV and bladder neck obstruction	?AR, ?XLD
Nephrosis, familial; hydrocephalus, thin skin, blue sclerae	Same, peculira facies, abnormal T-cell function	Steroid-resistant nephrosis, glomerulosclerosis, hypertension, renal failure	?AR; ?XL
Nephrosis with deafness, urinary tract and digital malformations	Same	Glomerulonephritis, hypertension	?AR ?XLD
Netherton disease	Congenital ichthyosis, "bamboo" hair, short stature, variable mental retardation	Selective or generalized aminoaciduria	AR
Neu-Laxova syndrome	Intrauterine growth retardation, microcephaly, abnormal facies	Unilateral renal agenesis	AR
Neuraminidase deficiency (sialidosis) Type II	Cherry red macular spots, loss of vision and intelligence, progressive myoclonus	Nephritis, nephrotic syndrome	AR

Syndrome, Disease, Condition	Main Features	Renal and Urinary Tract Abnormalities	Inheritance
Neurofibromatosis (von Recklinghausen's disease)	Café-au-lait spots, cutaneous neurofibromas, CNS tumors	Neurofibromatosis of urinary tract, renal vascular changes, renal artery involvement with hypertension	AD
Nevus sebaceous of Jadassohn (linear sebaceous nevus)	Linear sebaceous nevus, epilepsy, mental retardation	Renal hamartomas, nephroblastoma	?
Niemann-Pick disease, Type A (sphingomyelinase deficiency)	Hepatosplenomegaly, retarded mental and physical growth, severe neurological disturbances	Rare vacuolated glomerular cell, swollen glomerular epithelial cells	AR
Nipples, supernumerary	Accessory nipples and sometimes breast tissue	Double collecting system, hypoplastic, microcystic and polycystic kidneys; hydronephrosis,, UP junction stenosis, ureteral prolapse, Wilms' tumor	AD
Noduli cutanei, multiple with urinary tract abnormalities	Same	Hydronephrosis, double collecting system	?AD
Noonan syndrome	Short stature, webbed neck, pulmonary stenosis, mental retardation	Polycystic, malrotated and hydronephrotic kidneys; double collecting system	AD
Ochoa (urofacial) syndrome	Hydronephrosis, peculiar facial expression	Hydronephrosis, hydroureter, posterior urethral valves, VU reflux, neuropathic bladder	AR?
Oculo-auriculo-vertebral syndrome (OAV or Goldenhar)	Unilateral deformity of external ears, eye and vertebral anomalies	Unilateral agenesis and crossed ectopia of kidney, ureteral duplication, renal artery abnormality, unilateral cystic kidney	?AD
Oculo-cerebro-renal (Denys) syndrome	Hydrophthalmos with secondary glaucoma, mental retardation, short stature, renal tubular dysfunction	Renal tubular acidosis, hypercalciuria, hyperphosphaturia	?AR
Oculo-cerebro-renal (McCance) syndrome	Corneal opacities, nystagmus, brain abnormalities, mental retardation, failure to thrive, absence of testes, renal anomalies	Tubular dysfunction with acidosis, small glomeruli, chronic renal failure	?XL

Syndrome, Disease, Condition	Main Features	Renal and Urinary Tract Abnormalities	Inheritance
Oculo-reno-cerebellar syndrome	Tapetoretinal degeneration, choreoathetosis of upper limbs, spastic diplegia, mental retardation, glomerulopathy	Glomerular sclerosis, renal failure	AR
Oro-cranio-digital syndrome (Jeberg-Hayward)	Cleft lip/palate, abnormal thumbs, microcephaly	Horseshoe kidney	?AR
Oral-facial-digital syndrome (OFD I)	Malformation of oral cavity, face and digits; anomalies of anterior teeth, mental retardation	Polycystic kidney disease	XL
Osteogenesis imperfecta	Short, broad long bones, multiple fractures, blue sclerae	Aminoaciduria, cystinuria	AD; AR
Osteodysplasty of Melnick and Needles	Bowing of long bones, short upper limbs, ribbon-like ribs, typical facies, sclerosis of base of skull	Hydronephrosis, hydroureter, ureteral stenosis, dysplastic kidneys	?AD; ?XL
Osteolysis, hereditary, of carpal bones with nephropathy	Progressive osteolysis of carpal and tarsal bones, nephropathy	Chronic glomerulonephritis, hypertension, renal failure	AD
Osteopetrosis with renal tubular acidosis (carbonic anhydrase II deficiency)	Osteopetrosis, cerebral calcifications, stunted growth, pecular facies, renal tubular acidosis	Distal renal tubular acidosis	AR
Oto-palato-digital (OPD) syndrome	Short stature, characteristic craniofacial features, cleft palate, conductive deafness, bone dysplasia	Renal hypoplasia	XL
Pancreatic insufficiency and bone marrow dysfunction (Scwachman-Bodian)	Metaphyseal changes of femurs and ribs, short stature, bone marrow hypoplasia, exocrine pancreatic insufficiency	Renal glycosuria, aminoaciduria, renal acidosis, nephrocalcinosis	AR
Pernicious anemia, juvenile, due to selective intestinal malabsorption of vitamine B_{12} with proteinuria (Imerslund-Grasbach)	Megaloblastic anemia, weakness, failure to thrive, CNS symptoms, proteinuria	Proteinuria, aminoaciduria, mesangioproliferative glomerulonephritis, renal calculi, double collecting system, narrow calyces	AR
Photomyoclonus diabetes mellitus, deafness, nephropathy, cerebral dysfunction	Same	Hereditary nephropathy, aminoaciduria and other renal tubular defects	?AD

Syndrome, Disease, Condition	Main Features	Renal and Urinary Tract Abnormalities	Inheritance
Pneumothorax, spontaneous and/or pneumomediastinum, urinary tract anomalies	Same	Obstructive uropathy, polycystic kidneys	Sporadic
Poland syndrome	Unilateral aplasia of pectoralis major with ipsilateral symbrachydactyly and hypoplasia and aplasia of breast and nipple	Renal aplasia or hypoplasia, double collecting system	Sporadic
Polyarteritis nodosa	Fever, myalgia, arthralgia, abdominal pain, hypertension	Proteinuria, hematuria, fibrinoid arterial necrosis, renal failure	—
Polycystic kidneys, internal hydrocephalus, polydactilism	Same	Polycystic kidneys	AR
Polydactyly with neonatal chondrodystrophy, Type I (Saldino-Noonan type)	Hydrops fetalis, polydactyly, short limbs, metaphyseal dysplasia of tubular bones, death in neonatal period	Cystic, dysplastic and hypoplastic kidneys; cystic and hypoplastic ureters	AR
Polydactyly with neonatal chondrodystrophy, Type II (Majewski type)	Medial cleft lip, polydactyly, short limbs, genital abnormalities, death in perinatal period	Cystic kidneys	AR
Polydactyly with neonatal chondrodystrophy, Type III (Naurnoff type)	Thoracic narrowing, hypoplastic lungs, short cranial base, death in perinatal period	Dysplastic kidneys	?AR
Polyposis, intestinal II (Peutz-Jeghers)	Mucocutaneous pigmentation, GI polyposis	Polycistic kidneys, ureteral polyposis, urolithiasis	AD
Polyposis, intestinal III (Gardner)	Colon polyposis, epidermal cysts, osteomas	Hydronephrosis	AD
Proteinuria, low molecular weight, hyperlipoproteinemia, mental retardation	Same	Low molecular weight proteinuria, glomerulonephritis	?AR; ?XL
"Prune belly" syndrome	Congenital absence of abdominal musculature, urinary tract abnormalities, cryptorchidism	Dilated urinary tract, dysplastic, aplastic, multicystic and hydronephrotic kidneys	Sporadic
Pseudoaldosteronism (Liddle)	Hypertension, hypokalemic alkalosis	Hypertension	?AD

Syndrome, Disease, Condition	Main Features	Renal and Urinary Tract Abnormalities	Inheritance
Pseudohypoaldosteronism	Failure to thrive, severe dehydration, hyperkalemia, elevated plasmaq aldosterone	Glomerular sclerosis, tubular dilation	AD
Pseudoxanthoma elasticum	Xanthoma-like skin lesions, diminished vision and peripheral pulses, hypertension, hemangiomas	Renal artery stenosis	AR; AD
Pseudo-vitamin D-deficiency rickets	Hypocalcemia, hypotonia, rickets, growth retardation	Mild renal tubular acidosis, aminoaciduria	AR
Pulmonary stenosis and congenital nephrosis	Same	Congenital nephrotic syndrome	?AR
Pyloric stenosis	Hypertrophic pylorus, vomiting	Polycystic, horseshoe and hypoplastic kidney; double collecting system, hydronephrosis	Multifactorial
Radial-renal syndrome	Radial ray aplasia, short stature, renal anomalies	Unilateral renal agenesis, crossed ectopia	AD
Regional enteritis (Crohn)	Abdominal pain, diarrhea, weight loss, growth retardation	Nephrotic syndrome, nephrolithiasis, hydronephrosis, hydroureter, ileovesical fistulae	?
Renal and intestinal disease with tissue autoantibodies	Chronic diarrhea, villous atrophy of small intestine, chronic pancreatitis, elevated IgE and IgA levels, dermatitis	Tubulointerstitial and membranous nephritis	?AR
Renal disease (cystic), cataract, congenital blindness	Same	Polycystic, medullary; cystic and microcystic renal disease	?AR
Renal disease, deafness and ocular changes	Progressive deafness, cataracts, myopia, marfanoid habitus, renal disease	Proteinuria, renal insufficiency	?AD
Renal disease, deafness, myopia	Same	Proteinuria, hematuria, renal insufficiency	?AR
Renal disease (hereditary), neurosensory hearing loss, prolinuria, ichthyosis	Same	Proteinuria, hematuria, renal cysts and calculi, glomerular sclerosis, renal failure	?AR ?AD
Renal dysplasia and retinal aplasia (Loken-Senior)	Tapetoretinal degeneration, retinal dysplasia, renal anomalies	Nephronophthisis, renal dysplasia, uremia	AR

Syndrome, Disease, Condition	Main Features	Renal and Urinary Tract Abnormalities	Inheritance
Renal, genital and middle ear anomalies	Abnormal facies, low folded ears, renal abnormalities, vaginal atresia, deafness secondary to middle ear anomalies	Renal agenesis or hypoplasia, hemiatrophy of urinary bladder	?
Renal hamartomas, nephroblastomatosis, fetal gigantism (Perlman)	Large birth size, unusual facies, tendency to neoplasia, death in neonatal period	Large kidneys, immature glomeruli, renal hamartomas, hydronephrosis, nephroblastomatosis	AR
Renal, hepatic and pancreatic dysplasia	Hepatomegaly; hepatic, pancreatic and renal dysplasia	Renal dysplasia, pyelonephritis, renal failure	AR
Renal insufficiency, deafness, cataract, integument and skeletal abnormalities, susceptibility to infection, and mental retardation	Same	Chronic glomerulonephritis, renal failure	XL
Renal tubular acidosis with nerve deafness	Same	Distal renal tubular acidosis	AR
Retinal blindness, congenital polycystic kidneys, brain maldevelopment	Same	Polycystic kidneys, glomerular sclerosis	?AR
Retinal dysplasia, cataracts, cystic kidneys	Same	Polycystic kidneys, medullary cysts	?AR
Rheumatic fever	Fever, arthritis, carditis, other systemic involvement	Hematuria, focal or diffuse glomerulonephritis, rheumatic arteritis	—
Rheumatoid arthritis	Polyarthritis, joint stiffness, low-grade fever, organomegaly	Proteinuria (40%), hypertension (30%), hematuria (25%), urinary tract infection (20%), amyloidosis, glomerulonephritis, nephrosclerosis	?
Rieger (iridogoniodysgenesis with somatic anomalies)	Hypodontia, malformation of anterior chamber of eye, myotonic dystrophy	Hypospadias	AD
Roberts syndrome	Hypomelia, midfacial defect, severe growth retardation	Polycystic, horseshoe, or hydronephrotic kidney; ureteral stenosis	AR
Robinow dwarfism	Mesomelic dwarfism, hemivertebrae, characteristic facies, hypoplastic external genitalia	Duplication of urinary tract, hydronephrosis	AD

Syndrome, Disease, Condition	Main Features	Renal and Urinary Tract Abnormalities	Inheritance
Rubella, congenital	Small for date, microcephaly, cataracts, heart defects, hepatosplenomegaly	Polycystic and unilateral agenetic kidney, glomerular sclerosis, nephrocalcinosis, double collecting system, hypospadias	—
Rubinstein-Taybi syndrome	Broad thumbs and great toes, characteristic facial abnormalities, mental retardation	Renal calculi: nonfunctioning, aplastic or extra kidney, double renal pelvis dilated ureter, posterior urethral valves	?
Rudiger syndrome	Coarse facial features, lack of ear cartilage, bifid uvula, brachydactyly	UV junction obstruction	?AR
Typhoid fever (*Salmonella typhi*)	Fever, rose spots, stupor, splenomegaly, symptoms of other organ involvement	Occurs in 2–3% of patients; tubulointerstitial disease, oliguric renal failure, immune complex nephritis	—
Sarcoidosis	Feber, arthralgias, pulmonary hilar adenopathy on X-ray	Interstitial granulomas and inflammation, nephrocalcinosis, renal failure	?
Schinzel-Giedion midface retraction syndrome	Midface hypoplasia, brachymesomelia, hypoplasia of distal phalanges, clubfeet, hypertrichosis, seizures	Hydronephrosis, hypospadias	AR
Scleroderma	Morphea, progressive systemic sclerosis, organ system involvement	Rare in children; proteinuria, hematuria, renal failure	?
Schwartz-Jampel-Aberfeld syndrome (chondrodystrohic myotonia)	Myotonia, short stature, blepharophimosis, joint contractures, myopia, pigeon chest	Microcystic kidney disease	AR
Shprintzen syndrome	Dysmorphic facies, omphalocele, hypoplastic larynx, learning disabilities	Hypospadias	AD
Sickle cell disease	Characteristic anemia, fever, pain, infection	Papillary necrosis, cortical infarcts, nephrosis with minimal change or MPGN, hematuria, proteinuria	AR
Silver-Russell dwarfism	Prenatal-onset short stature, skeletal asymmetry, small incurved 5th finger	UP junction obstruction, VU reflux, pyelonephritis	?

Syndrome, Disease, Condition	Main Features	Renal and Urinary Tract Abnormalities	Inheritance
Sirenomelia	Fusion of limbs, incomplete development of caudal structures, absence of rectum and genitalia	Renal agenesis, absent bladder	Sporadic
Smith-Lemli-Opitz (RSH) syndrome	Growth retardation, microcephaly, mental retardation, abnormal facies, hypospadias, microphallus	Rotated, hypoplastic, dysplastic or multicystic kidney; cortical cysts, hypospadias	AR
Spherocytosis	Anemia, intermittent jaundice, splenomegaly	Polycystic kidneys	AD
Spina bifida	Asymptomatic or neurological symptoms, urinary incontinence	Ureteral duplication, neurogenic bladder	?
Spondylocostal dysplasia	Vertebral anomalies, barrel-shaped chest, rib defects, short neck	Unilateral agenesis and ectopia of kidney; hydronephrosis	AR
Sucrosuria, hiatus hernia and mental retardation	Same	Sucrosuria	?AR
Syndactyly, Type V	Metacarpal and metatarsal 3-4 or 4-5 fusion	Renal hypoplasia, bladder extrophy	AD
Syphilis	Rhinitis, rash, bone involvement, other protean and latent manifestations	Occurs in 0.3% of patients, nephrosis, rarely acute and interstitial nephritis, gumma of kidney	
Tachycardia, paroxysmal; hypertension, seizures	Same, microphthalmos, cataracts, hyperglycinuria	Urolithiasis	?
Takayasu's disease	Fever, hypertension, renal vascular lesions, weight loss, arthralgia	Hypertension (70%), renal vascular lesions (60%)	?
Telangiectasia, hereditary hemorrhagic of (Rendu, Osler and Weber)	Generalized telangiectasias, bleeding, liver disease	Telangiectasias of urinary bladder	AD
Testicular regression (XY gonadal agenesis)	Absence of gonads in an XY person	Interstitial nephritis, end-stage renal disease	?AR
Thalassemia B	Anemia, growth retardation, hepatomegaly	Distal renal tubular acidosis	AR
Thalidomide embryopathy	Limb defects	Renal agenesis, cystic dysplasia, hydronephrosis	—
Thanatophoric dwarfism	Short-limb dwarfism, narrow thorax, large cranium, respiratory distress, hypotonia	Hydronephrosis, horseshoe kidney	AD

Syndrome, Disease, Condition	Main Features	Renal and Urinary Tract Abnormalities	Inheritance
Thyro-cerebro-renal syndrome	Goiter, cerebellar ataxia, seizures, sensorineural deafness, muscle wasting, thrombocytopenia	Tubulointerstitial nephritis	?AR
Thyrotoxicosis, renal disease and absent frontal sinuses	Same	Proteinuria, hematuria, proliferative glomerulonephritis	?AR
Torticollis, keloids, cryptorchidism and renal dysplasia	Congenital muscular torticollis, multiple keloids, cryptorchidism, renal abnormalities	Renal dysplasia, pyelonephritis, hypertension, nephrosclerosis, urethral meatal stenosis, UP junction obstruction	?XL
Trichopoliodystrophy (Menkes)	Ceruloplasmin deficiency, copper malabsorption, peculiar hair, progressive neurological impairment	Hydronephrosis, hydroureter, VU reflux, neurogenic bladder, bladder diverticula	XL
Trichorhinophalangeal I	Thin, sparse hair, bulbous nose, protruding ears, peripheral dysostosis, variable mental retardation	Generalized aminoaciduria	AD
Trichorhinophalangeal syndrome, Type II (Langer-Giedion syndrome)	Thin, sparse hair, bulbous nose, multiple exostoses, mental retardation, microcephaly	Small scarred kidney, renal hypertension	?AD
Trimethadione, fetal	Small for date, microcephaly, malformed ears, irregular teeth	Hypospadias	—
Tuberculosis	Systemic manifestations or those related to specific site of infection	Sterile pyuria, hematuria, renal necrosis and caseating granulomas with destruction of collecting system, diffuse miliary renal parencymal lesions, glomerulonephritis, nephrosis	—
Tuberous sclerosis	Epilepsy, mental retardation, adenoma sebaceum, retinal phakomas	40–80% of patients have renal angiomyolipomas; cystic kidneys, adenomas or renal cell carcinoma	AD
Tyrosinemia, hereditary	Hepatosplenomegaly, rickets, failure to thrive	Proteinuria, tubular dysfunction	AR
Ulcerative colitis	Bloody diarrhea, abdominal cramps, weight loss	Nephrolithiasis	—

Syndrome, Disease, Condition	Main Features	Renal and Urinary Tract Abnormalities	Inheritance
Ulnar-mammary syndrome of Pallister	Abnormal development of ulnar rays, axillary apocrine glands and vertebral column	Unilateral renal agenesis, malrotation	?AD
Uterine anomalies with unilateral renal agenesis	Uterovaginal duplication, hematocolpos	Unilateral renal agenesis	Sporadic; AD
Vagina, absence of (Rokitansky-Kuster-Hauser syndrome)	Vaginal atresia, rudimentary uterus, primary amenorrhea	Renal agenesis and hypoplasia, double renal pelvis and ureters, pelvic and solitary fused kidney, caliectasis	Sporadic ?AR
VATER association	*V*ertebral anomalies, *A*nal atresia, *T-E* fistula, *Ra*dial dysplasia	Renal agenesis or ectopia; hydronephrosis; UP junction stenosis; hypospadias; rectourethral, vaginal and vesical fistulae	?
Von-Hippel-Landau syndrome	Cerebellar with retinal or spinal cord hemangioblastomas, pancreatic cysts and renal lesions; symptoms related to cerebellar or retinal tumors	67% of patients may have renal adenoma, carcinoma or cysts; pheochromocytoma; ureterocele	AD
Wegener's granuloma	Fever; cutaneous vasculitis; arthralgia; renal, cardiac and CNS involvement	Segmental necrotizing and crescentic glomerulonephritis, renal granulomas	—
Weyers' oligodactyly syndrome	Ulnar ray defects with oligodactyly, antecubital pterygia, sternal anomalies, cleft lip/palate	Horseshoe kidney, ureteral duplication	Sporadic
Williams-Beuren syndrome	Elfin face, supravalvular aortic stenosis, mental and growth deficiency, infantile hypercalcemia	Nephrosis, pyelonephritis, interstitial, nephritis, proteinuria, renal failure, renal artery stenosis, segmental renal hypoplasia	AD
Wilson's disease (hepatolenticular degeneration)	Ceruloplasmin deficiency, severe neurological abnormalities	Nephrocalcinosis, renal tubular acidosis, aminoaciduria	AR
Wohltman-Caglar syndrome	Polyuria, polydipsia, elevated renin, normotension	Juxtaglomerular apparatus hyperplasia	Sporadic
Wolcott-Rallison syndrome	Early-onset diabetes mellitus, multiple epiphyseal dysplasia	Renal insufficiency	AR

Syndrome, Disease, Condition	Main Features	Renal and Urinary Tract Abnormalities	Inheritance
Wolfram (Didmoad) syndrome	Diabetes insipidus and mellitus, sensory deafness, optic atrophy	Hydronephrosis, hydroureter, nephrosis, neurogenic bladder, sclerosis of bladder neck	AR
Xanthinuria (xanthine oxidase deficiency)	Increased urinary excretion of xanthine and hypoxanthine, hypouricemia	Urolithiasis	AR

Chromosomal Aberration	Renal and Urinary Tract Abnormalities
Autosomal trisomies	
Trisomy 8	75% of patients affected; hydronephrosis, horseshoe and nonfunctioning kidney, bifid pelvis, VU reflux
Trisomy 13	50–60% of patients affected; cystic, agenetic, horseshoe and hydronephrotic, kidney, duplication of urinary tract, fetal lobulation of kidney, megacystis, UV obstruction, bladder neck stenosis
Trisomy 18	Duplication of urinary tract (33–70%); horseshoe, cystic, hydronephrotic, ectopic, aplastic and hypoplastic kidney; glomerulosclerosis, Wilms' tumor, dysplasia, hamartoma, fetal lobulation and rotational anomalies of the kidney
Trisomy 21	Abnormalities occur in about 7% of cases: aplastic, hypoplastic, cystic and horseshoe kidney; hydronephrosis, hydroureter, ureteral stenosis, immature glomeruli, hypoplastic bladder, urethral valves
1q23 or 5→qter trisomy	Renal cysts and calcifications, hydronephrosis
2q21→qter trisomy	Ectopic, dysplastic and horseshoe kidney; ureteral atresia
2q3 trisomy	VU reflux
3q2 trisomy	Cystic dysplasia, calcification and duplication of kidney; accessory kidney
4p14→pter trisomy	Renal agenesis, rotated kidneys, intrarenal pelvis
4q2 or 3 trisomy	Cystic, aplastic, hypoplastic and horseshoe kidney; VU reflux, hydronephrosis, hydroureter
6p21→pter trisomy	Horseshoe and hypoplastic kidney, triple renal artery, double renal vein
6p2 trisomy	Proteinuria, small kidneys
6q21→qter trisomy	Renal dysplasia
7q3 trisomy	Hydronephrosis, hydroureter
8p trisomy	Ureteral stenosis, absent bladder

Chromosomal Aberration	Renal and Urinary Tract Abnormalities
8q2 trisomy	Hydronephrosis, hydroureter
9 trisomy	Cystic kidneys
9 trisomy mosaicism	Renal cysts
9p trisomy	Hydronephrosis, horseshoe kidney
9q3 trisomy	Hydroureter
10 trisomy mosaicism	Immature glomeruli
10p11→pter trisomy	Rotated, aplastic, cystic, dysplastic and double kidneys; megaplastic and aplastic ureter
10q2 trisomy	Renal failure; hypoplastic, dysplastic, cystic, hydronephrotic and double kidneys, double collecting system
11p15 trisomy	Large kidneys, Wilms' tumor
11q2 trisomy	Renal agenesis, VU reflux
12q2 trisomy	Hydronephrosis, ureterocele, pelvic kidney
12q24.1→qter	Ureterocele, hydronephrosis, ectopic and aplastic kidney
13q2 or 3 trisomy	Double renal artery, unspecified renal abnormalities
14 trisomy mosaicism	Renal failure
17q21→qter trisomy	Hypoplastic and cystic kidneys, hyperplastic urinary bladder
17q23→qter trisomy	Unspecified urinary tract malformations
18pter→18q21.2 trisomy	Multicystic kidneys, ureteral agenesis
18q2 trisomy	Polycystic and ectopic kidneys, VU reflux, hydroureter, unspecified renal malformations
19q13→pter trisomy	Hydronephrosis, hydroureter; ectopic, malrotated and cystic kidneys
20p trisomy	Hydronephrosis, polycystic kidneys, double collecting system
Partial 22 trisomy	Renal ectopia and hypoplasia
Autosomal monosomies	
4p-	33% of patients affected; agenetic, hypoplastic, hydronephrotic and nonfunctioning kidney; VU reflux, pyelonephritis, dilated collected system, hypospadias
5p- (Cri-du-chat)	40% of patients affected; ectasia of distal tubules, cystic and horseshoe kidney, duplication of urinary tract
8(q21→qter)	Hydronephrosis
18 q-	40% of patients affected; polycystic, aplastic, ectopic and horseshoe kidney; hydronephrosis, hydroureter
1q42 or 43→qter monosomy	Solitary kidney, VU reflux

Chromosomal Aberration	Renal and Urinary Tract Abnormalities
3p11→p14.2 monosomy	Horseshoe kidney
4q31→qter monosomy	Ectopic kidney, double collecting system
4q3 monosomy	Double collecting system, hydronephrosis, lobulated kidneys
5q13→q22 monosomy	Horseshoe kidney
6q13→q15 monosomy	Ectopic kidney
7p13→p21 monosomy	Hydronephrosis, renal dysplasia, ureteral diverticuli, ureterocele, double collecting system
10p13→pter monosomy	Cystic and segmental renal dysplasia, double collecting system, hydronephrosis, hydroureter
11p11 monosomy	Horseshoe kidney
11p13 monosomy	Wilms' tumor, malrotated kidney, pyelonephritis, hypertension
11q22 or 23→qter monosomy	Renal duplication, hydronephrosis
11q2 monosomy	Multicystic kidneys, double collecting system, hydronephrosis
13q monosomy	UV obstruction, hydronephrosis, hydroureter
13q3 monosomy	Hypoplastic kidneys
15q22→q24	Cystic renal dysplasia
17p11.2 monosomy	22% of patients may be affected; enlarged or solitary kidney, hydroureter, hydropelvis, malpositioned UV junction
18p monosomy	Unspecified renal malformations
21q monosomy	Aplasia, dysplasia and abnormal shape of kidney
22q12 monosomy	Dysplastic and cystic kidneys
Sex Chromosomes	
Turner syndrome (XO)	60–80% of patients affected; horseshoe kidney (commonest); duplications and rotational anomalies; hydronephrotic, ectopic, ptotic, aplastic, hypoplastic and cystic kidney; urethral meatal stenosis; hypertension, double renal artery, UP and UV junction stenosis
Klinefelter's syndrome (XXY)	Renal cysts, hydronephrosis, hydroureter, ureterocele, chronic glomerulonephritis
49,XXXXX	Renal hypoplasia and dysplasia
Fragile X syndrome	UP junction stenosis
Other chromosomal aberrations	
Triploidy (69 chromosomes)	Cystic renal dysplasia and hydronephrosis (50%), fetal lobulations, pelvic kidney

Chromosomal Aberration	Renal and Urinary Tract Abnormalities
Tetraploidy (92 chromosomes)	50% of patients affected; renal hypoplasia and dysplasia, pyelonephritis, megaureter, VU reflux, urethral stenosis
Cat-eye syndrome	60–100% of patients affected; renal agenesis, hypoplasia and cystic dysplasia; horseshoe and pelvic kidney; UP junction obstruction; VU stenosis and reflux; hypoplastic urinary bladder, chronic pyelonephritis
2q3 trisomy/7p22 monosomy	Renal hypoplasia
9p tetrasomy	Renal hypoplasia
18p tetrasomy	Malrotated and horseshoe kidney, double ureter
r(10)	Renal failure, hydronephrosis, hydroureter
r(13)	Aplastic, hypoplastic or ectopic kidney
r(15)	Incomplete duplication of kidney
r(18)	Ectasia of proximal tubules, hydronephrosis, megaureter, VU obstruction
r(21)	Renal agenesis, ureteral anomaly
Small marker chromosome of unknown origin	Hypoplastic kidney, hydronephrosis, VU reflux

Bibliography

Barakat AY, Butler MG (1987) Renal and urinary tract abnormalities associated with chromosome aberrations. Intern J Pediatr Nephrol 8: 215–226

Barakat AY, Dakessian B (1986) The kidney in heart disease. Intern J Pediatr Nephrol 7: 153–160

Barakat AY, Der Kaloustian VM, Mufarrij AA, et al (1986) The Kidney in Genetic Disease. Churchill Livingstone, Edinburgh

Barakat AY, Noubani H (1986) The kidney in hematologic disease. A review. Intern J Pediatr Nephrol 7: 207–212

Barakat AY, Seikaly MG, Der Kaloustian VM (1986) Urogenital abnormalities in genetic disease. J Urol 136: 778–785

de Grouchy J, Turleau C (1984) Clinical Atlas of Human Chromosomes, 2nd edn. John Wiley and Sons, New York

Gilli G, Berry AC, Chantler C (1987) Syndromes with a renal component. In: Holliday MA, Barratt TM, Vernier RL (eds) Pediatric Nephrology, 2nd edn. McGraw-Hill, New York, pp 384–404

Holliday MA, Barratt TM, Vernier RL (eds) (1987) Pediatric Nephrology, 2nd edn. Williams and Wilkins, Baltimore

Jones KL (1988) Smith's Recognizable Patterns of Human Malformation, 4th edn. WB Saunders, Philadelphia

Mc Kusick VA (1988) Mandelian Inheritance in Man, 8th edn. Johns Hopkins University Press, Baltimore

Stanbury JB, Wyngaarden JB, Fredrickson DS, et al (eds) (1983) The Metabolic Basis of Inherited Disease, 5th edn. McGraw-Hill, New York

Suki WN, Eknoyan G (eds) (1981) The Kidney in Systemic Disease. John Wiley and Sons, New York

Zonona J, Di Liberti JH (1983) Congenital and hereditary urinary tract disorders. In: Emery AEH, Rimoin DL (eds) Principles and Practice of Medical Genetics. Churchill Livingstone, Edinburgh, pp 987–1001

Index